PROGRESS IN BRAIN RESEARCH

VOLUME 43

SOMATOSENSORY AND VISCERAL RECEPTOR MECHANISMS

# PROGRESS IN BRAIN RESEARCH

## ADVISORY BOARD

PROGRESS IN BRAIN RESEARCH

VOLUME 43

# SOMATOSENSORY AND VISCERAL RECEPTOR MECHANISMS

Proceedings of an International Symposium held in
Leningrad, U.S.S.R. on October 11–15, 1974

EDITED BY

A. IGGO

AND

O. B. ILYINSKY

*University of Edinburgh, Royal (Dick) School of Veterinary Studies, Edinburgh (Great Britain)*
*The Pavlov Institute of Physiology, Leningrad (U.S.S.R.)*

ELSEVIER SCIENTIFIC PUBLISHING COMPANY

AMSTERDAM/OXFORD/NEW YORK

1976

ELSEVIER SCIENTIFIC PUBLISHING COMPANY
335 JAN VAN GALENSTRAAT
P.O. BOX 211, AMSTERDAM, THE NETHERLANDS

AMERICAN ELSEVIER PUBLISHING COMPANY, INC.
52 VANDERBILT AVENUE
NEW YORK, NEW YORK 10017

ISBN 0-444-41342-1

WITH 145 ILLUSTRATIONS AND 9 TABLES

PRINTED IN THE NETHERLANDS

# List of Contributors

G. N. Akoev, Laboratory of General Physiology of Reception, I. P. Pavlov Institute of Physiology, Academy of Sciences of the U.S.S.R., Leningrad, U.S.S.R.

E. P. Anyukhovsky, Cardiological Institute, Academy of Medical Sciences of the U.S.S.R., Moscow, U.S.S.R.

L. A. Baraz, Institute of Normal and Pathological Physiology, Academy of Medical Sciences of the U.S.S.R., Moscow, U.S.S.R.

G. G. Beloshapko, Cardiological Institute, Academy of Medical Sciences of the U.S.S.R., Moscow, U.S.S.R.

P. R. Burgess, Department of Physiology, University of Utah College of Medicine, Salt Lake City, Utah 84132, U.S.A.

W. T. Catton, Physiology Department, Medical School, The University, Newcastle upon Tyne, Great Britain.

N. Cauna, Department of Anatomy and Cell Biology, The School of Medicine, University of Pittsburgh, Pittsburgh, Pa., U.S.A.

N. I. Chalisova, Laboratory of General Physiology of Reception, I. P. Pavlov Institute of Physiology, Academy of Sciences of the U.S.S.R., Leningrad, U.S.S.R.

Yu. A. Chelyshev, Kazan State Medical Institute, Kazan, U.S.S.R.

V. L. Cherepnov, Institute of Applied Mathematics and Cybernetics, N. I. Lobachevsky State University, Gorky, U.S.S.R.

V. N. Chernigovsky, I. P. Pavlov Institute of Physiology, Academy of Sciences of the U.S.S.R., Leningrad, U.S.S.R.

P. E. Chernilovskaya, Institute of Normal and Pathological Physiology, Academy of Medical Sciences of the U.S.S.R., Moscow, U.S.S.R.

Ch. N. Chouchkov, Department of Anatomy and Histology, Medical Academy, Sofia 31, Bulgaria.

D. Cormier, Department of Psychology and the Psychobiology Research Center, Florida State University, Tallahassee, Fla., U.S.A.

N. Danilova, I. P. Pavlov Institute of Physiology, Academy of Sciences of the U.S.S.R., Leningrad, U.S.S.R.

E. D. Efes, Department of Biocybernetics of the Institute of Applied Mathematics and Cybernetics, N. I. Lobachevsky State University, Gorky, U.S.S.R.

S. I. Elman, Laboratory of General Physiology of Reception, I. P. Pavlov Institute of Physiology, Academy of Sciences of the U.S.S.R., Leningrad, U.S.S.R.

L. R. Gavrilov, Acoustical Institute, Academy of Sciences of the U.S.S.R., Moscow, U.S.S.R.

G. V. Gersuni, Sechenov Institute of Evolutionary Physiology and Biochemistry, Academy of Sciences of the U.S.S.R., Leningrad, U.S.S.R.

N. F. Glebova, O. V. Kuusinen State University, Petrozavodsk, U.S.S.R.

R. C. Goris, Department of Physiology, Tokyo Medical and Dental University, Tokyo, Japan.

H. Hensel, Institute of Physiology, University of Marburg/Lahn, Marburg/Lahn, G.F.R.

A. Iggo, Department of Physiology, Faculty of Veterinary Medicine, University of Edinburgh, Edinburgh EH9 1QH, Great Britain.

O. B. Ilyinsky, Laboratory of General Physiology of Reception, I. P. Pavlov Institute of Physiology, Academy of Sciences of the U.S.S.R., Leningrad, U.S.S.R.

K. Ivanov, I. P. Pavlov Institute of Physiology, Academy of Sciences of the U.S.S.R., Leningrad, U.S.S.R.

P. Kenins, Department of Physiology, School of Medicine, University of North Carolina, Chapel Hill, N.C. 27514, U.S.A.

D. R. Kenshalo, Department of Psychology and the Psychobiology Research Center, Florida State University, Tallahassee, Fla., U.S.A.

E. B. Khaisman, B. I. Lawrentiew Neurohistological Laboratory, Institute of Normal Physiology, Academy of Medical Sciences of the U.S.S.R., Moscow, U.S.S.R.

V. M. Khayutin, Institute of Normal and Pathological Physiology, Academy of Medical Sciences of the U.S.S.R., Moscow, U.S.S.R.

V. Konstantinov, I. P. Pavlov Institute of Physiology, Academy of Sciences of the U.S.S.R., Leningrad, U.S.S.R.

T. L. Krasnikova, Laboratory of General Physiology of Reception, I. P. Pavlov Institute of Physiology, Academy of Sciences of the U.S.S.R., Leningrad, U.S.S.R.

B. V. Krylov, Laboratory of General Physiology of Reception, I. P. Pavlov Institute of Physiology, Academy of Sciences of the U.S.S.R., Leningrad, U.S.S.R.

T. Kumazawa, Department of Physiology, School of Medicine, Nagoya University, Nagoya, Japan.

Yu. I. Levkovich, Laboratory of Scientific Cinematography, I. P. Pavlov Institute of Physiology, Academy of Sciences of the U.S.S.R., Leningrad, U.S.S.R.

U. Lindblom, Department of Neurological Rehabilitation, Karolinska Sjukhuset, 104 01 Stockholm, Sweden.

E. V. Lukoshkova, Institute of Normal and Pathological Physiology, Academy of Medical Sciences of the U.S.S.R., Moscow, U.S.S.R.

B. Lynn, Department of Physiology, University College London, London, Great Britain.

L. Malinovský, Department of Anatomy, Faculty of Medicine, J. Ev. Purkynie University, Brno, Czechoslovakia.

N. Malovichko, I. P. Pavlov Institute of Physiology, Academy of Sciences of the U.S.S.R., Leningrad, U.S.S.R.

G. I. Malysheva, Department of Biocybernetics of the Institute of Applied Mathematics and Cybernetics, N. I. Lobachevsky State University, Gorky, U.S.S.R.

V. N. Mayorov, Laboratory of Functional Neuromorphology, I. P. Pavlov Institute of Physiology, Academy of Sciences of the U.S.S.R., Leningrad, U.S.S.R.

M. Mellos, Department of Psychology and the Psychobiology Research Center, Florida State University, Tallahassee, Fla., U.S.A.

B. A. Meyerson, Department of Neurosurgery, Karolinska Sjukhuset, 104 01 Stockholm, Sweden.

O. P. Minut-Sorokhtina, O. V. Kuusinen State University, Petrozavodsk, U.S.S.R.

B. Y. Nilsson, Department of Physiology, Karolinska Institutet, Stockholm, Sweden.

E. R. Perl, Department of Physiology, School of Medicine, University of North Carolina, Chapel Hill, N.C. 27514, U.S.A.

E. K. Pletchkova, The B. I. Lawrentiew Neurohistological Laboratory, Institute of Normal Physiology, Academy of Medical Sciences of the U.S.S.R., Moscow, U.S.S.R.

L. A. Podoljskaya, Laboratory of Functional Neuromorphology, I. P. Pavlov Institute of Physiology, Academy of Sciences of the U.S.S.R., Leningrad, U.S.S.R.

V. L. Shaposhnikov, Department of Biocybernetics of the Institute of Applied Mathematics and Cybernetics, N. I. Lobachevsky State University, Gorky, U.S.S.R.

E. E. Shchekanov, Sechenov Institute of Evolutionary Physiology and Biochemistry, Academy of Sciences of the U.S.S.R., Leningrad, U.S.S.R.

M. G. Sirotyuk, Sechenov Institute of Evolutionary Physiology and Biochemistry, Academy of Sciences of the U.S.S.R., Leningrad, U.S.S.R.

L. N. Smolin, Institute of Normal and Pathological Physiology, Academy of Sciences of the U.S.S.R., Moscow, U.S.S.R.

R. S. Sonina, Institute of Normal and Pathological Physiology, Academy of Sciences of the U.S.S.R., Moscow, U.S.S.R.

S. Terashima, Department of Physiology, Tokyo Medical and Dental University, Tokyo, Japan.

E. M. Tsirulnikov, Sechenov Institute of Evolutionary Physiology and Biochemistry, Academy of Sciences of the U.S.S.R., Leningrad, U.S.S.R.

V. Trusova, I. P. Pavlov Institute of Physiology, Academy of Sciences of the U.S.S.R., Leningrad, U.S.S.R.

N. K. Volkova, Laboratory of General Physiology of Reception, I. P. Pavlov Institute of Physiology, Academy of Sciences of the U.S.S.R., Leningrad, U.S.S.R.

J. G. Widdicombe, Department of Physiology, St. George's Hospital Medical School, Tooting, London SW17 OQT, Great Britain.

F. P. Yasinovskaya, Cardiological Institute, Academy of Medical Sciences of the U.S.S.R., Moscow, U.S.S.R.

J. Zelená, Institute of Physiology, Czechoslovak Academy of Sciences, 142 20 Prague 4 — Krč, Czechoslovakia.

A. V. Zeveke, Department of Biocybernetics of the Institute of Applied Mathematics and Cybernetics, N. I. Lobachevsky State University, Gorky, U.S.S.R.

# Preface

This volume records the proceedings of an International Symposium organised under the auspices of the I. P. Pavlov Institute of Physiology, Academy of Sciences of the U.S.S.R., and held in Leningrad in October 1974. The symposium provided a welcome opportunity for scientists in the U.S.S.R. and the West to present their work on sensory receptor mechanisms at a meeting of specialists drawn from many active research centres of the world. The programme reflects this situation in making available concise reviews of "tissue receptor" research by the active groups of investigators in the U.S.S.R., in which their hypotheses and results can be seen in conjunction with parallel studies in western laboratories.

The formal programme was supplemented by often vigorous discussion, which is reported briefly in this volume. As in all such meetings there was a development of ideas arising from informal discussion and some of this is reflected in the published articles.

The topics selected for presentation inevitably reflect the interests of the organisers and, as Academician Chernigovsky points out in his introductory article, it was a feature of the symposium that the original intention to give prominence to "tissue receptors" gradually broadened out to become a wide-ranging treatment of the morphology and physiology of cutaneous, joint and visceral receptor mechanisms, the transducer processes, possible central regulation of the receptors in the periphery and the central nervous system, and a consideration of the central actions of the receptors.

The rapid publication of the Proceedings was made possible by the discipline shown by the contributors whose articles are included, and in particular by the very great efforts made to transcribe and edit the recorded discussions on the part of Dr. Ilyinsky and his colleagues. It is hoped that these efforts will be appreciated by those who now have the opportunity to inform themselves of the contemporary state of knowledge of "tissue receptors" in many parts of the world.

A. IGGO
*Edinburgh (Great Britain)*

# Introduction

During recent years studies on the sensory systems and, in particular, on primary processes occurring in individual sensory elements, have been carried out very actively. This might be explained by several reasons, and perhaps the most significant of all is that studies on sensory systems bear a direct relationship on the activity of the central nervous system — a subject receiving the attention of many physiologists. There is no need, I believe, to go into details and adduce too many arguments to affirm this assumption. It should be readily apparent that the nervous system without its sensory "inputs" would be a mass of neurones completely or almost inactive. Other reasons lie, if I may say so, outside physiological science and result from the rapid development of technology. The progress in this direction began from the time of the appearance of oscillographs in physiological laboratories and the application of electronic amplifiers. These technical devices provided an opportunity to study the processes originating in the individual sensory elements and single nerve fibres. Later, processes occurring within these nerve cells and individual receptors were made accessible by the advent of microelectrodes. Finally, the electron microscope was developed and very rapidly became not only a tool for morphological studies, but also an essential device for physiologists.

Owing to different combinations of all these technical procedures real progress in the physiology of sensory systems was achieved, and the abundant new data permitted several important conclusions to be reached and also the formulation of useful hypotheses.

The wide use of precise methods and new techniques led to the generalisation of discussions at several symposia from some narrow subjects of the physiology of sensory systems into the broader discussion and evaluation of general physiological problems. Of course this is inevitable, because the main problems of physiology of sensory systems are common not only for this field, but for many others. To a certain degree this was also true of our Symposium, held in Leningrad, 11–15, October, 1974, which was originally planned as a meeting to discuss only the physiology of tissue receptors.

Perhaps the widening of the fields of discussion could be explained by the fact that the definition of "tissue receptors" should be more precise and exact, but to find such a definition is a complicated task. Indeed, all receptors belong to some tissue, even the most specialised ones, such as, for instance, Pacinian corpuscles, but they could be found in various tissues, in the mesentery near the blood vessels, in the pancreas and even situated near the tendons of the extremities (in cats).

Finally, we know other receptors of different structures which were found by morphologists in practically all tissues and organs of the body. The definition of "tissue receptor" is so wide that almost all receptors belong to this category. Therefore, to define these receptors we should mainly use the characteristics of their physiological parameters rather than the tissue localisation. Additional difficulties in classification of the receptors create the fact of the existence of polysensory receptors.

However, it seems to me that we should not regret the widening of the discussion during the Symposium. The participants had a chance to consider different concepts of reception, including the evaluation of properties and peculiarities of numerous kinds of receptors located in visceral organs and firstly described by Sir Charles Sherrington as "interoceptors".

Thus, detailed discussion was held not only on interoceptor systems but also on the properties of somatosensory systems. The proprioceptors of muscles and such specialised receptors as visual, auditory, vestibular, olfactory and taste receptors were not included in the programme. It was the right decision because it would have been impossible for the participants to cover all varieties of sensory systems, and would have transformed the Symposium into a Congress.

An important advantage of this meeting was in the possibility for the physiologists and morphologists from various countries of the world — Great Britain, U.S.S.R., Sweden, Poland, Czechoslovakia, Italy, Bulgaria, U.S.A., Japan and others — to meet each other informally and to exchange their opinions and experiences.

Extensive discussions were followed by the establishment of very important scientific contacts and informal agreements for future cooperation.

In spite of the fact that all the participants knew each other from the literature, I believe that all will agree that direct and informal communication and personal contact are most important for the progress of science and the stimulation and creation of new scientific ideas.

I hope, that such meetings will be continued. Of course, we could not solve all of the scientific problems, but the common and pleasant law of science is that scientific achievements and solutions lead to new problems and new aims.

V. N. CHERNIGOVSKY
*Leningrad (U.S.S.R.)*

# Contents

# GENERAL PROBLEMS OF SENSORY RECEPTOR MECHANISMS

# Tissue Receptors. Historical Scope. Modern View. Perspectives

V. N. CHERNIGOVSKY

*I. P. Pavlov Institute of Physiology, Academy of Sciences of the U.S.S.R., Leningrad (U.S.S.R.)*

It is rather difficult to give a clear definition of "tissue reception" on the basis of present knowledge. Strictly speaking, almost all receptors, with the possible exceptions of the retina, the organ of Corti and some others, could be placed into the category of tissue receptors since all of them are, to some extent, connected with one or another tissue and themselves constitute a part of neural tissue located at a distant periphery. Among these are the receptors described by Leek (1972) as "abdominal visceral receptors". I think that sufficient evidence is available to refer to the "receptors of lungs and airways", as described by Widdicombe and Fillenz (1972) as tissue receptors.

The morphology of tissue receptors is extremely varied and is represented by free nerve endings of varying structure as well as by complex-built encapsulated bodies such as Pacini, Herbst and Golgi–Mazzoni corpuscles and so on. Sherrington in his famous book "Integrative action of the nervous system" (1911) shrewdly suggested a division into three categories, as follows: *exteroceptive, proprioceptive* and *interoceptive*. The first group comprised receptors of the "inner surface", that is, in the digestive tract proper. He believed that the receptors of the third group are mainly adapted to receive chemical stimulations since the chemical processing, splitting and absorption of food substrates takes place precisely in the digestive tract. Sherrington thought that the interoceptive field is much less saturated with receptors in comparison with the other two fields. Further investigations have shown that this assumption was unlikely. In any case, the neuromorphologists have discovered and described a great variety of nerve endings of different structure and form in all tissues and organs. These receptors should be considered, if only conditionally, as *tissue receptors*.

Perhaps Pavlov had these receptors in mind when, in his address at the Fifth Conference of Russian Physicians (1894) he said: "These endings pervade all organs and all tissues. These endings must be visualized as extremely diverse, specific ones, each individually adapted, like the nerve endings of sense organs, to its own specific irritant of mechanical, physical or chemical nature . . . Hence it is clear that many substances introduced into the organism disturb its equilibrium as a result of their interaction in one form or another with the peripheral endings which are predominantly sensitive and in readily responsive parts of the animal body".

Before I describe the data obtained by myself and my colleagues I would like to point out one essential detail: the majority of these results were obtained in the period from 1938 to 1949. At that time, electrophysiological techniques were just being

*References p. 13–14*

introduced to the laboratories of physiology for the study of receptors, and the cathode ray oscillograph had not yet become such a common device, as for instance the kymograph in the second half of the nineteenth century. We started our electrophysiological investigations much later. Nevertheless, in spite of non-perfected techniques, numerous data obtained in our laboratory were later confirmed and some of them, as I shall demonstrate here, were "newly" discovered.

Our articles were published mainly in Russian, and unfortunately remained almost unknown to our colleagues abroad. Later on, in 1967, my principal monograph "Interoceptors" was fully translated in the United States with the help of Dr. D. B. Lindsley to whom I am very much obliged.

In this report I shall use such a classification where four categories of interoceptors are defined as follows: *chemoreceptors*, *mechanoreceptors*, *thermoreceptors* and *osmoreceptors*. I shall consider only the first two categories since the physiology of thermoreceptors will be discussed separately in this Symposium. Osmoreceptors will not be discussed at our meetings.

There is another remark I would like to make. It seems to me there are no grounds for a definition as a separate group of "baroreceptors" as was done by Paintal (1972). I believe the term mechanoreceptors to be more universal and allow the investigator

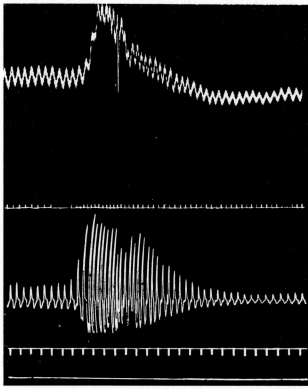

Fig. 1. Reflex changes in arterial pressure and respiration following introduction of 20 μg of nicotine into the vessels of the intestinal segment. Recordings from top: arterial pressure (arteria carotis) (mm Hg); drops of perfusate from vein; respiration; time scale —5 sec; signal marker for nicotine, Cat.

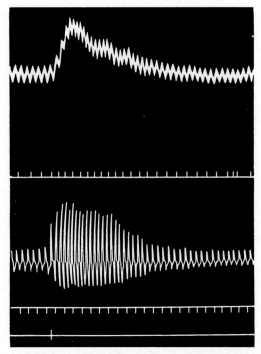

Fig. 2. Reflex changes in arterial pressure (arteria carotis) and respiration following introduction of 20 $\mu$g of acetylcholine into the vessels of the intestinal segment. Recordings from top: arterial pressure (mm Hg); drops of perfusate from vein; respiration; time scale —5 sec; signal marker for acetylcholine. Cat.

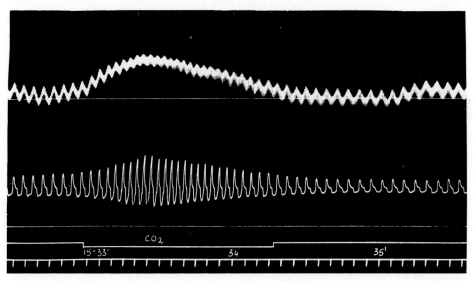

Fig. 3. Changes in arterial pressure and respiration during the perfusion of the intestinal segment with Tyrode solution saturated with $CO_2$. Recordings from top: arterial pressure (arteria carotis, mercury manometer); respiration, zero line of the mercury manometer; signal marker for introduction of the solution containing $CO_2$; time scale —5 sec. Cat.

a wider choice. Furthermore, *the baroreceptors* respond not to pressure as such, but
to the mechanical deformation of tissues resulting from any influence. Therefore,
the division of mechanoreceptors into *baroreceptors* and *pseudobaroreceptors*, which
includes, according to Paintal, stretch receptors of lungs and Pacinian corpuscles,
also does not look very convincing to me. Finally, my last remark. We used in our
investigations mainly the technique of perfusion of individual organs with oxygenated
Tyrode solution; sometimes some blood was added. The Tyrode solution was
circulated through the vascular system of an organ connected to the body only by
neural connections. All experimental conditions were carefully controlled. The perfusion technique has been used for many years, particularly by Heymans (1958), in
chemoreceptor studies on the glomus caroticum.

The principal chemical stimulants used in our studies were nicotine, acetylcholine
and carbon dioxide; the latter was dissolved in Tyrode solution beforehand. For
mechanoreceptor stimulation changes in the pressure of the perfusion solution were
used. In the experiments where electrophysiological recordings were used the potentials
were recorded from the small nervous trunks *in toto*. The electrical activity of single
nerve fibers was not recorded. The effects of substances used as stimulants were
estimated by the alterations in the systemic arterial pressure and respiration. In the
majority of experiments we used cats anesthetized with urethane or chloralose
(Chernigovsky, 1943).

Figs. 1 and 2 show the effects of introduction into the perfused intestinal segment
of various, but usually very low, concentrations of nicotine or acetylcholine. As far
as I know these levels could be correlated with those used by Heymans (1958) and his
colleagues and followers in studies on glomus caroticum chemoreception. Fig. 3
shows the results of other experiments with perfusion of intestinal vessels with
Tyrode solution saturated with $CO_2$. In these experiments the pH of the perfusion
solution was kept in the range from 7.24 to 7.28 by means of special buffer solution.
All attempts to use anoxic solutions as stimulants proved to be successful only in
50% of all experiments, and changes in arterial pressure and respiration were much
less pronounced. We shall discuss these data later. The data on reflex changes in
blood pressure and respiration following the delivery of chemical stimulants to tissue
receptors were confirmed by Matthies *et al.* (1956) as well as by Frank (1964, 1971).

The experiments which I carried out in 1941 showed that the administration of
low doses of nicotine into the rabbit pericardial cavity, or application to the epicardial
surface of the ventricle of filter paper soaked in nicotine solution, produced, in a
very short latent period (1–1.5 sec), a fall in blood pressure, bradycardia and hyperpnea
(Fig. 4A). Section of the vagus nerves eliminated the response. The increase of bioelectrical discharges in the branches of vagal nerves in similar experiments was shown
by my associate Kulaev (1962). Later, similar results were obtained by Sleight (1964)
and Sleight and Widdicombe (1964a, b, 1965a, b) who studied this phenomenon in
detail and confirmed its reflex origin.

The correlation of recordings made in my experiments in 1941 with a figure re-
produced from the article of Sleight is shown in Fig. 4B. It is safe to say that they are
identical. Finally, it must be taken into account that not only chemical agents —

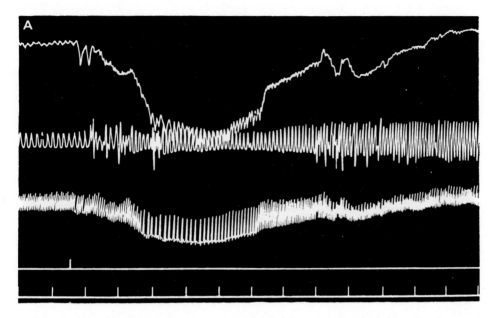

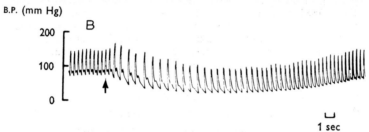

B.P. (mm Hg)

200

100

0

1 sec

Fig. 4. A: reflex changes in arterial pressure and respiration following introduction of 200 mg of nicotine into pericardial cavity. Recordings from top: blood pressure (arteria carotis, mercury manometer); respiration; blood pressure (membrane); signal mark for nicotine; time scale, −5 sec. Intact thorax, local anesthesia. Rabbit. (From Chernigovsky, 1941.) B: anesthetized open chest dog. Aortic blood pressure in mm Hg. At the arrow 100 mg of nicotine were injected into pericardial sac. (From Sleight, 1964.)

nicotine, acetylcholine, $CO_2$ and some others — can produce reflex changes in blood pressure and respiration following their action upon tissue receptors. Changes in blood pressure in the range of 30–40 mm Hg in the vascular system of the intestinal segment can also produce the reflex changes in systemic blood pressure and respiration. Fig. 5 shows that these changes progress relatively slowly, with a latency of about 5–10 sec, and look like prolonged tonic waves.

After this incomplete account of the most essential facts I would like to turn to the interpretation of these data. First of all I would like to point out that the reflexes observed in our experiments should not be considered as responses able to compete with those produced by stimulation of reflexogenic areas of the aorta, sinus caroticus and chemoreceptors of glomus caroticum. Nevertheless, it should be noted that the sensitivity to the same doses of chemical stimulants (acetylcholine and nicotine) of

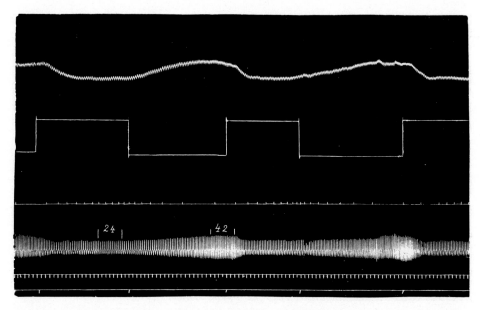

Fig. 5. Reflex changes in arterial pressure and respiration during fluctuations in perfusion pressure in vessels of the perfused intestinal segment. Recordings from top: arterial pressure (mercury manometer); perfusion pressure (elevated part of line corresponds to an increase in perfusion pressure by 38 mm Hg, lower part indicates its return to the initial values); drops of perfusate; respiration (the number of respirations per minute); time scale, —5 sec. Signal mark for fluctuations in perfusion pressure. Cat.

receptors of the glomus caroticum and the tissue receptors studied in our experiments is comparable. However, any analogy here would be unjustified. It seems to me that precisely this fact was the cause of an underestimation of our data by Heymans and Neil in the well known book "Reflexogenic areas of the cardiovascular system" (1958). More important, however, is to give an explanation of those questions which arise during the discussion of data.

The first problem is to locate as precisely as possible the receptors which respond to the stimulation of chemical substances. It seems to me that we are able to give a convincing answer to this question: receptors could be located either in the tissues in the capillary bed area or on the borderline between tissues and capillaries. This assumption was confirmed in special experiments. These experiments were performed using two kinds of the perfusion techniques of the intestinal segment vessels. In the first series of experiments the perfusion was carried out "in the direct way", i.e., artery → capillaries → vein, and in the second one it was performed "backwards"; vein → capillaries → artery. Calculations, measurements and the use of a dye with the perfusion solution have demonstrated that reflexes following the introduction of chemical substances did not appear until these agents reached the capillaries.

Perhaps there was no special need for these experiments since as early as in 1887 Heger published a paper, almost forgotten now, where he demonstrated that the introduction of chemical substances into the arteria femoralis could produce a reaction in animals only at the moment the substances reached the capillaries.

It is more difficult to clarify a question of location of the source of a reflex producing the changes in systemic arterial pressure and respiration during the periodical increase of blood pressure in the vessels of an isolated intestinal loop.

It could be suggested that the changes in systemic arterial pressure and respiration resulted in this case from the hypoxia produced by a decrease in supply of tissue receptors with oxygenated Tyrode solution. Such a hypothesis cannot be ruled out completely, but considering that in our experiments hypoxia or anoxia produced relatively small reflex reactions, this hypothesis seems to us improbable. More preference has been given to the concept which relates the changes in systemic arterial pressure to the stimulation of mechanoreceptors at the level of arteries.

Further, I shall try to provide an interpretation for all of the observations described in my report. Perhaps it would be advisable to consider my interpretation as a fairly reliable hypothesis.

First of all, is it possible to consider the reflex reactions observed in our experiments as an apparatus ensuring the local regulation of the vascular tone? Such an assumption seems to be logical since the reflexes observed were less pronounced than those produced by the stimulation of the mechanoreceptors in sinocarotid and cardio-aortic areas and by stimulation of chemoreceptors of the glomus caroticum. However, this assumption contradicts the facts accumulated and does not explain the distinct changes in systemic arterial pressure and respiration following the action of chemical agents on tissue receptors as well as the responses of systemic arterial pressure and respiration recorded during the fluctuations of the blood pressure in the vascular system of the perfused intestinal segment.

At the same time, how can we explain the reduced sensitivity to hypoxia or anoxia of tissue receptors demonstrated in our experiments? It is common knowledge that chemoreceptors of the glomus caroticum are noted for their high sensitivity to $pO_2$ and hypoxic poisons.

It seems to me that both the special features of glomus caroticum chemoreception and those of tissue receptors could be better understood if we use a comparative physiological, evolutionary approach. The glomus caroticum and sinus caroticus alike develop in animals in parallel with the switch from branchial to pulmonary respiration. An identical process, even now, can also be traced in studies of gradual changes in the axolotl vascular system — a neotenic form — to a definitive one — amblystoma.

A paleontologist, Bystrov (1939), has reconstructed the vascular system of a fossil — Bentosuchus, one of the representatives of the labyrinthodonts, and its neotenic form, dvinosaurus — and suggested that during the evolutionary process the vascular labyrinth appeared when the animal switched from branchial to pulmonary respiration. Actually, it was shown (Chernigovsky, 1962) that both mechanical and chemical stimulation of the vascular labyrinth could produce the reflex reactions.

Samoilov and Chernyakov in a recently published paper (1974) demonstrated that the perfusion of the vascular labyrinth of the frog *Rana temporata* with solutions of different pH values, "acidic" as well as "alkaline", resulted in reflex changes in cardiac activity.

Earlier, Kravtchinsky (1945a–d) demonstrated a high sensitivity of branchial vessels of fishes to lobeline. Application of a solution of cocaine to the branchial vessels of fishes resulted in an irreversible arrest of respiration.

Such data permit one to suggest that a high sensitivity of the chemoreceptors of the glomus caroticum to anoxia reflects the aquatic period of existence of living organisms when an acquired sensitivity to fluctuations in oxygen tension in the water was vitally important.

After the transition of animals to air-breathing, the sensitivity to a lack of oxygen in the blood was retained by the glomus caroticum. Apparently the reduced sensitivity of tissue receptors to a lack of oxygen in the arterial blood was a regular reaction since tissue receptors have lost the sensitivity with the transition of animals to pulmonary respiration: air-breathing. Moreover, the $O_2$ content in the arterial blood of different organs is usually constant. At the same time the sensitivity of *tissue* receptors to $pCO_2$ had to remain unchanged, or even increased, since $CO_2$ represents the most constant and common product of *tissue metabolism*. This hypothesis accepted it would account for the low sensitivity of tissue receptors to anoxia as well as for their considerably higher sensitivity to fluctuations of $CO_2$ tension. The assumption I put forward in 1947, that the sensitivity of tissue receptors to nicotine, acetylcholine and some other chemical substances is likely to be non-specific and is, perhaps, related to other metabolic cycles, was later developed in studies performed in our laboratory by Lebedeva (1965). However, our original hypothesis, perhaps, would be less preferable than another one forwarded by Khayutin who related the effects of chemical agents to nociceptive reflexes (see Chapter 29 of this Symposium).

In conclusion I have to discuss the possible significance and the role of the reflexes from tissue receptors which are not produced by the chemical stimulants, but are related to the maintenance of the vascular tone.

It seems to me that I had already adduced the arguments to support the idea that reflexes observed during the fluctuations of the blood pressure in the vessels of the intestinal loop (and, I can safely add now, in the vascular system of the spleen) could not be considered as the apparatus ensuring the local, regional regulation of the vascular tone.

Now I presume it is essential to present new arguments supporting the assumption that reflexes from tissue receptors (at present I can not name them) participate in regulation of *general vascular tonus*. I do not consider these arguments as decisive for the solution of this problem, but they appear important enough to confirm this point of view.

One of these arguments refers to epicardial receptors. The administration of low doses of cocaine into the pericardial cavity resulting in passive but reversible inhibition of all receptors, produces a rapid and pronounced increase of systemic blood pressure. The increase in the arterial pressure following the cocaine administration was not very significant and developed slowly, but nevertheless was distinct enough. This effect was more pronounced after the introduction of Novocain solution into the vessels of the perfused intestinal segment, which temporarily blocked all impulses in the

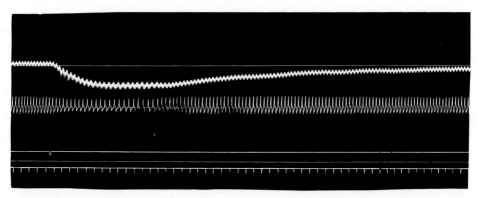

Fig. 6. Prolonged drop of arterial pressure and decrease in respiration rate following introduction of 2 ml of 1 % Novocain solution into the vessels of a perfused intestinal segment. Recordings from top: arterial pressure (mercury manometer, arteria carotis); respiration; signal marker for Novocain; zero line of the mercury manometer; time scale, −5 sec. Cat.

nerves connected with the segment and prevented the appearance of reflexes following the administration of chemical stimulants.

As can be seen from Fig. 6, a prolonged and considerable fall in the arterial pressure as well as a pronounced inhibition of the respiration was observed after 2 ml of 1 % Novocain administration. Both responses were reversible. These and several other experiments not described here, suggest that tissue receptors participate, perhaps, in the reflex maintenance of the essential and, if I may say so, of the basal tone of the blood vessels. Perhaps these influences develop slowly with time and, therefore, in no way compete with rapidly developing changes in the tone of the blood vessels following the stimulation of mechanoreceptors of the sinus caroticus, aortal zone or even following the stimulation of appropriate nerves — sinus caroticum nerves or the depressor nerve, with electrical current. These rapid and urgent responses overlap those I have described earlier and represent the mechanisms of the urgent adaptation of the cardiovascular system. I think these considerations do not minimize the significance of slow changes in the tone just as, for instance, rapidly developing and quickly disappearing primary responses do not diminish the importance of slow and "superslow" fluctuations of the potentials in the central nervous system.

I have presented in this report the data obtained (some years ago) in our laboratory. It was motivated by the fact that the investigations performed in our laboratory were, for some years, and still are, almost unknown to our colleagues abroad.

In conclusion I would like to mention some possible trends in future scientific developments. But in no case would I make any predictions, since the rapid development of science makes any prediction unreliable. In my opinion the following directions are promising and could be developed in the future.

(1) Investigation, mainly with electrophysiological techniques, of primary processes occurring in sensory elements.

(2) Investigation of the role of tissue receptors and reflexes evoked by their stimulation in the regulation of physiological processes.

*References p. 13–14*

(3) A search for chemical substances which could be considered as adequate, physiological stimulants for chemoreceptors of tissues and organs.

(4) Correlation between structure and functions of tissue receptors.

(5) Studies on the role of tissue receptors in the organization of such motivated behavioral activities as hunger, thirst and specific forms of the appetite.

(6) Comparative physiological aspects of studies on tissue receptors.

## SUMMARY

The responses elicited by stimulation of tissue receptors were studied in numerous earlier experiments (1938–1949) on adult anesthetized (urethane or chloralose) cats during perfusion with oxygenated Tyrode solution of various organs (small intestine segments, stomach, spleen and kidney) connected to the body only with neural connections. Systemic arterial pressure, respiration and summated bioelectrical activity in afferent fibers were recorded and responses evoked by tissue receptors' stimulation with acetylcholine and nicotine were studied. In some experiments Tyrode solution saturated with carbon dioxide (pH 7.24–7.28) and added buffer solution was used.

Nicotine, acetylcholine (10 $\mu$g and above) and $CO_2$-containing Tyrode solution caused an increase in systemic arterial pressure, respiratory stimulation and an enhancement of summated bioelectrical activity in afferent fibers. These effects could be abolished by previous administration of Novocain or cocaine into the vessels of the perfused organs. The responses were restored when the perfused organs were washed with Tyrode solution. Anoxic solutions produced similar but less pronounced effects in 50% of animals.

Introduction of nicotine (20 $\mu$g and above) into the rabbit pericardial cavity produced a fall in systemic arterial pressure, bradycardia and respiratory stimulation. These effects could not be produced if Novocain or cocaine were introduced beforehand into the pericardial cavity. Afferent discharges in vagal nerves were recorded during the nicotine administration.

Changes in perfusion pressure in the vessels of the intestinal segment in the range from 30 to 40 mm Hg resulted in the reflex changes in the systemic arterial pressure and respiration. An increase in the perfusion pressure produced a reflex fall in the systemic arterial pressure, and respiration inhibition. A fall in the perfusion pressure caused a reverse effect.

Introduction of Novocain or cocaine solutions into the perfused vessels of the intestinal segment inhibited the reflexes evoked by simultaneous administration of nicotine or acetylcholine and resulted in a prolonged fall in the systemic arterial pressure and inhibition of respiration. Introduction of Novocain or cocaine into the pericardial cavity produced a slow rise in the systemic arterial pressure. Changes in respiration rate were not observed or were insignificant.

A possible role of the reflex tissue receptors' responses in the regulation of physiological functions studied is discussed. The low sensitivity of tissue receptors to hypoxia and high sensitivity to $CO_2$ might be explained in terms of evolutionary development.

## REFERENCES

BYSTROV, A. P. (1939) Blutgefassystem der Labyrinthodonted (Gefasse des Kopfes). *Acta zool.*, **20**, 125–155.

CHERNIGOVSKY, V. N. (1941) The receptors of the pericardium. In *Neurohumoral Regulation of the Activity of Organs and Tissues*. Naval Medical Academy Press, Leningrad, pp. 54–79.

CHERNIGOVSKY, V. N. (1943) *The Afferent Systems of the Internal Organs*. Naval Medical Academy Press, Kirov.

CHERNIGOVSKY, V. N. (1947) The receptors of the cardiovascular system. *Advanc. mod. Biol.*, **23**, 215–240 (in Russian).

CHERNIGOVSKY, V. N. (1960) *Interoceptors*. Medgiz, Moscow.

CHERNIGOVSKY, V. N. (1962) Evolutionary aspect in the study of chemoreception of the glomus caroticum. *Arch. int. Pharmacodyn.*, **140**, 20–29.

CHERNIGOVSKY, V. N. (1967) *Interoceptors. Russian Monographs on Brain and Behavior*, No. 4. American Physiological Association, Washington, D.C.

FRANK, M. H. (1964) *Receptor Function of Perfused Innervated Intestinal Segments in Reflex Regulation of Blood Pressure*. Ph.D. Thesis, Ohio State University.

FRANK, M. H. (1971) Neural origin of cardiovascular reflexes from the intestine. In *Proc. XXV Int. Congr. Union Physiol. Sci. Vol. 9*. German Physiological Society, Munich, p. 184 (abstract).

HEGER, P. (1887) Einige Versuche über die Empfindlichkeit der Gefasse. In *Beitr. zur Physiol*. Verlag von F. C. W. Vogel, Leipzig, pp. 193–199.

HEYMANS, C. AND NEIL, E. (1958) *Reflexogenic Areas of the Cardiovascular System*. Churchill, London.

KRAVCHINSKY, B. D. (1945a) The evolution of reflex connections of the respiratory center in vertebrate animals. I. The role of branchial nerves in the regulation of respiration in fishes. *Sechenov physiol. J. U.S.S.R.*, **21**, 11–24 (in Russian).

KRAVCHINSKY, B. D. (1945b) The evolution of reflex connection of the respiratory center in vertebrate animals. II. The role of the aortic reflexogenic zone in the regulation of respiration in amphibians (frogs). *Sechenov physiol. J. U.S.S.R.*, **21**, 25–42 (in Russian).

KRAVCHINSKY, B. D. (1945c) The evolution of reflex connections of the respiratory center in vertebrate animals. III. Reflex connections of the respiratory center in reptiles (tortoises). *Sechenov physiol. J. U.S.S.R.*, **30**, 120–136 (in Russian).

KRAVCHINSKY, B. D. (1945d) The evolution of reflex connections of the respiratory center in vertebrate animals. IV. Reflex connections of the respiratory center in mammals. *Sechenov physiol. J. U.S.S.R.*, **31**, 137–150 (in Russian).

KULAEV, B. S. (1962) Characteristics of afferent impulse activity evoked in cardiac nerves by chemical stimulation of epicardial receptors. *Sechenov physiol. J. U.S.S.R.*, **48**, 1350–1358 (in Russian).

LEBEDEVA, V. A. (1965) *The Mechanism of Chemoreception*. Nauka, Leningrad.

LEEK, B. F. (1972) Abdominal visceral receptors. In *Handbook of Sensory Physiology, Vol. III/I. Enteroceptors*, Springer-Verlag, Berlin, pp. 113–160.

MATTHIES, H., WIEDERSHAUSEN, B., OTTO, G. UND SCHOLTZ, G. (1956) Pharmakologische Untersuchungen an Interoceptoren. *Naunyn-Schmiederberg's Arch. exp. Path. Pharmak.*, **229**, 544–555.

PAINTAL, A. S. (1972) Cardiovascular receptors. In *Handbook of Sensory Physiology, Vol. III/I. Enteroceptors*, Springer-Verlag, Berlin, pp. 1–45.

PAVLOV, I. P. (1894) (1940) On the incompleteness of modern physiological analysis of drug effects. In *Complete Works, Vol. 1* U.S.S.R. Academy of Sciences Press, Moscow, pp. 323–325.

SAMOILOV, V. O. AND CHERNYAKOV, G. M. (1974) The heart reflexes of the frog carotid labyrinth receptors. *Sechenov physiol. J. U.S.S.R.*, **60**, 784–788 (in Russian).

SHERRINGTON, C. S. (1911) *The Integrative Action of the Nervous System*. Constable, London.

SLEIGHT, P. (1964) A cardiovascular depressor reflex from the epicardium of the left ventricle in the dog. *J. Physiol. (Lond.)*, **173**, 321–343.

SLEIGHT, P. AND WIDDICOMBE, J. G. (1964a) Action potentials in nerve fibres from left ventricular receptor in the dog. *J. Physiol. (Lond.)*, **171**, 34p–35p.

SLEIGHT, P. AND WIDDICOMBE, J. G. (1964b) Action potentials in afferent fibres from receptors in the pericardium of the dog. *J. Physiol. (Lond.)*, **175**, 63p–64p.

SLEIGHT, P. AND WIDDICOMBE, J. G. (1965a) Action potentials in fibres from receptors in the pericardium and myocardium of the dog's left ventricle. *J. Physiol. (Lond.)*, **181**, 235–258.

SLEIGHT, P. AND WIDDICOMBE, J. G. (1965b). Action potentials in afferent fibres from pericardial mechanoreceptors in the dog. *J. Physiol. (Lond.)*, **181**, 259–269.

WIDDICOMBE, J. G. AND FILLENZ, M. (1972) Receptors of the lungs and airways. In *Handbook of Sensory Physiology*, *Vol. III/I. Enteroceptors*, Springer-Verlag, Berlin, pp. 81–112.

# Is the Physiology of Cutaneous Receptors Determined by Morphology?

A. IGGO

*Department of Physiology, Faculty of Veterinary Medicine, University of Edinburgh, Edinburgh EH9 1QH (Great Britain)*

One way to start this paper is by posing a question — to what extent is the morphology of receptors a decisive factor in determining the functional activity of sensory receptors?

Cutaneous receptors are present at several depths in the skin but are principally concentrated near the boundary of the dermis and epidermis. In general, receptors have a specialised structure that distinguishes them from the tissues in which they are embedded, although such distinctiveness was, and is, not invariably accepted by morphologists (see, for example, Montagna and Macpherson, 1973). Electron microscopy has, however, established this specialisation beyond reasonable doubt (see Andres and Von Düring, 1973). The basic ground plan for sensory receptors is:

(1) an afferent nerve cell body,

(2) an extension of which (either axon in vertebrates, or a dendrite in some invertebrates) enters the skin and

(3) forms a terminal region that is modified in varying degree and is associated with

(4) non-nervous tissue elements which enclose or encapsulate the morphologically specialised nerve terminal, and

(5) a centrally directed branch of the axon which enters the central nervous system and there, often forming several collateral branches, makes synaptic contact with interneurones or, in some special cases, motoneurones of the central nervous system.

This ground plan is subject to considerable variation in particular instances, but the essential elements detailed above are always recognisable.

Vertebrate cutaneous receptors conform most generally to the plan, since in all cases the nerve cell bodies are in cranial or spinal ganglia remote from the receptors in the skin in contrast to invertebrates in which the sensory cell may be in the periphery. There is one significant difference in the organisation of the receptors that has been revealed by ultrastructural studies. In some receptors the nerve terminal ends in special relation to an accessory cell, *the receptor cell* (Grundfest, 1971) as in the Merkel cell (Fig. 4) and lateral line organs. In others, such as the Ruffini ending (Fig. 5), the primary sensory neurones have no intermediary cellular element between the nerve terminal and collagen fibrils. This difference in structure has a functional correlation since it is probable that the physiological processes of stimulus detection are fundamentally different in the two kinds of receptor — in the former the transduction of the physical input to a biological signal occurs in the accessory cell, by analogy with photoreceptors, whereas in the latter the transformation must occur in the nerve terminal itself, as is also the case in olfactory cells.

The general morphological plan can be paralleled by a functional framework which can be used to focus attention on morphological features with a known or predicted functional role. The sequence of events as it occurs during normal afferent excitation is the following:

(1) physical input impinges on skin and

(2) is transmitted via intervening epidermal (and dermal) tissue to

(3) the transducer element where it initiates a chemical or physicochemical transformation that

(4) leads to depolarization of the nerve terminal (generator potential) which, by current flow in the nerve terminal,

(5) causes depolarization at a sensitive spike-initiation site in the preterminal nerve, which if sufficiently large will

(6) cause the generation of nerve impulses that are conducted orthodromically along the afferent nerve fibre to enter the central nervous system and alter the excitability of second order neurones in the afferent pathway.

In morphological studies to be reviewed these various functional aspects should be kept in mind to assess the significance of the structural elements. This basic functional framework is further extended by the phenomenon of *selectivity sensitivity* or *specificity* of the receptors in responding to natural stimuli. Once again the detailed account to be given will be anticipated and summarised by stating that there are four main classes of cutaneous receptor: (a) *mechanoreceptors* that detect physical displacement of, and perhaps physical pressure or tension in, the skin; (b) *thermoreceptors* that can register skin temperature; (c) *chemoreceptors* of various kinds responding to chemicals in solution on or in the skin and (d) *nociceptors* that are activated by potentially harmful stimuli or by chemicals released as a sequel to tissue damage or inflammatory responses.


DIVERSITY OF RECEPTORS


There is a rich variety of receptors in the skin of any given species and even greater diversity when different orders and phyla of animals are considered. This present paper will place an emphasis on mammalian receptors.

Recent work in several laboratories has drawn attention to the high degree of biophysical specificity that is such a striking feature of vertebrate cutaneous receptors (see Iggo, 1966; Burgess and Perl, 1973; Hensel, 1973 for reviews). The specialisation extends beyond a differentiation into mechanoreceptors, thermoreceptors, etc., since it is now firmly established that within each of these major groupings there is a further subdivision into subclasses, *e.g.* the thermoreceptors include cold receptors and warm receptors. In parallel with these electrophysiological studies of cutaneous afferent units, there has been a revival of interest in the morphology of cutaneous receptors now that the electron microscope and associated techniques have made it possible to see so much more clearly their fine cellular structure. I shall endeavour to bring the two streams of new information together and consider whether it is possible to sustain the proposal that there is a necessary relation between structure and function.

At the outset I must exclude any consideration of the internal structure of excitable membranes since the present techniques applied to afferent units do not yield detailed information on the structure of the cell membranes, although they can indicate regions of special contact, e.g. synapses, desmosomes, tight junctions. Nevertheless, it should be mentioned that even in peripheral nerves and spinal roots, the myelinated axons can be shown to have different physiological characteristics at their nodes of Ranvier (Stämpfli, personal communication) although no structural counterpart has yet been described.

I shall discuss those cutaneous mechanoreceptors for which the initial step of relating general physiological characteristics to gross morphological features has been taken successfully. There are now several examples of proven correlation, these are the *Pacinian corpuscle;* the *Golgi–Mazzoni corpuscle;* the *Merkel "touch-spot"* (Tastfleck); the *Ruffini endings;* and the *Herbst* and *Grandry corpuscles* in birds. In each of these examples a particular kind of mechanoreceptor response has been correlated with the receptor and the question to be asked is whether the physiological characteristics are dependent on, or determined by, the observed morphological characteristics. If this is the case, then a method is available for an extension of knowledge of receptor function, based on either physiological or morphological data.

### The Pacinian corpuscle (Pacini, 1840)

This corpuscle responds to a sudden mechanical displacement with the discharge of a single action potential (Gray and Matthews, 1951) but will follow a vibratory displacement with a threshold that is frequency-dependent with maximal sensitivity between 400 and 800 Hz. This typical property of the Pacinian corpuscles depends on the presence of the lamellated encapsulation of the centrally placed nerve terminal by non-nervous tissue. The lamellae of the outer core (derived from the perineural sheath) act as a high-pass mechanical filter, allowing the high frequency components of the applied displacement to reach the central core containing the nerve terminal, but preventing any steady displacement from doing so (Loewenstein and Skalak, 1966). Detailed electrophysiological experiments, in which the generator potential has been recorded at the nerve terminal, in response to localised small displacements of the isolated central core (tightly packed Schwann cell lamellae and nerve terminal) of the corpuscle, reveal a graded depolarisation which can outlast the action potential generated more proximally along the afferent axon. The morphological studies have not so far identified the actual transducer sites at which these generator potentials arise. It is likely that there is a molecular specialisation of the membrane not yet made visible by contemporary techniques. The action potentials arise from the distal (terminal) node of Ranvier (Diamond et al., 1956) which is embedded in the corpuscle, but once again no distinctive ultrastructural features have been reported. The site of

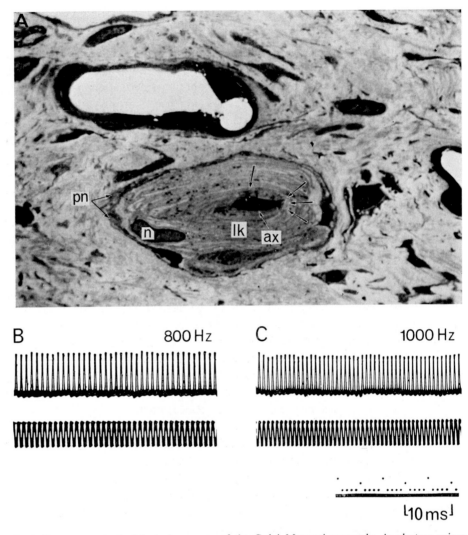

Fig. 1. Structure and physiological response of the Golgi–Mazzoni corpuscle. A: electron micrograph of a Golgi–Mazzoni corpuscle — the axonal ending (ax) is surrounded by the non-nervous lamellar cell (lk); n, lamellar cell nucleus; pn, perineural sheath from Andres (1966). B and C: afferent discharge in response to high-frequency vibratory movement of a sinus hair; upper traces, discharge of impulses in a single afferent fibre; lower traces, sine wave stimulus (from Gottschaldt et al., 1973).

spike initiation may have an important influence on the characteristics of the spike trains that leave the receptor.

Finally, individual normal Pacinian corpuscles appear to be supplied by separate afferent nerve fibres, and each fibre supplies only one corpuscle, so that the afferent discharge entering the central nervous system can be entrained by a vibratory stimulus and interference effects that could arise from impulses being initiated in several branches of an axon are absent. It can be seen from this example that morphology can have a strong influence on physiology, but that membrane effects (for which no morphological features have been described) are also important (see also the contributions from the Pavlov Institute of Physiology to this Symposium).

In other mammalian mechanoreceptors there is circumstantial evidence that lamellation of the corpuscle has a function similar to that in the Pacinian corpuscle. These other receptors are smaller and have a much simpler structure, with fewer lamellae, *e.g.* the *Golgi–Mazzoni receptor* (Fig. 1A) (Andres and Von Düring, 1973) in which the lamellae of the outer core of the Pacinian corpuscle with a large capsule space are absent. Schwann cell lamellae are, however, numerous and relatively tightly packed. This kind of corpuscle is present in the centre of the sinus hair follicle (Andres, 1966).

In physiological experiments Gottschaldt *et al.* (1973) recorded a high-frequency discharge in certain afferent fibres from facial sinus hairs in response to sinusoidal oscillations at frequencies up to 1000 Hz delivered to the hair (Fig. 1B, C), but not when similar displacements were applied to the adjacent epidermis. The carpal sinus hairs, described in detail by Nilsson (1969), do not respond in exactly the same way to vibratory stimuli. Although high-frequency-locked discharges similar to those from facial sinus hairs can be recorded from nerves to the carpal hairs, the responses originate from Pacinian corpuscles that are clustered around the hair follicle (Nilsson, 1969; Gottschaldt *et al.*, 1973). Lamellated corpuscles of the simple Golgi–Mazzoni type are found elsewhere in the body of mammals, but it is not yet confirmed by electrophysiological recording that they are high-frequency mechanoreceptors. Even simpler lamellated receptors have also been described (von Düring, 1973).

### Hair follicle receptors

Lamellation may be a morphological prerequisite to high-frequency responsiveness acting in the way established for Pacinian corpuscles by Loewenstein and Skalak (1966). The capacity to act as velocity detectors is not, however, limited to lamellated corpuscles since ordinary *hair follicle receptors* are well-known to act physiologically in this way. They differ structurally from the lamellated corpuscles; there is a highly organised circumferential array of "palisade" nerve terminals, parallel to and surrounding the hair follicle in monotrich hairs (Yamamoto, 1966; Cauna, 1969; Andres and Von Düring, 1973). The nerve terminals are enclosed by Schwann cells except at their inner and outer edges (Fig. 2A). At the inner edge the nerve terminals are in contact with the glassy membrane of the hair follicle, but at the outer edge they appear to be unattached or to make contact with the dermis of the hair follicle. This quite different morphological arrangement is associated with a different kind of physiological response from the Pacinian corpuscles. A train of impulses is present in the axon during *movement* of the hair (Fig. 3A), but the discharge does not follow vibration of the hair at frequencies greater than about 300 Hz. This latter difference can be attributed to the absence of lamellation from the hair follicle palisade endings. With rigorous control of the mechanical conditions the interspike interval of the iterative discharge during constant velocity displacement of the hair can be very regular (Fig. 3A) and is related to the velocity of movement by a power function

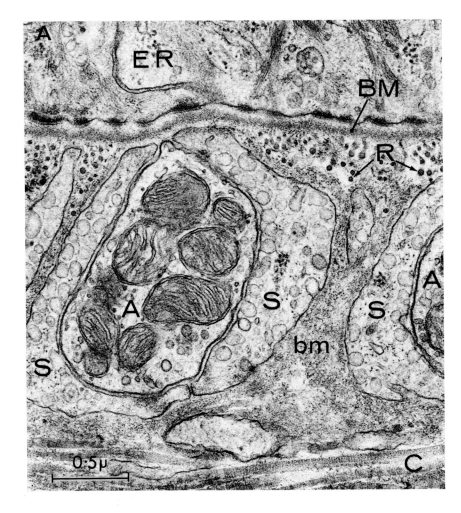

(Brown and Iggo, 1967). This feature implies the existence of a mechanism for the
proportional conversion of the constant velocity displacement to a steady transducer
potential (first order differential) but no hint as to the mechanism is evident from
existing morphological studies. Several kinds of hair follicle receptor have been
described — types D, $G_{1+2}$, T (Brown and Iggo, 1967; Burgess and Perl, 1973). These
differ in several respects, especially since the associated hair follicles (down hairs,
guard hairs and tylotrichs respectively) and afferent fibres (small and large diameter
axons) are of different kinds. Their "velocity" threshold and sensitivity also differ
and it may be possible, by a detailed correlative study, to establish if there are any
specific morphological characteristics underlying these forms of physiological behaviour.

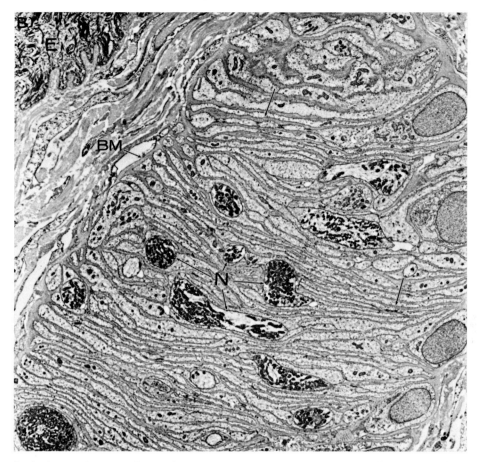

Fig. 2. A: neural receptor elements in a hair follicle from the ear of a rat. The fine nerve filaments (A) lie parallel to and encircle the hair and epithelial root sheath (ER), separated from them by the basement membrane (bm). C, collagen; R, fine collagen fibrils; S, Schwann cells encasing the nerve terminals (from Cauna, 1969). B: internal structure of a Meissner's corpuscle from human glabrous skin, in a longitudinal section of the apical part of a corpuscle. BM, basement membrane; E, epidermal cell; N, nerve endings (from Cauna, 1966).

## The Meissner corpuscle (Meissner, 1853)

The Meissner corpuscle is another putative rapidly adapting mechanoreceptor, *i.e.* velocity detector, and is present in glabrous skin in primates (Lindblom, 1965). These afferent units also respond with a velocity-dependent stream of impulses when the skin is displaced mechanically at a constant velocity (Fig. 3B). Like the palisade endings in hair follicles, the receptor terminals are in the form of flat plates sandwiched between Schwann cell tissue (Fig. 2B) (Cauna, 1966) and parallel to the epidermis. The functional significance of this arrangement requires to be investigated. A further specialisation of the Meissner corpuscle is that the collagen fibres of the dermis are continuous with the tonofibrils of the epidermal cells on one hand, and enter the

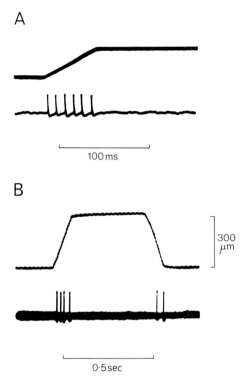

Fig. 3. Afferent discharges from A, guard hair follicle receptor (type $G_2$) in cat and B, a presumed Meissner corpuscle in monkey glabrous skin. In each record the upper trace shows the mechanical stimulus and the lower trace the afferent discharge. (A from Brown and Iggo, 1967; B from Iggo and Ogawa, unpublished).

Meissner corpuscle on the other, where they may fuse with the fibrils of the inter-cellular substance (Andres and Von Düring, 1973). These collagenous bundles thus provide a physical linkage of the mechanical displacement of the skin surface with the internal structural elements of the receptor.

*Merkel "touch-spot" (Tastfleck) (Merkel, 1875)*

This receptor which has been rediscovered several times and thus is rich in synonyms, is a slowly-adapting receptor, in which the afferent discharge persists for several minutes under constant displacement of the skin (Iggo and Muir, 1969). The receptors, which consist of Merkel discs, Merkel cells and associated tissue elements, are scattered over the hairy surface of the skin, often in association with large hairs (tylotrichs of Straile) and in some species (*e.g.* the cat) can be seen at the skin surface, where they appear as small red dome-shaped spots. In glabrous skin the Merkel cells are at the base of intermediate ridges of the epidermis and the individual receptors cannot, therefore, be seen at the skin surface. Distinctive morphological features of the receptor complex (Fig. 4A, B) are the cluster of Merkel cells at or close to the base of the epidermis within 30–40 μm of the skin surface, with each element in the

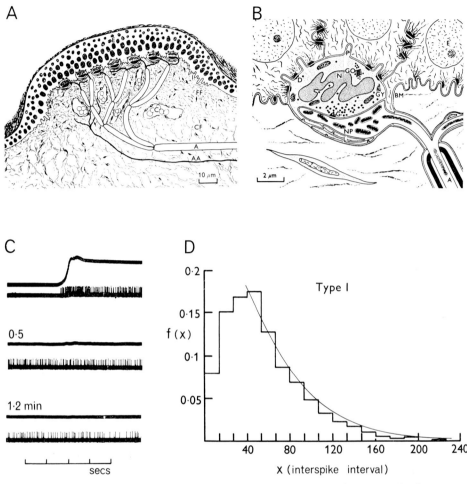

Fig. 4. Slowly adapting type I mechanoreceptor in cat skin. A: detail of the Merkel cell. B: cross-sectional diagram of a Merkel Tastfleck (touch-spot). A, myelinated axon; AA, non-myelinated axons; BM, basement membrane; C, capillary; CF, coarse collagen; D, desmosome; E, epidermis; FF, fine collagen; G, osmiophilic granules; GO, Golgi apparatus; GY, glycogen; L, laminae beneath the Merkel disc; N, polylobulated nucleus of the Merkel cell; NP, nerve plate or Merkel disc; T, tactile cell (from Iggo and Muir, 1969). C: afferent discharge in a type I afferent unit of monkey before and during steady displacement of the skin (from Iggo, 1963b). D: frequency distribution of the interimpulse intervals during the adapted discharge of a type I unit in cat (from Iggo and Muir, 1969).

cluster supplied by a branch of a single myelinated afferent axon, a thickened epidermis overlying the Merkel cells, a dense collagenous core to the receptor and a circumferential ring of epidermodermal invaginations. The expanded nerve-endings (Merkel discs) are enclosed by the overlying Merkel cells and specialised junctional regions are found between the cell and the nerve disc. The Merkel cell, which in Grundfest's terminology is a "receptor cell", also displays cytological specialisation in the form of an extensively polylobulated nucleus, osmiophilic dense-cored vesicles subjacent to the nucleus and rod- or finger-like extensions penetrating invaginations

*References p. 29–31*

of the overlying epidermal cells (Fig. 4) (Andres, 1966; Iggo and Muir, 1969). Electro-physiological evidence (Brown and Iggo, 1963; Burgess and Horch, 1973; Burgess *et al.*, 1974) indicates that the slow-adapting characteristic of the afferent units is dependent on the presence of the Merkel cells. When the cutaneous nerve is cut or crushed the afferent fibres lose their characteristic distinctive physiological responses, and the regenerating nerve tips respond non-specifically to natural stimuli. Regenerating cutaneous axons lack an ability to generate a sustained discharge on mechanical stimulation until the Merkel cell–nerve terminal complex has been restored during regeneration.

The Merkel Tastfleck is the receptor terminal for the slowly adapting type I (SAI) afferent unit (Iggo, 1966), which has several physiologically distinctive features. *First*, the receptive field is spot-like, and the spots are Merkel Tastflecken. If the stimulus probe is moved off the visible spot in hairy skin to adjacent epidermis, the mechanical displacement becomes ineffective. This highly localised sensitivity is attributed to the mechanical insulation afforded by the circumferential finger-like processes of the touch-spot and its dense collagenous core, so that the morphological organisation is a significant factor in deciding the functional capacity. *Second*, the afferent discharge, during controlled ramp and plateau mechanical indentation, typically and characteristically becomes irregular during the adaptation after the end of the ramp displacement. The irregularity is most conspicuous at low rates of discharge (Fig. 4C, D), but can also be revealed by numerical analysis as high discharge rates (Iggo and Muir, 1969). The interimpulse intervals are very variable in length and may be as short as 2 msec and as long as 100 msec in a given set of conditions. The frequency distribution of such a discharge is Poisson-like (Fig. 4D), except for the absence of very short intervals and indicates that a random process determines the likelihood of a spike discharge. This randomness can be accounted for if it is assumed that there are multiple independent spike generators (Iggo and Muir, 1969; Horch *et al.*, 1974). The morphological organisation of the Merkel touch-spot is consistent with this hypothesis if it is assumed that the Merkel disc is a spike generator, or at least that the impulses arise within the branched terminal arborisation of the single myelinated axon that innervates a touch-spot. The lack of very short impulse intervals is attributable to interactions within the arborisation, arising from antidromic invasion and collision, and to resetting of impulses discharges (Chambers *et al.*, 1972).

These two features: (1) localised mechanical sensitivity and (2) Poisson-like distribution of impulse intervals, can be attributed to structural causes, and can also be used as an aid in identifying the origin of spike discharges in situations where it is not possible with the same degree of certainty to recognise the receptor by visual means, as in glabrous primate skin and in the sinus hairs (Gottschaldt *et al.*, 1973).

### *The Ruffini ending (Ruffini, 1891)*

This ending is present in the dermis and in its original description was reported in the subcutaneous tissue of human fingers, and has since been found in hairy skin (see Chambers *et al.*, 1972, where there has been a detailed electrophysiological study),

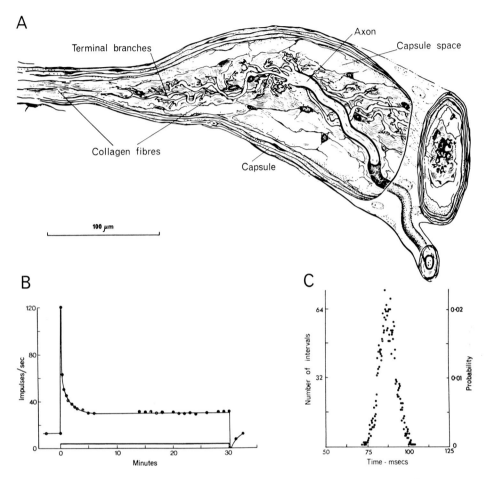

Fig. 5. Ruffini ending. A: diagrammatic reconstruction based on serial sections of a Ruffini ending in cat hairy skin. The myelinated axon penetrates the capsule, loses its myelin sheath to break up into numerous terminal branches which are in intimate contact with fine collagen fibrils which fuse to form fibres that emerge at the pole of the receptor. B: impulse discharge from a type II afferent unit. There is a maintained discharge (●——●) in response to steady displacement (solid bar at bottom) (from Iggo, 1963a). C: the frequency distribution of interimpulse intervals is Gaussian (from Chambers et al., 1972).

in joints (see Skoglund, 1973) and in periodontal tissues. The receptor in the cat is an encapsulated fusiform structure, with a thinly lamellated capsule enclosing a fluid-filled capsule space, at the centre of which lies the profusely branched receptor terminal (Fig. 5A). The single large myelinated axon penetrates the capsule before losing its myelin sheath. Small processes on fine subdivisions of the terminal are in close contact with collagenous fibrils that run through the central core of the receptor to emerge at the poles as collagen fibres that fuse with collagenous bundles in the subcutaneous and cutaneous layers. No specialised intermediary transducer cell is interposed between the collagen fibrils and the nerve terminal processes and it must be concluded that the biophysical transducer processes occur in the nerve terminal in this receptor — i.e., it is a primary sensory neurone. There are no certain morphological signs of these transducer elements. The structural arrangements account for the high sensitivity of these Ruffini endings (slowly-adapting type II (SAII) receptors (Iggo, 1966)) to stretch of the skin, since the collagen fibres form an effective mechanism for transmitting stretch to the interior of the receptor. The transducer action is, on analogy with other mechanoreceptors, likely to be a localised change in ionic permeability of the membrane, and hence of an ionic current change. The small changes, generated widely over the receptor terminals, would cause passive voltage changes more proximally in the non-myelinated part of the receptor, which would eventually reach the myelinated part of the axon and there, if sufficiently large, generate action potentials.

Another morphological feature of the Ruffini ending now becomes of interest. Each ending is supplied by one myelinated axon which only loses its myelin sheath on entering the capsule. It is probable that in Ruffini endings impulse initiation occurs in the myelinated part of the axon. The afferent discharge, therefore, in contrast to the SAI mechanoreceptor, arises from only one or, if the parent axon supplies several Ruffini endings, a limited number of spike generators. In cat hairy skin, each SAII axon appears to supply a single Ruffini ending. A typical feature of the cat SAII afferent units is that the discharge is very regular, and the frequency distribution of impulse intervals is Gaussian (Fig. 5C) (Chambers et al., 1972). Such a property is consistent with a single spike-generating site that is subject to normal variability in the processes leading to the discharge of impulses.

Once again a number of features in the functional activity of a mechanoreceptor, viz. (1) sensitivity to stretch, and (2) impulse discharge pattern, can be seen to have a structural determination, and, as with the Pacini, Golgi–Mazzoni and Merkel receptors, this information can provide a tool to identify the receptors morphologically in situations where it is otherwise difficult, as in the sinus hair follicle.

### The Herbst corpuscle (Herbst, 1848)

The Herbst corpuscle is the avian equivalent of the Pacinian corpuscle, although it is much smaller. It is structurally distinctive since there is a regular orientation of "sentinel" nuclei (Quilliam, 1966) which are present in the inner core, aligned parallel with the centrally located nerve terminal. A further specialisation of the Herbst corpuscle is the large vesicle in which the nerve terminal ends. Physiological studies of this corpuscle have been less detailed than for the Pacinian corpuscle, but it is established that it functions as a high-frequency detector (Dorward and McIntyre, 1971), presumably because of its lamellation.

### The Grandry corpuscle (Grandry, 1869)

This corpuscle provides an instance of a receptor which, on general morphological grounds, was mistyped functionally. There is a resemblance between Grandry corpuscles and Merkel cells, at least when the simplest Grandry is the basis of comparison. In both cases there is a nerve plate enclosed by a non-nervous cell or cells, and for this reason the suggestion was made that the Grandry corpuscle was a slowly adapting mechanoreceptor. Recent combined histological and electrophysiological studies by Gottschaldt (1974) have brought new information. First, the Grandry corpuscles are the receptor terminals of rapidly adapting afferent units, with a velocity dependence but no static discharge. Second, the Grandry cells have several morphological features that distinguish them from Merkel cells, and, in fact, they are more similar to Meissner corpuscles and hair follicle palisade endings. (1) They have a dermal, and not epidermal, location; (2) even in the simplest Grandry the nerve plate is sandwiched between two satellite cells and in more complex receptors there is a stack of interleaved nerve plates and satellite Schwann cells. Gottschaldt (1974)

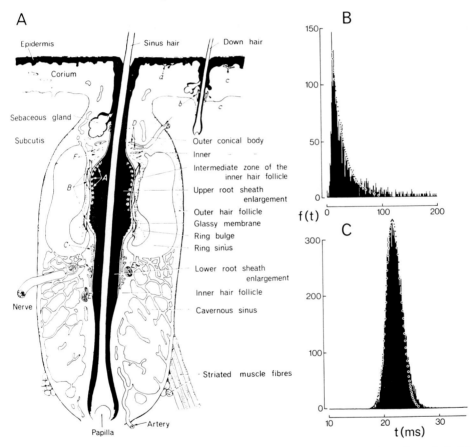

Fig. 6. A complex sense organ — the sinus hair. A: diagrammatic reconstruction of a cat's facial sinus hair (vibrissa), showing the highly organised structure and four distinct kinds of neural receptor: $A$, Merkel cells and discs in the root sheath; $B$, straight lanceolate endings adjacent to the glassy membrane; $C$, branched lanceolate endings in the lower root sheath enlargement; $D$, circular lanceolate endings and $E$, Golgi–Mazzoni corpuscles. There are also fine nerve endings $(F)$ in the conical body (from Andres, 1966). B and C: theoretical (encircled dots) and observed frequency distributions for the discharge of impulses in sinus hair afferent fibres, in 2 different units. B: St I unit, which fits an exponential relation (*i.e.*, Poisson distribution) and C: St II, a unit which satisfies a normal (Gaussian) distribution (from Gottschaldt *et al.*, 1973, to which reference should be made for further details).

*References p. 29–31*

reports that there may be as many as six, a degree of lamination that is reminiscent of the Meissner corpuscle. The extent to which any of these features are necessary for the functional properties of Grandry corpuscles are open questions.

COMPLEX CUTANEOUS SENSORY ORGANS

The receptors considered so far are, for the most part, simple encapsulated elements. In several places in the skin of mammals there are more complex arrays of receptors such as glabrous skin in primates, Eimer's organ in the mole (Halata, 1972a and b), sinus hair follicles (Andres, 1966) and the bill tip organ in aquatic birds (Gottschaldt, 1974). In each of these situations the morphology is complex but it is possible, on the basis of the detailed single unit studies of the kind reviewed above, to predict the functional role of various morphological elements (Iggo and Gottschaldt, 1974). One interesting feature of these complex sensory units is the combination, in a single organ, of mechanoreceptors that detect a wide range of stimulus parameters, especially frequency and maintained distortion. This is achieved by incorporating several kinds of receptor elements, each separately innervated, not by requiring a single receptor to have multiple analysers, *i.e.* to be polymodal.

The morphology of the complex structure imposes a further constraint on the functional characteristics of the receptors. The facial sinus hairs (vibrissae) (Gottschaldt *et al.*, 1973) are a good example (Fig. 6). *First*, individual large myelinated afferent fibres pass to single follicles, without branching to other follicles, thus permitting more accurate spatial localisation. *Second*, within each follicle there are representatives of all the major kinds of mechanoreceptor, so that each follicle is capable of providing information of all available parameters (frequency, displacement, amplitude, velocity and direction). *Third*, the mechanoreceptors within the follicle are insulated mechanically, by the blood sinus which encloses them, from movements other than those transmitted via the hair shaft. *Fourth*, the location of receptor terminals within the follicle, especially the Merkel cells, is a deciding factor in determining the directional sensitivity that the receptors exhibit.

In the complex cutaneous sensory units, therefore, the individual distinctive physiological characteristics of the receptors may be further modified by the morphology of the whole sensory structure.

CONCLUSION

This review of some mechanoreceptors indicates that some features of the structure of receptors can account for certain aspects of their functional characteristics, but also shows that existing structural information is insufficient to account for all. In particular, the morphological studies throw little light on the actual transducer mechanisms, although they do provide useful indicators for future work — for example, the Merkel cells are obvious candidates as transducers, whereas in the

Ruffini ending it is likely that the transducer mechanisms are located in the nerve terminals.

Finally, it is now clear from physiological experiments (*e.g.*, Nakajima and Onodera, 1969; Ringham, 1971) that the temporal characteristics of the impulse discharge leaving receptors may be strongly influenced by the site on the axon from which the impulses arise. The discharge of self-propagating impulses, although it depends on a membrane depolarisation arising in the specialised nerve terminals, is initiated more proximally along the axon. In several receptors (Pacinian corpuscle, crayfish stretch receptor), the persistence of a discharge is determined by the characteristics of the spike-initiation site but, as Ringham (1971) reports, there is no evident structural difference at the place from which the impulses arise, or at least none has yet been reported in ultrastructural studies.

## SUMMARY

The general morphological and physiological principles governing the sensory mechanisms of cutaneous receptors are outlined and the extent to which morphology determines physiology is analysed. Particular attention is given to the organised mechanoreceptors — Pacinian and Golgi–Mazzoni corpuscles; hair follicle receptors; the Meissner corpuscle; Merkel "touch-spot"; the Ruffini ending in mammals and the Herbst and Grandry corpuscles in birds. In each case the distinctive morphology revealed in fine detail by electron microscopy is associated with a specific physiological responsiveness, which may be evident as a "selective sensitivity" to certain parameters of the physical stimulus and/or in the output discharge "code" of impulses in the afferent nerve fibre.

A complex sense organ, the sinus hair, is then considered to test the hypothesis that the general principles enunciated for individual kinds of mechanoreceptor can be applied to more elaborate systems.

No morphological elements responsible for the specific transducer mechanisms or membrane permeability can yet be identified. Nevertheless, it is evident that the morphological elements do determine, to a degree, the physiological characteristics of the peripheral sensory receptors.

## REFERENCES

ANDRES, K. H. (1966) Über die Feinstruktur der Rezeptoren an Sinushaaren. *Z. Zellforsch.*, **75**, 339–365.

ANDRES, K. H. AND VON DÜRING, M. (1973) Morphology of cutaneous receptors. In A. IGGO (Ed.), *Handbook of Sensory Physiology, Vol. II.* Springer-Verlag, Heidelberg, pp. 3–28.

BROWN, A. G. AND IGGO, A. (1963) The structure and function of cutaneous "touch corpuscles" after nerve crush. *J. Physiol. (Lond.)*, **165**, 28–29P.

BROWN, A. G. AND IGGO, A. (1967) A quantitative study of cutaneous receptors and afferent fibres in the cat and rabbit. *J. Physiol. (Lond.)*, **193**, 707–733.

BURGESS, P. R. AND HORCH, K. W. (1973) Specific regeneration of cutaneous fibers in the cat. *J. Neurophysiol.*, **36**, 101–114.

BURGESS, P. R. AND PERL, E. (1973) Cutaneous mechanoreceptors and nociceptors. In A. IGGO (Ed.), *Handbook of Sensory Physiology, Vol. II*. Springer-Verlag, Heidelberg, pp. 29–78.

BURGESS, P. R., ENGLISH, K. B., HORCH, K. W. AND STENSAAS, L. J. (1974) Patterning in the regeneration of type I cutaneous receptors. *J. Physiol. (Lond.)*, **236**, 57–82.

CAUNA, N. (1966) Fine structure of the receptor organs and its probable functional significance. In E. V. S. DE REUCK AND J. KNIGHT (Eds.), *Touch, Heat and Pain, CIBA Foundation Symp.* Churchill, London, pp. 117–127.

CAUNA, N. (1969) The fine morphology of the sensory receptor organs in the auricle of the rat. *J. comp. Neurol.*, **136**, 81–98.

CHAMBERS, M. R., ANDRES, K. H., VON DUERING, M. AND IGGO, A. (1972) The structure and function of the slowly adapting type II mechanoreceptor in hairy skin. *Quart. J. exp. Physiol.*, **57**, 417–445.

DIAMOND, J., GRAY, J. A. B. AND SATO, M. (1956) The site of initiation of impulses in Pacinian corpuscles. *J. Physiol. (Lond.)*, **133**, 54–67.

DORWARD, P. K. AND McINTYRE, A. K. (1971) Responses of vibration-sensitive receptors in the interosseous region of the duck's hind limb. *J. Physiol. (Lond.)*, **219**, 77–87.

GOTTSCHALDT, K.-M., IGGO, A. AND YOUNG, D. W. (1973) Functional characteristics of mechanoreceptors in sinus hair follicles of the cat. *J. Physiol. (Lond.)*, **235**, 287–315.

GOTTSCHALDT, K.-M. (1974) Mechanoreceptors in the beaks of birds. In J. SCHWARTZKOPFF (Ed.), *Mechanorezeption*. Westdeutscher Verlag, Düsseldorf. pp. 109–113.

GRANDRY, M. (1869) Recherches sur les corpuscules de Pacini. *J. Anat. (Paris)*, **6**, 390–395.

GRAY, J. A. B. AND MATTHEWS, P. B. C. (1951) A comparison of the adaptation of the Pacinian corpuscle with the accommodation of its own axon. *J. Physiol. (Lond.)*, **144**, 454–464.

GRUNDFEST, H. (1971) The general electrophysiology of input membrane in electrogenic excitable cells. In W. R. LOEWENSTEIN (Ed.), *Handbook of Sensory Physiology, Vol. I*. Springer-Verlag, Heidelberg, pp. 136–165.

HALATA, Z. (1972a) Innervation der unbehaarten Nasenhaut des Maulwurfs *(Talpa europaea)* I. Intraepidermale Nervenendigungen. *Z. Zellforsch*, **125**, 108–120.

HALATA, Z. (1972b) Innervation der unbehaarten Nasenhaut des Maulwurfs *(Talpa europaea)* II. Innervation der dermis (einfache eingekapselte Körperchen). *Z. Zellforsch.*, **125**, 121–131.

HENSEL, H. (1973) Cutaneous thermoreceptors. In A. IGGO (Ed.), *Handbook of Sensory Physiology, Vol. II*. Springer-Verlag, Heidelberg, pp. 79–110.

HERBST, G. E. F. (1848) *Die Pacinischen Körper und ihre Bedeutung*. Badenhoech und Ruprecht, Göttingen.

HORCH, K. W., WHITEHORN, D. AND BURGESS, P. R. (1974) Impulse generation in type I cutaneous mechanoreceptors. *J. Neurophysiol.*, **37**, 267–281.

IGGO, A. (1963a) An electrophysiological analysis of afferent fibres in primate skin. *Acta neuroveg. (Wien)*, **24**, 225–240.

IGGO, A. (1963b) New specific sensory structures in hairy skin. *Acta neuroveg. (Wien)*, **24**, 175–180.

IGGO, A. (1966) Cutaneous receptors with a high sensitivity to mechanical displacement. In E. V. S. DE REUCK AND J. KNIGHT (Eds.), *Touch, Heat and Pain, CIBA Foundation Symposium*. Churchill, London, pp. 237–256.

IGGO, A. AND MUIR, A. R. (1969) The structure and function of a slowly adapting touch corpuscle in hairy skin. *J. Physiol. (Lond.)*, **200**, 763–796.

IGGO, A. AND GOTTSCHALDT, K.-M. (1974) Cutaneous mechanoreceptors in simple and in complex sensory structures. In J. SCHWARTZKOPFF, (Ed.), *Mechanorezeption*. Westdeutscher Verlag, Dusseldorf, pp. 153–176.

LINDBLOM, U. (1965) Properties of touch receptors in distal glabrous skin of the monkey. *J. Neurophysiol.*, **28**, 966–985.

LOEWENSTEIN, W. R. AND SKALAK, R. (1966) Mechanical transmission in a Pacinian corpuscle. An analysis and a theory. *J. Physiol. (Lond.)*, **182**, 346–378.

MEISSNER, G. (1853) *Beiträge zur Anatomie und Physiologie der Haut*. Voss, Leipzig.

MERKEL, F. (1875) Tastzellen und Tastkorperchen bei den Hausthieren und beim Menschen. *Arch. mikr. Anat.*, **11**, 636–652.

MONTAGNA, W. AND MACPHERSON, E. (1973) Similarities in cutaneous nerve receptors. *Arch. Derm.*, **107**, 383–385.

NAKAJIMA, S. AND ONODERA, K. (1969) Adaptation of the generator potential in the crayfish stretch receptors under constant length and constant tension. *J. Physiol. (Lond.)*, **200**, 187–204.

NILSSON, B. Y. (1969) Hair discs and Pacinian corpuscles functionally associated with the carpal tactile hairs in the cat. *Acta physiol. scand.*, **77**, 417–428.

PACINI, F. (1840) Nuovi organi Scorperti nel corpo umano. Ciro, Pistoia.

QUILLIAM, T. A. (1966) Unit design and array patterns in receptor organs. In E. V. S. DE REUCK AND J. KNIGHT (Eds.), *Touch, Heat and Pain, CIBA Foundation Symposium*. Churchill, London, pp. 86–116.

RINGHAM, G. L. (1971) Origin of nerve impulse in slowly adapting stretch receptor of crayfish. *J. Neurophysiol.*, **34**, 773–784.

RUFFINI, A. (1891) Di un nuovo organo nervoso terminale e sulla presenza dei corpuscoli Golgi-Mazzoni nel connettivo sottocutaneo dei polpastrelli delle dita dell'uomo. *Mem. Accad. Lincei.*, **7**, 398–410.

SKOGLUND, S. (1973) Joint receptors and kinaesthesis. In A. IGGO (Ed.), *Handbook of Sensory Physiology*, *Vol. II*. Springer-Verlag, Heidelberg, pp. 111–136.

VON DÜRING, M. (1973) The ultrastructure of lamellated mechanoreceptors in the skin of reptiles. *Z. Anat. Entwickl.-Gesch.*, **143**, 81–94.

YAMAMOTO, T. (1966) The fine structure of the palisade-type sensory endings in relation to hair follicles. *J. Electron Micr.*, **15**, 158–166.

## DISCUSSION

SANTINI: If I understood Dr. Iggo correctly, he said there is no specialization between the sensory ending and the Pacinian corpuscle. (Demonstration of 3 of his own slides). I would like to propose a new term "receptrice" defined as follows: a desmosome-like junction between the sensory endings and an adjacent cell of non-neuronal origin, as we have seen in the case of the Pacinian corpuscles and Dr. Iggo showed in the core of Merkel cells. These are interneuronal junctions by which the external world can communicate with the neurons.

IGGO: I made a comment at the start of my paper that at this meeting we would come with some ideas and go away with others. I think your proposal is a good example of the kind of information which continues to come forward. It is very interesting that you have evidence for some morphological specialization between the Pacinian corpuscle and the adjacent cell, which would become even more interesting if it turns out that these are not desmosomes but actually some kind of synaptic junction.

ILYINSKY: In connection with your report I would like to ask a question. What is the basic difference between the two groups of the receptors: those with specialized sensory cells and those without them? I suggest that there is a difference between them which can be formulated as follows: for the more sensitive strength ranges there are receptors, such as in the sense organ with intermediate cell, which possess specialized elements. If this assumption is accepted the details of the general organization of tissue receptors become more clear and the possibility appears to make a correlation between primary receptors in tissue and secondary receptors of the sense organs. It concerns the efferent regulation of inhibitory nature; while in tissue receptors which are less sensitive we may often observe facilitatory as well as excitatory effects as in the case of muscle spindles.

IGGO: I think this is an interesting question that you raise. Why do some afferent units have the receptor cell? There may be an opportunity to modify receptor action at the synapses and in Merkel cells there seem to be a number of synaptic-like junctions where such changes could occur. I do not know of any good evidence for the modulation of cutaneous receptors by some direct central process as, for example, in the muscle spindle, although it is quite possible. It may occur but may be more general in action than in the muscle spindle.

# MORPHOLOGY, DEVELOPMENT AND HISTOCHEMISTRY OF RECEPTORS

# Morphological Basis of Sensation in Hairy Skin

NIKOLAJS CAUNA

*Department of Anatomy and Cell Biology, The School of Medicine, University of Pittsburgh, Pittsburgh, Pa. 15261 (U.S.A.)*

In the present study of the hairy skin, particular attention has been paid to the non-nervous tissue elements that are associated with the nerve terminals and to the microtopography of the receptor organs. An external stimulus can only reach the cutaneous nerve ending through the intervening non-nervous tissues. Therefore, these tissues may reveal features that either facilitate the transmission of a specific stimulus to the appropriate receptor or restrain inappropriate stimuli from reaching a particular ending. Morphological data of this kind, together with electrophysiological and psychophysical findings should enlarge the basis for functional evaluation of the sensory end organs.

## MATERIAL AND METHODS

The material of this study includes human hairy skin from the shoulder and upper arm region, the hairy skin from the nose of the bat and the hairy skin of the rat's auricle. Electron microscopical studies were carried out on serial and semiserial sections of osmium fixed material (Cauna, 1969, 1973). Histochemical distribution of cholinesterase activity was demonstrated in frozen sections using a modified Koele technique (Cauna, 1968).

## RESULTS

The results of this and earlier studies showed that there were no naked axon terminals in the skin of man and other mammals. Even the simplest nerve endings consisted of neural and non-neural components, the latter ranging from modified Schwann sheath elements to epithelial and connective tissue cells including some extracellular material. All endings were separated from the tissues of the corium by a basal lamina (basement membrane).

### Innervation of the hair

The hair has been considered to be a mechanoreceptor since the experimental studies

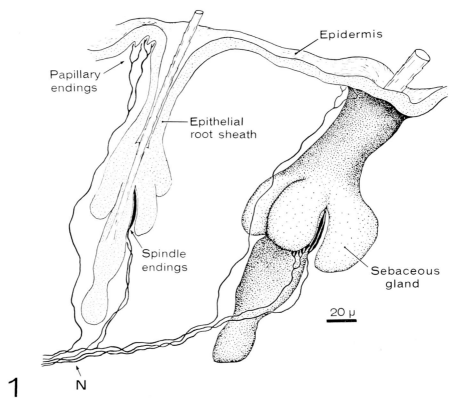

Fig. 1. Wax plate reconstruction of two adjacent fine hairs of the rat's auricle. A corial nerve fascicle (N) carries myelinated axons that either end on the hair in terminal spindles or produce papillary endings next to the hair orifice. ×400.

of Von Frey (1897), but the exact organization of its nerve supply has not yet been adequately described. We were able to bridge the gap in respect to the finest hairs of the cutaneous areas listed above. It was found that the myelinated nerve fibers that proceeded to the hair were accompanied by similar fibers that bypassed the hair and ended in the papillary endings around the hair orifice (Fig. 1 and arrows in Fig. 4). When the axons proceeding to the hair lost their myelin sheaths and started to divide, the branches of each axon did not diverge but remained enfolded within a common Schwann sheath of the stem axon and resembled regular non-myelinated nerve fibers. After some further divisions and splitting into smaller fascicles they ended in terminal spindles which formed a semicircle against the surface of the epithelial root sheath of the hair (Sp in Fig. 2, *cf.* with Fig. 1). Each set of preterminal and terminal branches, including the terminal nerve spindles was enfolded by a single branching Schwann cell which constituted the terminal cell of the Schwann sheath (Fig. 3). The perikaryon of the terminal Schwann cell (T Sch in Fig. 3) remained some distance removed from the hair shaft while long cytoplasmic processes of this cell carried sets of terminal axons towards the hair shaft (B and C in Fig. 3). By further division, processes of the terminal Schwann cell provided separate sheaths for smaller sets of fine axonal branches, until the spindles were reached. In this region, the Schwann cell processes ended in bulky flaps which flanked the terminal spindles in a rather regular manner (F and Sp in Figs. 2 and 3). Distally, the flaps extended beyond the spindles for a short distance. The endings were asymmetrically covered by a basal lamina that was an extension of the basal lamina of the preterminal nerve segments. In the spindle region, the basal lamina was thick and irregular over the outer surfaces of the endings. It extended from one ending to the next and also filled the gaps between the endings (BL in Fig. 2), enclosing in its substance some fine collagen fibers. The basal lamina also extended into the adventitia over the external aspect of the endings partly enclosing the adjacent collagen fibers (Fig. 2). The basal lamina was deficient over the inner aspect of the endings where the latter faced the basal lamina of the hair (BL in Fig. 2).

The endings exhibited strong acetyl- and butyrocholinesterase activity (Fig. 4) while the preterminal nerve fibers gave a negative reaction for both enzymes (Cauna,

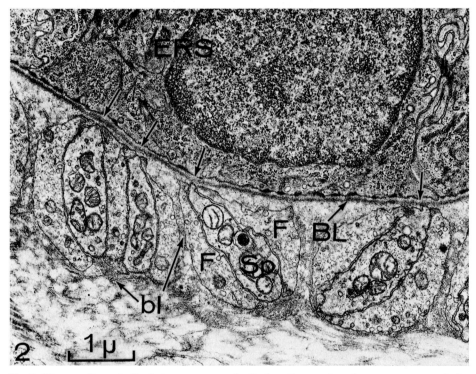

Fig. 2. Nerve endings of a fine hair cut transversely. Each ending consists of one or two axon spindles (Sp) flanked by cytoplasmic flaps (F) derived from the terminal Schwann cell (*cf.* with Fig. 3). The external surfaces of the endings are covered with a basal lamina (bl) which also fills the spaces between the endings where it encloses some fine collagen fibers. It also extends into the adventitia over the external aspect of the endings enclosing the adjacent collagen fibers (unstained in this preparation and therefore appearing as blank spots against the background of the surrounding basement membrane material). The axoplasm of the spindles contains accumulations of mitochondria and some agranular vesicles. The axolemma is exposed to the basal lamina (BL) of the epithelial root sheath of the hair (ERS) through a longitudinal gap formed by the Schwann sheath flaps (unlabeled arrows). Skin of the bat's nose. ×20,000.

*References p. 44–45*

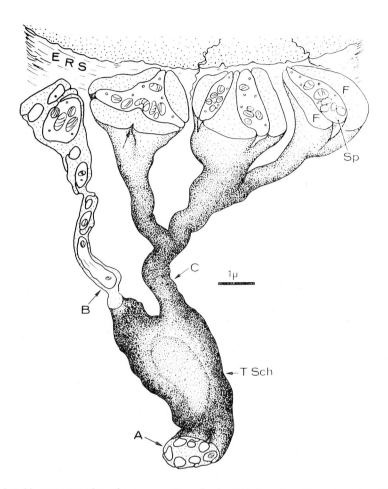

Fig. 3. Graphic reconstruction of a nerve ending of a fine hair based on 26 semiserial sections. The terminal Schwann cell (T Sch) enfolds seven non-myelinated axons (at A) which are branches of a single myelinated nerve fiber. The terminal Schwann cell splits into two branches. The one on the left (B) is a tracing from a single electron micrograph and reveals winding preterminal axons enfolded by the Schwann cell process. The termination of this branch has not been followed. The branch on the right (C) is traced to its three endings shown in transverse sections against the surface of the epithelial root sheath (ERS). The ending on the right consists of a terminal spindle (Sp) filled with mitochondria and microvesicles, and flanked by two flaps (F) of the Schwann sheath. The ending in the middle contains two spindles which are flanked by three Schwann sheath flaps. The ending on left contains one axon terminal that is about to split into two spindles. The Schwann sheath flap backing the axon terminal will protrude between the two daughter spindles and will itself split along the plane of the unlabeled arrow. The axolemma of each spindle is exposed to the basal lamina of the hair sheath through a narrow gap formed between the Schwann cell flaps. The gap extends for about 20 $\mu$m along the hair shaft. Basal laminae of the hair sheath and of the nerve endings have been omitted (*cf.* with Fig. 2). Skin of the rat's auricle. $\times 10,000$.

1961, 1969). The axoplasm of the spindles contained accumulations of mitochondria and agranular vesicles which resembled those found in cholinergic nerves. The axolemma of each spindle was exposed to the basal lamina of the hair sheath through a narrow longitudinal gap formed by the Schwann sheath flaps (unlabeled arrows

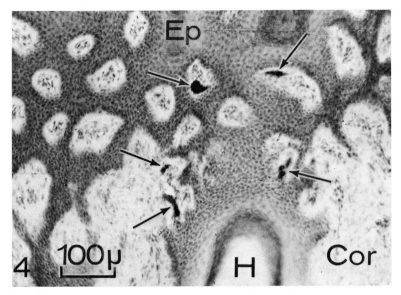

Fig. 4. Oblique section of human hairy skin through the epidermis (Ep) and the superficial corium (Cor) showing a hair (H) and the surrounding dermal papillae, some of which contain nerve endings (arrows). The papillary endings are derived from myelinated nerve fibers, and their presence has been demonstrated by the cholinesterase technique with hematoxylin as a counterstain. Male, 19 years old. ×150.

in Fig. 2). A degree of separation was sometimes observed between the hair basal lamina and the endings, apparently due to shrinkage during processing of the tissues. The cleavage plane appeared to permit movement and friction between the relatively rigid hair sheath and the interconnected semicircle of the endings, signifying the probable locus of mechanical stimulation. The position of the spindle endings in relation to the whole hair was found to be constant in hairs of all sizes. The semicircle of spindles was located against the deep aspect of the sloping hair shaft just below the openings of the sebaceous glands. This area corresponds to the lower end of the keratinized hair shaft where the epithelial root sheath is thinnest and is attached to the shaft. Here, the lever action of the hair seemed to be most effective. Below this point, the hair root was soft and could not effectively serve in the transmission of mechanical stimuli to the nerve endings (Fig. 1).

Merkel corpuscles were not observed in the vicinity of the fine hairs except in the skin of infants.

### The free nerve endings

The free nerve endings are present in nearly all tissues, yet they have attracted relatively little attention from morphologists. In the hairy skin, they are composed of relatively simple axon terminals invested by the Schwann sheath and by the nerve basal lamina.

We have carried out morphological and microtopographical studies of two kinds of superficial free endings in the hairy skin of man and rat, and propose to term them penicillate and papillary endings, respectively.

*The penicillate endings*

The penicillate endings showed a plexiform distribution. In the literature, they are usually referred to as the subepidermal nerve net. It was found that the endings gave a negative cholinesterase reaction and they appeared to be derived from non-myelinated nerve fibers in a tuft-like manner (Cauna, 1973). The point of origin of each penicillus was marked by the perikaryon of a modified Schwann cell (T Sch in Fig. 5) at which point the primary ramification occurred. This cell was the only source of the cyto-plasmic sheaths which it provided for all its endings. The branches of each penicillus were distributed over large overlapping areas and they exchanged axons with branches of the same and neighboring penicilli (Com in Fig. 5). The endings were located close to the corioepidermal junction, and they ended without undergoing any notice-able morphological change apart from progressive ramification. Occasionally they sent axonal twigs into the epidermis (Int in Fig. 5). These proceeded obliquely towards

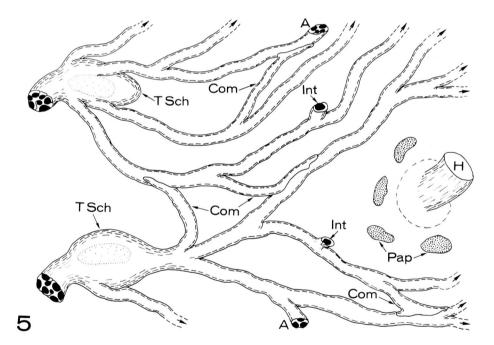

Fig. 5. Diagram showing the distribution pattern of the penicillate and the papillary nerve endings of the human skin and their relationship to the hair (H). The origin of each penicillus from non-myelinated nerve fibers is marked by the perikaryon of the terminal Schwann cell (T Sch). The latter supplies cytoplasmic sheaths for all its endings. Communicating branches (Com) between adjacent endings provide ample exchange of axons along the course of the endings. These extend far beyond the field of the diagram (indicated by dotted outlines and arrowheads at the edges of the diagram). Some endings are shown in transverse sections (A) indicating that each contains several axon ter-minals (black). Two intraepidermal branches (Int) are also shown in transverse sections prior to their entrance into the epidermis. The papillary endings (Pap) derived from myelinated nerve fibers are concentrated next to the hair orifice.

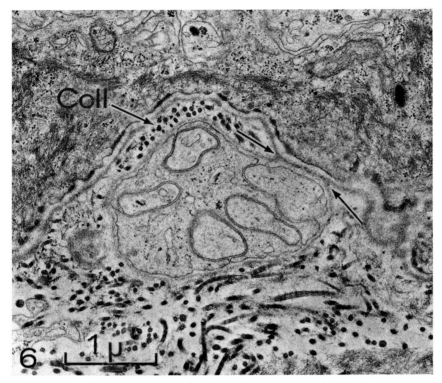

Fig. 6. Distal segment of a penicillate ending cut transversely, containing five axon terminals. The ending is accommodated within a groove on the deep aspect of the epidermis. The zone of collagen fibers (Coll) that accompany the nerve ending has been reduced. The basal laminae of the ending and of the epidermis have fused in the area between the unlabeled arrows. Note the paucity of organelles in the axon terminals and in the Schwann sheath. Male, 11 months old. × 25,000.

the stratum corneum enwrapped by keratinocytes which replaced the Schwann envelope. The axoplasm of the penicillate endings contained few mitochondria or other morphologically distinct components (Fig. 6), probably a feature that signifies rapidly adapting receptors. During most of their subepidermal course, the endings were surrounded by a distinct zone of collagen fibers oriented in the same direction as the axons. It became reduced only around the finer segments of the penicillate endings (Coll in Fig. 6). These were attached to the undersurface of the epidermis by connections that extended between the basal lamina of the nerve and that of the epidermis, or by fusion of the two basal laminae (area between arrows in Fig. 6).

*The papillary endings*

The papillary endings were scattered in the immediate vicinity of the hair orifices and could best be demonstrated by the use of the cholinesterase reaction (arrows in Fig. 4). The endings were derived from myelinated nerve fibers that ascended from the deep corium in the company of those that supplied the hairs. Each ending consisted of several axon terminals enclosed by the Schwann sheath and surrounded by a basal lamina (Fig. 7). The latter was frequently connected to or fused with the basal

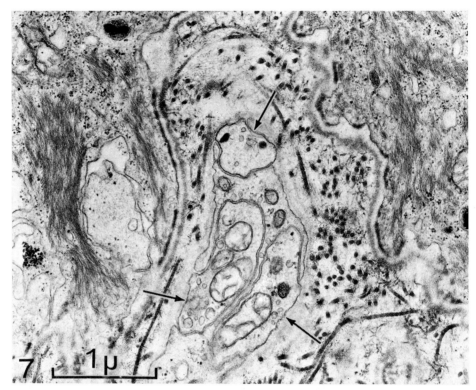

Fig. 7. Papillary ending cut obliquely, in a dermal papilla next to the hair orifice (*cf.* with Fig. 4, arrows). The Schwann sheath enfolds three axon terminals (arrows) which contain mitochondria and some pinocytotic vesicles. Male, 11 months old. ×25,000.

lamina of the epidermis. In contrast to the penicillate endings, the axoplasm of the papillary endings usually contained mitochondria and some microvesicles (Fig. 7, *cf.* with Fig. 6). Its Schwann sheath also contained mitochondria as well as vesicles. The latter were usually aligned along the plasmalemma and appeared to signify pinocytosis.

## DISCUSSION

The hair and its typical nerve endings constitute a functional unit designed for effective mechanical stimulation. It illustrates most conspicuously the principle of transmission of mechanical stimuli to the nerve endings by leverage. In this way the neural component of the end organ (1) can be concentrated in a confined space, thus forming a "corpuscular" receptor and (2) can be situated relatively deep in the corium, where the endings are shielded from external thermal or painful stimuli. The sebaceous glands approach the hair from all directions and join the hair sheath just above the spindle endings, thus creating a fixed point or a fulcrum for lever action of the shaft (Fig. 1). In addition, the compact dome of the sebaceous glands as well as the overlying keratinized shaft of the hair provide thermal insulation that is about three times as effective as the water-containing tissues elsewhere.

The principle of mechanical stimulation by leverage can usually be demonstrated in most "corpuscular" receptors (Cauna, 1966). These include Meissner corpuscles (Cauna, 1954); all forms of Merkel corpuscles (Cauna, 1954; Iggo and Muir, 1969); lingual, genital corpuscles, Eimer organ (Cauna, 1968) and the various forms of the hair. Experimental evidence shows that the lamellar corpuscles of the mesentery are also mechanoreceptors (Loewenstein, 1966). The large Vater–Pacini corpuscles of the digital tissues of man are linked with the glomerular arteriovenous anastomoses and probably respond to the pulsating stimuli when the anastomosis opens (Cauna and Mannan, 1958).

While it is generally agreed that the hair in its various forms constitutes a mechano-receptor, the functions of the various kinds of the free nerve endings still remain unresolved.

Concerning the penicillate endings, several morphological features are of particular interest in relation to their probable function or functions. The collagen fibers that faithfully enwrap each penicillate ending throughout most of its winding course and the links between the epidermis and the terminal segments of the endings appear to guard the receptor organ against acute deformation or friction. Therefore, the endings are not designed for effective mechanical stimulation. Should they respond to a mechanical stimulus, the threshold would be high. On the other hand, they appear to be highly efficient in collecting the appropriate non-mechanical stimuli because they possess large neural surface areas that are evenly distributed in the corium next to and inside the epidermis overlapping with areas of adjacent penicilli. While this arrangement secures the reception of appropriate external stimuli, it also renders the receptors inefficient in precise localization of a stimulus or in two point discrimination. Therefore, the penicillate endings may be associated with sensory modalities that do not have punctate representation in the skin. It is important to remember that each penicillus is a collection of non-myelinated axons that originate not from a single sensory nerve cell but from several and perhaps different kinds of nerve cells in the dorsal root ganglion. Furthermore, there is no way to exclude the possibility that some of the penicilli may be derived from, or may receive contribu-tions from, branches of originally myelinated axons. Therefore, each of the penicillate endings, such as seen in Fig. 6, is a multiaxon receptor, and it may represent a *multi-modal sensory package* rather than a single receptor associated with one modality. There is experimental evidence in support of this idea (see Perl *et al.*, Chapter 27 in this volume).

The papillary endings are closely associated with the hairs with respect to their localization and with respect to the course of their myelinated preterminal nerve fibers. For this reason, their function could be masked by that of the hair endings and *vice versa*, presenting problems in experimental work. Since application of a cold stimulus to the skin over a hair sometimes results in an apparent response from the hair nerves (Hensel and Boman, 1960), it may be a possibility that the response is actually coming from the papillary endings.

SUMMARY

The hairy skin of man, rat and bat was investigated electron microscopically and histochemically, paying particular attention to the non-nervous components of the nerve endings and to the microtopography of the receptor organs.

In the fine hairs, terminal branches of each myelinated axon, including the terminal spindles, were invested by a single branching Schwann cell. The endings exhibited strong cholinesterase activity. They were shielded from non-mechanical stimuli by their deep position and by the overlying hair shaft and sebaceous glands.

The hairy skin contained free endings of two kinds. The papillary endings were derived from myelinated axons. They occupied the dermal papillae next to the hair orifices and gave a positive cholinesterase reaction. These endings may be involved in the reception of cold stimuli.

The penicillate endings were primarily derived from non-myelinated axons. They gave a negative cholinesterase reaction and were poor in axoplasmic organelles. Each penicillus ramified over a large subepidermal area overlapping the area of adjacent penicilli. These endings appear to be associated with modalities that do not have punctate representation in the skin. Since each penicillus is composed of a number of axons derived from several nerve cells, it may constitute a multimodal sensory package rather than a receptor associated with a single modality.

ACKNOWLEDGEMENT

This study was supported by U.S. Public Health Service Grant 2RO1 NS04147.

REFERENCES

CAUNA, N. (1954) Nature and functions of the papillary ridges of the skin. *Anat. Rec.*, **119**, 449–468.
CAUNA, N. (1961) Cholinesterase activity in cutaneous receptors of man and some quadrupeds. *Bibl. anat. (Basel)*, **2**, 86–96.
CAUNA, N. (1966) Fine structure of the receptor organs and its probable functional significance. In A. V. S. DE REUCK AND J. KNIGHT (Eds.), *Touch, Heat and Pain, Ciba Foundation Symposium.* Churchill, London, pp. 117–136.
CAUNA, N. (1968) Light and electron microscopical structure of the sensory end-organs in human skin. In D. R. KENSHALO (Ed.), *The Skin Senses, Proc. First Int. Symp. Skin Senses, Florida State University, Tallahassee.* Thomas, Springfield, Ill., pp. 15–37.
CAUNA, N. (1969) The fine morphology of the sensory receptor organs in the auricle of the rat. *J. comp. Neurol.*, **136**, 81–98.
CAUNA, N. (1973) The free penicillate nerve endings of the human hairy skin. *J. Anat. (Lond.)*, **115**, 277–288.
CAUNA, N. AND MANNAN, G. (1958), The structure of human digital Pacinian corpuscles (corpuscule lamellosa) and its functional significance. *J. Anat. (Lond.)*, **92**, 1–20.
HENSEL, H. AND BOMAN, K. K. A. (1960) Afferent impulses in cutaneous sensory nerves in human subjects. *J. Neurophysiol.*, **23**, 564–578.
IGGO, A. and MUIR, A. R. (1969) The structure and function of a slowly adapting touch corpuscle in hairy skin. *J. Physiol. (Lond.)*, **200**, 763–796.

LOEWENSTEIN, W. R. (1966) Input and output ends of a transducer process. In A. V. S. DE REUCK AND J. KNIGHT (Eds.), *Touch, Heat and Pain, Ciba Foundation Symposium.* Churchill, London, pp. 186–202.

VON FREY, M. (1897) Untersuchungen über die Sinnesfunktionen der menschlichen Haut. *Abhandl. math.-phys. Classe d.k. Sächs. Ges. d. Wiss.*, **23**, 169–266.

## DISCUSSION

ZELENA: In various nerve terminals, we frequently observe vesicles. May I ask you if you have observed some vesicles with dense cores, especially in the spindle endings round the hair?

CAUNA: No, these investigations especially apply to the finer nerves and their structure is simple. These hairs indeed can be traced from one to another electron microscopically. So, we can see their continuity up to whole preterminal segments, but I have not seen granular vesicles inside the axon spindle.

ANDRES: I would ask you what kind of method you used for the preparation of your electron microscopic material fixation. I think your material in some places is brighter than mine, and I think this is the question of fixation. Do you use Epon or Araldite for embedding?

CAUNA: Various processing methods are used; the routine method is osmium fixation, but I have used glutaraldehyde, and also formalin fixation, especially for electron microscopic material. I used an Epon–Araldite mixture for embedding. It was used for the procedure before, but there is a difference, especially in revealing cytoplasm or in staining or not staining collagen fibers, or revealing different numbers clearly or not clearly; so of course, all methods have to be compared in order to judge the structure. We have to have reservations anyway. We have seen these granulated vesicles which Dr. Zelena asked about, I think that was in cat and rat normal hair.

ANDRES: In reptiles skin I found sprays or penicillate-like endings such as you described here. They are very common in the surroundings of special touch papillae of crocodile and I wonder are they similar receptors to those you have seen?

CAUNA: No, I think I have seen the basket type of endings related to the epidermis.

ANDRES: In the touch papillae of crocodile several different types of the receptors are seen and one type with unmyelinated endings, and we think this is very similar to your receptors. Many axons come up to these endings.

# Process of Regeneration and Development of the Tissue Receptors Specificity

N. I. CHALISOVA AND O. B. ILYINSKY

*Laboratory of General Physiology of Reception, I. P. Pavlov Institute of Physiology, The Academy of Sciences of the U.S.S.R., Leningrad (U.S.S.R.)*

Development of the receptors is one of the most important but unsolved problems of sensory physiology. It is well known that the growth of afferent nerve fibres produces nerve endings specific to the given tissue. However, it is not clear what determines the development of such receptors: the properties of nerve fibres or just the specificity of tissue elements. It is quite possible that a differentiated neurone possesses the specificity which allows the growing nerve fibres to develop a selective connection with a tissue of certain biochemical nature at the periphery. Thus, the nerve fibres play the main role in the development of tissue receptors (Kadanoff, 1925; Zazybin, 1936). Other authors consider that the tissue develops specific receptors when innervated by any sensory fibres (Dijkstra, 1933; Lavrentjev, 1937; Saxod, 1972; Burgess and Horch, 1973). Tissue receptor specificity could easily be traced in studies on peripheral nerves regeneration. When studying the process of receptor development, using not only morphological but also functional methods, it is very important to perform continuous observation of a single sensory element at various stages of its development. Thus, the Pacinian corpuscles of cat mesentery are well suited for a study of this kind (Ilyinsky *et al.*, 1973).

METHODS

In chronic experiments on 35 adult cats and 15 one-month-old kittens nervus saphenous and/or nervus femoralis was dissected at the femur; then, the proximal end of the nerve preserving a connection with the spinal cord, was guided under the ligamentum pupartum into the abdominal cavity. The ends of the nerve were dissected to produce thin bundles and then were led between the two layers of mesocolon and omental mesentery in the region where the Pacinian corpuscles were either absent or had been extirpated. Animals were sacrified 1–8 months after the operation. Total preparations of the mesentery were silver-impregnated according to the method of Billshovsky-Gross. Functional properties of receptors were studied as reported previously (Ilyinsky, 1963)

RESULTS

After transplantation of the nervus saphenous to the mesentery tissue, neuromas developed at the end of the nerve (Fig. 1a). A chaotic growth of the nerve fibres in all directions was observed; typical anastomoses appeared between fibres. The neuroma, as well as the grafted nerve trunk, produced various collaterals in the form of slightly myelinated fibres, which expanded in the mesenteric tissue. A part of the fibres ended by the growth cone and free nerve endings could sometimes be observed. These elements could be seen at all stages of the development of the nerve. However, within 3 months of nerve transplantation its terminals produced new Pacinian corpuscles (Fig. 1a), from 2 to 14 in each animal (Ilyinsky *et al.*, 1973). There are both early- and fully-formed receptors. As a rule, one of the greater nervus saphenous collaterals produced the smaller ones, with the Pacinian corpuscles and their endings.

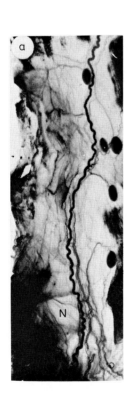
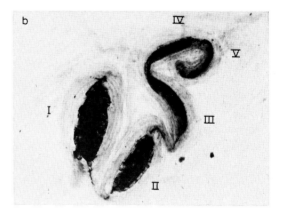
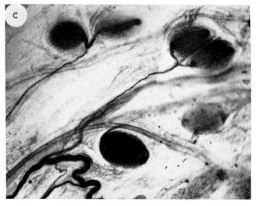

Fig. 1. a: newly formed receptors after transplantation of nervus saphenous (N) at 4 months after operation. × 10. b: the development of newly formed (I–V) receptors at a dichotomically ramified nerve ending in kitten 4 months after the operation. × 50. c: 5 bead-like Pacinian corpuscles 4.5 months after the operation. × 70.

Young animals had a higher speed of formation of the corpuscles. Thus, in one-month-old kittens 45 days after the transplantation of the nerve to the mesentery new Pacinian corpuscles at various stages of development could be found; 22 newly formed receptors could be observed in one animal (Fig. 1c).

Therefore, during the regeneration of Pacinian corpuscles normal development phases of the normal histogenesis were repeated (Chalisova *et al.*, 1974). Newly formed Pacinian corpuscles often showed a nerve fibre going through the receptor. The proximal end diameter of such a fibre (15 $\mu$m) significantly exceeded the diameter of slightly myelinated fibres from the distal receptor end (5 $\mu$m). It may be assumed that these forms of receptors produced the so-called bead-like Pacinian corpuscles in parts of the skin with a greater functional stretch (Otelin, 1953), though they might be rarely seen in an intact cat mesocolon. The bead-like Pacinian corpuscles are one of the stages of their development. This stage was often observed in the newly formed receptors (Fig. 1b). From Fig. 1b it will be seen that the forming receptors (III–V) have a common outer capsule, whereas two fully formed Pacinian corpuscles have separate outer capsules and transplantation of a nerve fibre from one receptor to another is clearly seen (I–II).

Transplantation of a sensory nerve does not necessarily lead to the formation of receptors. If the grafted nerve is placed in such parts of the mesentery (omental mesentery) that did not naturally produce Pacinian corpuscles, and where only free nerve endings could be observed (Torskaya, 1953), the nervus saphenous did not form any encapsulated endings.

The pattern of nerve fibres was as important as the pattern of the mesentery tissue (Taylor, 1944). When grafted to mesocolon both cutaneous and motor nerves (nervus femoralis) that possessed not only efferent but also afferent fibres (muscle spindles), did not form Pacinian corpuscles. Functional characteristics of fully formed Pacinian corpuscles appear to be the same as those of the normal ones. However, the undeveloped Pacinian corpuscles had after-hyperpolarisation and were more slowly adaptative in comparison with the mature forms (Fig. 2). The effect of mechanical stimulus duration was correlated with the increase of the duration of receptor potential, off-responses being absent. This is conditioned by insufficient development of the mechanoreceptor capsule and by the transmission of a static component of the stimulus to the nerve terminal, which is in line with the well known facts concerning the adaptation phenomena in the Pacinian corpuscle (Loewenstein and Mendelson, 1965; Ilyinsky, 1965).

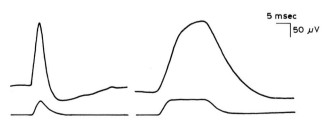

Fig. 2. Adaptation properties in early forms of Pacinian corpuscles.

*References p. 50–51*

It is only with the ontogenetic development of receptors that their conversion from a slow- to a fast-adaptive receptor, and their normal functions become possible.

Formation of tissue receptors might be described as follows. The cells of connective tissue receive non-specific stimuli from the nerve fibres growing into the tissue and, thus, stimulated cells in their turn can exert a specific influence on the somatic sensory nerve fibres and surrounding cells. The nerve endings can then induce the surrounding cells, which in their turn form an accessory receptor structure, corresponding to the pattern of the particular innervated tissue.

The changes in the inner core after denervation (Lee, 1936; Chouchkov, 1971; Schiff and Loewenstein, 1972) show, though indirectly, the influence of the nerve on surrounding cells. It is also known that a normally functioning tissue receptor releases biochemically active substances (Habgood, 1950; Dmitrieva et al., 1973). One of the morphological characteristics of the related biochemical activity is the availability of the pinocytosis vesicles seen both in accessory structures (Pease and Quilliam, 1957; Cherepnov, 1968), and in nerve endings of tissue receptors (Pease and Quilliam, 1957; Cherepnov, 1968). But this question requires further studies.

SUMMARY

It is yet to be seen what determines the development of receptors specific to a given tissue; whether it be the properties of nerve fibres or just the specificity of tissue elements. For a study of this kind the effect of additional innervation of cat mesentery tissue by the somatic sensitive nerve and motor nerve was investigated. The sensitive nerve foreign to mesentery develops the type of sensory endings characteristic of the mesentery tissue (Pacinian corpuscles) when making contact with it. According to the histological and physiological investigation, Pacinian corpuscles newly- and normally-formed in the same cat's mesentery showed no differences in their morphological and functional properties. However, early forms of Pacinian corpuscles were slowly adaptive, contrary to mature forms. Therefore, it is necessary to produce the determinative nerve–tissue situation to make it possible to develop mechanoreceptors.

REFERENCES

BURGESS, P. AND HORCH, K. (1973) Specific regeneration of cutaneous fiber in the cat. J. Neurophysiol., 26, 101–114.
CHALISOVA, N. I., KUZNETSOV, V. F. AND VOLKOVA, N. K. (1974) Peculiarities in the formation of Pacinian corpuscles with additional somatic innervation of mesentery. Bull. exp. biol., Med., 99, 99–101 (in Russian).
CHEREPNOV, V. L. (1968) The ultrastructure of the inner core of Pacinian corpuscles. J. comp. biochem., Physiol., 4, 91–96 (in Russian).
CHOUCHKOV, H. N. (1971) Ultrastructure of Pacinian corpuscles after the section of nerve fibers. Z. mikr.-anat. Forsch., 83, 33–46.
DIJKSTRA, C. (1933) Die De- und Regeneration der sensiblen Endkörperchen des Entensehnabels (Grandry- und Herbst-Körperchen) nach Durchschneidung des Nerven, nach Fortnahme der ganzen Haut und nach Transplantation des Hautstückchens. Z. mikr.anat. Forsch., 34, 75–158.

DMITRIEVA, T. M., ESAKOV, A. I. and NISTRATOVA, S. N. (1973) Humoralis factors in lateral inhibition of skin receptors. *Sechenov physiol. J. U.S.S.R.*, **59**, 558–564 (in Russian).

HABGOOD, J. S. (1950) Sensitization of sensory receptors in the frogs skin. *J. Physiol. (Lond.)*, **111**, 195–213.

ILYINSKY, O. B. (1963) Properties of single mechanoreceptors (Vater–Pacinian corpuscles). *Sechenov physiol. J. U.S.S.R.*, **29**, 201–207 (in Russian).

ILYINSKY, O. B. (1965) Processes of excitation and inhibition in single mechanoreceptors (Pacinian corpuscles). *Nature (Lond.)*, **208**, 351–353.

ILYINSKY, O. B., CHALISOVA, N. I. AND KUZNETSOV, V. F. (1973) Development of new Pacinian corpuscles; studies on the foreign innervation of mesentery. *Experientia (Basel)*, **29**, 1129–1131.

KADANOFF, D. (1925) Histologische Untersuchungen über die Regeneration sensibiler Nerven endingungen in Hauttransplantaten. *Klin. Wschr.*, **4**, 1266–1288.

LAVRENTJEV, B. I. (1937) Some studies on the structure of nervous tissue. *Arch. biol. sci.*, **48**, 194–213 (in Russian).

LEE, F. C. (1936) A study of the Pacinian corpuscle. *J. comp. Neurol.*, **64**, 497–522.

LOEWENSTEIN, W. R. AND MENDELSON, M. (1965) Components of receptor adaptation in a Pacinian corpuscle. *J. Physiol. (Lond.)*, **177**, 377–397.

OTELIN, A. A. (1953) Relation between structure and function in capsulated mechanoreceptors. *Probl. Physiol.*, **8**, 140–145 (in Russian).

PEASE, D. C. AND QUILLIAM, T. A. (1957) Electron microscopy of the Pacinian corpuscle. *J. biophys. biochem. Cytol.*, **3**, 331–342.

SAXOD, R. (1972) Rôle du nerf et territoire cutané dans le développement des corpuscles de Hêrbst et de Grandry. *J. Embryol. exp. Morph.*, **27**, 277–289.

SCHIFF, J. AND LOEWENSTEIN, W. R. (1972) Development of receptor on a foreign nerve fiber. *Science*, **177**, 712–715.

TAYLOR, A. C. (1944) Selectivity of nerve fibers from the dorsal and ventral roots in the development of the frog limb. *J. exp. zool.*, **96**, 159–185.

TORSKAYA, I. V. (1953) Experimental studies on innervation of big omental in Mammalis. *Probl. Physiol.*, **3**, 177–186 (in Russian).

VOLKOVA, N. K. (1972) Forming of some Pacinian corpuscle structures in ontogenesis. *Proc. Acad. Sci. U.S.S.R., Biol. Sci.*, **204**, 717–720 (in Russian).

ZAZYBIN, N. I. (1936) Embryogenesis of peripheral nervous system. *Ivanovo* (in Russian).

## DISCUSSION

OTELIN: The paper is very impressive and confirms the plasticity of Pacinian corpuscles. We have observed that these mechanoreceptors may appear as a result of changing circumstances in such places where they were normally absent. For instance, we made the amputation of limbs in dogs and when the locomotion was restored numerous new Pacinian corpuscles in the skin of the amputated limb were found. In healthy human subjects we found that the palmar skin of the right hand contains a greater number of Pacinian corpuscles than the skin of the left hand. At the same time in blind persons we found a greater number of Pacinian corpuscles in the palmar skin than in healthy subjects. We considered this fact as evidence that mechanoreceptors adapt themselves for increased functional requirements.

BURGESS: Do you think that the saphenous nerve does not form receptors in skin, or do you think that there is much more specificity in this process and the same fibers that make the Pacinian corpuscles in the saphenous nerve now make the Pacinian corpuscles in mesentery? This is an important question because if a saphenous nerve normally does not have Pacinian corpuscles, then it's reappearance in mesentery is a case where formation of endings is determined by the tissue and not by the specific capacity of the fibers themselves. We have evidence that in other conditions, when the regeneration of nerve was in same tissue, it was very specific. For example the nerve fibers innervated Merkel cells before the cut. After regeneration the nerve fibers return back to the location of Merkel cells.

ILYINSKY: Practically every tissue innervated by somatic nerves (muscles, joints, hair skin) contains Pacinian corpuscles. Probably, then, only acoustic nerves do not form Pacinian corpuscles. The experiments with this nerve create many technical difficulties. At the same times, nervus saphenous forms a minimal number of Pacinian corpuscles in the hair skin of limb, but when it innervates mesentery the massive formation of this mechanoreceptor can be seen. This is evidence of the importance of tissue factor. However, the experiments with the muscle nerve which does not form Pacinian corpuscles, emphasize also the role of nerve specificity. Thus, when receptors are being formed there is a correlation between tissue and nerve factors.

ZELENA: There is a preexisting specialization of nerve terminals because the differentiation and induction of the Pacinian corpuscles was observed only in some cases, but not when muscle nerves were transposed to the mesentery. A similar finding has already been described in the case of mammalian taste buds. Only gustatory nerves were differentiated in taste buds. No other sensory endings are able to induce the taste buds in mammalians. However, it appears that in low vertebrates (anurans and amphibians) non-gustatory fibers may also induce the differentiation of taste buds. I wonder if it would be interesting to make such experiments in lizards and amphibians to see whether non-gustatory fibers could induce the differentiation of taste buds and Pacinian corpuscles. In other words, it is interesting if, in cold blooded animals, the specialization of nerve terminals is of a low degree and they are pluripotential in their capacity.

# Ultrastructural Features of Pacinian Corpuscles in the Early Postnatal Period

L. MALINOVSKÝ

*Department of Anatomy, Faculty of Medicine, J. Ev. Purkynie University, Brno (Czechoslovakia)*

## INTRODUCTION

Many authors have studied the development of Pacinian corpuscles in mammals by means of the light microscope (for a survey of the existing literature see Malinovský, 1970; Malinovský and Sommerová, 1972; Volkova, 1972). On the other hand, there are few data available in the literature on the development of Pacinian corpuscles examined with the aid of electron microscopy, although Pease and Quilliam (1957) described the ultrastructure of Pacinian corpuscles in the mesentery of newborn kittens. Honde (1959) followed the ultrastructural changes of Pacinian corpuscles in the cat mesentery in the adult animals and in young animals 30, 50 and 80 days after their birth. Poláček and Mazanec (1966) mention some characteristic features in the ultrastructure of immature Pacinian corpuscles in their paper on the ultrastructure of Pacinian corpuscles from the cat mesentery. The development of simple encapsulated corpuscles in the nasolabial region of the cat was studied by means of the electron microscope by Poláček and Halata (1970). In our previous paper (Malinovský and Sommerová, 1972) we reviewed our study of the postnatal development of Pacinian corpuscles in foot pads of the domestic cat by means of the light microscope. We have shown that at the time of birth the Pacinian corpuscles are not yet mature. In view of the limited data in the literature concerning the ultrastructure of developing Pacinian corpuscles we have decided to complete our previous examinations by electron microscope investigations.

## MATERIAL AND METHODS

The postnatal ultrastructural changes of Pacinian corpuscles were followed in the foot pads of the domestic cat (*Felis silvestris f. catus* L.) The investigation was carried out in eight cats of ages between 2 hr after birth and maturity. After anaesthetization of the animals with ether, 3% glutaraldehyde solution in 0.1 $M$ phosphate buffer (pH 7.4) was injected into the foot pads. Small pieces from the middle pad were then prefixed in the injection solution for a further 2 hr period. The fixation was

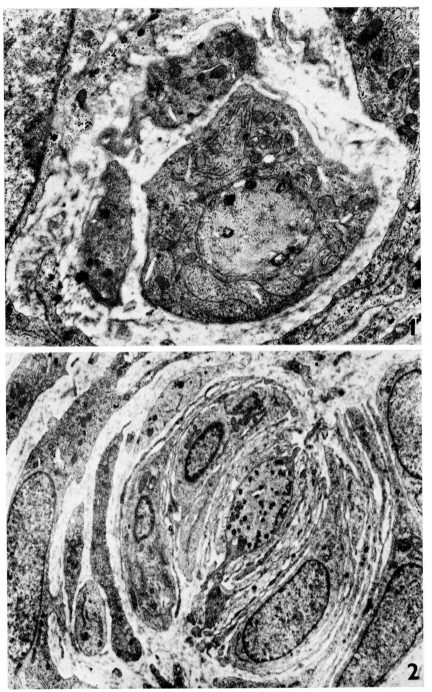

Fig. 1. The first stage of Pacinian corpuscle development. Cross-section. The axon is enveloped by an inner core cells. The other inner core cells are in the surroundings. Kitten, 18 hr after birth. Tesla BS 500, × about 12,000.

Fig. 2. The second stage of Pacinian corpuscle development. Cross-section. Around the axon there is a small number of lamellae. Around the lamellae there is an accumulation of inner core cells which are elongated in form. Kitten, 18 hr after birth. Tesla BS 500, × about 5200.

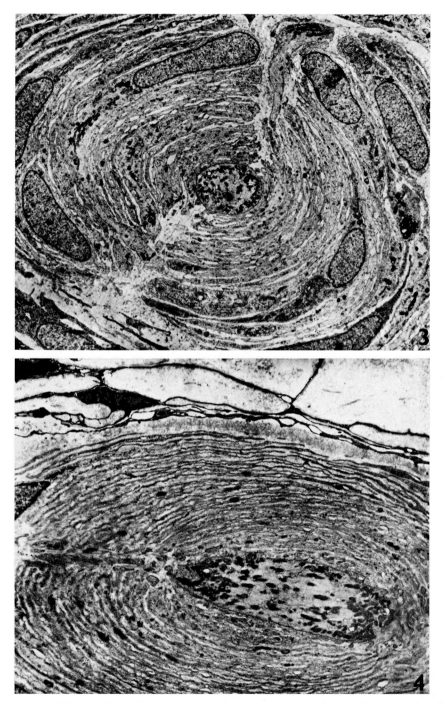

Fig. 3. The third stage of Pacinian corpuscle development. An accumulation of inner core lamellae around the axon. Note the plasmatic arm penetrating the cleft of the inner. Kitten, 18 hr after birth. Tesla BS 500, × about 3500.

Fig. 4. Oblique section of Pacinian corpuscle of the adult cat. The inner core is formed by a great number of thin lamellae, between the inner core and the capsule there is a typical boundary space. The lamellae of capsulae are thin, the interlamellar spaces are filled with collagenous fibres. Tesla BS 500, × about 4000.

References p. 58

completed in 2% $OsO_4$ solution with phosphate buffer. The material was then dehydrated with acetone and alcohols and embedded in Durcupan. The semithin sections for light microscopy and the ultrathin sections for electron microscopy were cut with the Tesla BS 490A ultramicrotome. The sections were stained with aqueous uranyl acetate and lead citrate and examined and photographed in the Tesla BS 500 electron microscope.


OBSERVATIONS


The first stage of the Pacinian corpuscle development has been characterized to date by the irregular accumulation of cells around the axon and the formation of a concentrically arranged capsule around these cells. The inner core in the impregnated specimens was not visible in the first postnatal period. The first sign of the inner core existence was observed at the end of the first week of life.

Our observations of the ultrastructure show that at about the time of birth it is possible to find Pacinian corpuscles in various stages of development.

(1) Firstly, corpuscles (Fig. 1) which lack an inner core are evident. The axon is enveloped by a cell of the inner core; other cells of this type are concentrated in the surroundings of the axon. The plasma of these cells is dark in colour, with well-formed organelles. The nucleus of some of these cells is lobular in shape. These young cells resemble the fibrocytes on the corpuscles surface.

(2) In other corpuscles of the same kitten (Fig. 2) we could observe the origin of the inner core formed by several cell lamellae. The axon is oval (but at the same time in some cases still circular) in shape and sends off finger-like processes to both the clefts. The mitochondria are distributed irregularly throughout the whole axon. Around the lamellae of the inner core there are concentrically arranged cells, some of them forming lamellae; the other cells are only elongated or oval in shape. The boundary space, which is typical of the mature corpuscles, is not distinct here.

(3) In some corpuscles we observed a greater number of inner core lamellae. The elongated cells form a circle between the axon and the surface of the corpuscles. Some of these cells send off plasmatic arms into the clefts of the inner core (Fig. 3). The lamellae are thinner towards the surface of the corpuscle, and form a capsule on the corpuscle surface.

(4) The final structure of the inner core and the capsule is shown in Fig. 4. The capsule lamellae are very thin and the interlamellar spaces are wide and filled with collagenous fibres. On the surface there are typical fibrocytes.


DISCUSSION


Our findings can be compared only with those obtained by Pease and Quilliam (1957) and Poláček and Mazanec (1966). Pease and Quilliam described an irregular arrangement of the mitochondria in the axon, a prominent cellular growth zone

between the inner core and the capsule and a smaller number of fibrils of collagen
in the newborn kitten, which is in accord with our findings. According to Poláček
and Mazanec (1966) the typical features of a young corpuscle are: regular inner core
rich in lamellae, two regular clefts in the inner core, and one axon. We cannot confirm these findings concerning the first two items. Honde's description (1959) of
ultrastructural changes in the Pacinian corpuscles does not concern the first postnatal
days, since the youngest group investigated by him are kittens 30 days old.

It is very interesting to compare our observations with the description of the development of Herbst corpuscles given by Saxod (1970) in his electron microscope study.
There is an analogy to a certain degree. The stage of Pacinian corpuscle development
in which the axon is still enveloped by the inner core cell, was not described by
Saxod. While the structure development of the axon and the inner core in the Herbst
corpuscles is finished by the hatching time, as suggested by Saxod (1970), in the
Pacinian corpuscles of the foot pads of the domestic cat the maturation of all structures
occurs in the postnatal period.

The origin of the inner core and the capsule cells remains open to investigation.
Saxod (1970) is of the view that it is difficult to solve the problem now. In this respect
we agree with his opinion since the inner core cells during the first development stage
resemble fibrocytes on the capsule surface. According to Martinez and Pekarthy
(1974), the capsule cells of simple corpuscles in the rat gingiva are of fibroblast
origin. We leave this question without answer. A solution to this problem could be
contributed by the ultrahistochemical investigations which will be the object of our
next work.

## SUMMARY

Ultrastructural features of the Pacinian corpuscles in the foot pads of eight cats
between the age of 2 hr after birth and adulthood were followed by means of the
electron microscope. According to the results the Pacinian corpuscles are not yet
mature in this region at the time of birth. At birth three different development stages
were found.

(a) Corpuscles without inner core. The axon is enveloped in a polygonal inner
core cell, the other cells are accumulated in the surroundings.

(b) Corpuscles with a small number of inner core lamellae. The other inner core
cells are arranged irregularly about the inner core basis. Their plasma gradually
forms the inner core lamellae.

(c) Corpuscles with a greater number of inner core lamellae. The nuclei of these
cells are in periphery of the inner core (growth zone). These corpuscles in no way
correspond to the mature ones. Only in the later period of postnatal life is it possible
to find a final structural picture of the Pacinian corpuscles: a great number of the
inner core lamellae, a distinct boundary space, thin capsule lamellae and wide interlamellar spaces filled with collagenous fibres.

The cells of the inner core in the postnatal period resemble the cells on the capsule surface. The problem of the origin of the inner core and the capsule cells is left open for further investigation to which the author intends to contribute ultrahistochemical studies.

## REFERENCES

HONDE, S. (1959) Electron microscopy of the Pacinian corpuscle in the cat mesentery, especially of its development. *Arch. jap. Chir.*, 28, 3330–3347.

MALINOVSKÝ, L. (1970) Ein Beitrag zur Entwicklung einfacher sensibler Körperchen bei der Hauskatze (*Felis silvestris f. catus* L.). *Acta anat. (Basel)*, **76**, 220–235.

MALINOVSKÝ, L. AND SOMMEROVÁ, J. (1972) Die postnatale Entwicklung der Vater-Pacinischen Körperchen in den Fußballen der Hauskatze (*Felis silvestris f. catus* L.). *Acta anat. (Basel)*, **81**, 183–201.

MARTINEZ, R. AND PEKARTHY, J. M. (1974) Ultrastructure of encapsulated nerve endings in rat gingiva. *Amer. J. Anat.*, **140**, 135–138.

PEASE, D. C. and QUILLIAM, T. A. (1957) Electron microscopy of the Pacinian corpuscle. *J. biophys. biochem. Cytol.*, **3**, 331–342.

POLÁČEK, P. AND HALATA, Z. (1970) Development of simple encapsulated corpuscles in the nasolabial region of the cat. Ultrastructural study. *Folia morph. (Warszawa)*, **18**, 359–368.

POLÁČEK, P. AND MAZANEC, K. (1966) Ultrastructure of mature Pacinian corpuscles from mesentery of adult cat. *Z. mikr.-anat. Forsch.*, **75**, 343–354.

SAXOD, R. (1970) Etude au microscope électronique de l'histogénèse du corpuscule sensorial cutané de Herbst chez le canard. *J. Ultrastruct. Res.* **33**, 463–482.

VOLKOVA, N. K. (1972) Formirovanie nekotorych struktur telca Pačini v ontogeneze. *Dokl. Akad. Nauk SSSR, Otd. Biokh.*, **204**, 717–719.

## DISCUSSION

ULUMBEKOV: Does the basal membrane exist around the cell with the mesoaxon, that is at the early stage of development of the corpuscles that you have observed? Second question: do the basal membranes exist at the later stages of development around those cells which you believe synthesize collagen? Third question: may I assume from your data that the inner core cells can synthesize collagen?

MALINOVSKÝ: These corpuscles are very large. I cannot tell with confidence that the basal membrane exists. Many serial sections are to be made. I studied only the postnatal stage of development and observed collagen at this stage. I did not investigate the prenatal stages of development. I am planning to carry out such experiments. I cannot answer your third question either.

# The Role of Sensory Innervation in the Development of Mechanoreceptors

JIŘINA ZELENÁ

*Institute of Physiology, Czechoslovak Academy of Sciences, 142 20 Prague 4 – Krč (Czechoslovakia)*

The essential component of peripheral receptors is the sensory nerve terminal of the primary sensory neuron. As regards perception, the sensory neuron is polarized so that it receives messages at the periphery and transmits then to the nerve centers. However, the sensory neuron may also act in the reverse direction, inducing the differentiation and ensuring the maintenance of specialized cells constituting the peripheral receptor. Such a neural effect of sensory terminals upon specialized cells was observed in various types of receptors, both primary and secondary (for review, see, for example, Zelená, 1964; Jacobson, 1971; Guth, 1971, 1975). In our experiments, we have studied the neural influence upon the development of mechanoreceptors, mainly rat muscle spindles (Zelená, 1957, 1962, 1964; Zelená and Hník, 1960, 1963a, b; Zelená and Soukup, 1973, 1974, 1975).

## Development

Skeletal muscles in which muscle spindles are localized develop, initially, in the absence of nerves. Peripheral nerves grow into the muscle primordia when uninucleated myoblasts fuse to form myotubes. The large majority of myotubes receives motor innervation and develops into extrafusal muscle fibers which remain under the trophic control of motor nerve fibers (for review, see, for example, Guth, 1968; Gutmann, 1968). Muscle spindles differentiate from a small number of myotubes contacted by IA sensory nerve terminals.

In the rat, the onset of spindle differentiation is observed in 18–19-day-old fetuses, *i.e.* about 3 days before birth (Kalugina, 1956; Zelená, 1957; Landon, 1972; Milburn, 1973a, b). In each nascent spindle, primary sensory terminals encircle a single myotube, and a thin capsule is formed around the innervated region from an extension of the perineurium. Additional intrafusal fibers develop subsequently by proliferation and fusion of intracapsular myoblasts. At birth, spindles usually consist of two intrafusal myotubes; a full complement of about four intrafusal fibers is reached by the fourth postnatal day. The first two developing myotubes differentiate into nuclear bag fibers, typical and intermediate, both containing an accumulation of nuclei in the equatorial region innervated by sensory terminals; the other two myotubes develop into nuclear chain fibers with a single file of nuclei in the equatorial zone (Fig. 1).

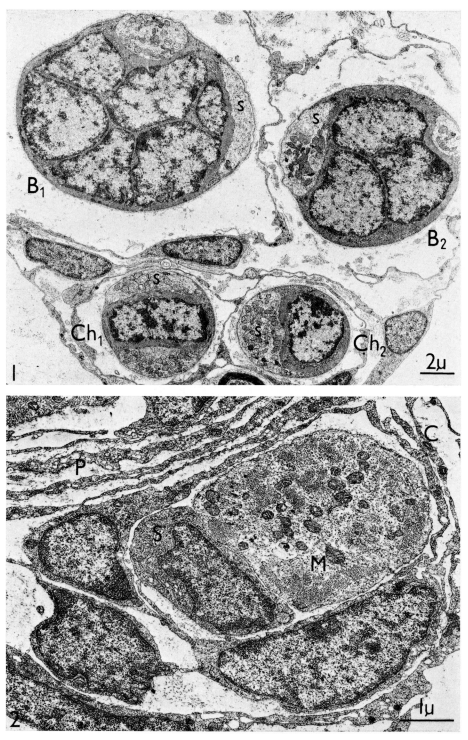

Fig. 1. A transverse section through the equatorial region of a rat muscle spindle, showing two nuclear bag fibers (B$_1$ and B$_2$) and two nuclear chain fibers (Ch$_1$ and Ch$_2$) innervated by primary sensory terminals (s). The external capsule is not shown in the picture.

Fig. 2. A transverse section through a denervated spindle from the soleus muscle 10 days after neonatal neurotomy. The spindle consists of a dedifferentiated intrafusal myotube (M) and of a satellite myoblast (S). Two layers of the spindle capsule (C) are in continuity with the perineurium (P) of an adjacent nerve.

However, the differentiation of polar zones into fiber types and the development of the complex innervation pattern formed by two types of sensory fibers and by three types of fusimotor fibers are only completed two to three weeks after birth. (For further details on structure and function see Barker, 1974; Matthews, 1972.)

## The effect of denervation

When developing limb muscles of the rat are denervated by sectioning the sciatic nerve in 19-day-old embryos, the differentiation of muscle receptors is arrested before it begins, and no spindles are subsequently found in denervated muscles (Zelená, 1957). The immature spindles of newborn rats also disintegrate rapidly after nerve section performed at birth. It is seen in the electron microscope that sensory terminals degenerate first and are phagocytozed by Schwann cells within 12 hr after neurotomy (Zelená and Soukup, 1975). The myotubular nuclei become reduced in number in the equatorial region, so that the characteristic nuclear bags disappear from denervated spindles during the first two days after nerve section (Milburn, 1973b). The de-differentiated intrafusal myotubes either atrophy or degenerate. The spindle capsule ceases to develop and is reduced to one or two discontinuous layers. Therefore, it becomes increasingly difficult to detect spindle remnants in denervated muscles. Only occasional encapsulated myotubes of disarranged myofibrillar ultrastructure can be found in denervated muscles after careful search (Fig. 2). The spindle content of hind limb muscles decreases nearly to zero values 10 days after neonatal neurotomy, whereas normally innervated muscles contain a characteristic number of spindles at that time (Zelená, 1964; Fig. 3).

Similarly, Golgi tendon organs of denervated rat muscles disintegrate within 10 days after nerve section at birth (Zelená and Hník, 1963b; Zelená, 1964). Pacinian corpuscles, localized on the interosseous membrane, also disintegrate and disappear from denervated hind limbs within 10 days when the sciatic nerve is transected in

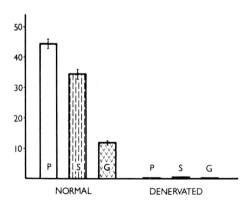

Fig. 3. Number of receptors in normal and denervated hind limbs of 10-day-old rats after nerve section of the right sciatic nerve at birth. P, Pacinian corpuscles on the interosseous membrane; S, muscle spindles, G, Golgi tendon organs in the extensor digitorium longus muscles. (Columns represent mean number ± S.E. of 8, 5 and 8 animals respectively.)

newborn rats, whereas contralateral control limbs contain, on the average, 44.5 Pacinian corpuscles in the same localization (Fig. 3).

In contrast to the rapid disintegration of immature spindles after neonatal neurotomy, the fully differentiated spindles of young and adult rats survive denervation and are reinnervated again after nerve regeneration (Zelená and Hník, 1963b). When denervation is prolonged and maintained, intrafusal fibers undergo atrophy and dedifferentiation (Tower, 1932). However, the characteristic number of spindles per muscle remains unchanged in the rat up to two years after nerve section (Gutmann and Zelená, 1962).

## Reinnervation

If muscle nerves are allowed to regenerate after crushing the sciatic nerve in newborn rats, limb muscles become reinnervated several days later. In the gastrocnemius muscle, the average number of spindles may become increased after a rapid re-innervation (Zelená and Hník, 1963b; Zelená, 1964; Werner, 1973). In other limb muscles, however, only occasional spindle remnants become reinnervated; such spindles remain small and atypical, and their average number per muscle is greatly reduced (Zelená and Hník, 1960, 1963a, b; Hník and Zelená, 1961). If the denervation period is prolonged by repeated crushing of the sciatic nerve, reinnervated limb muscles become completely devoid of muscle receptors (Zelená, 1964).

## The effect of de-efferentation

Polar zones of intrafusal fibers, which represent more than two-thirds of the total spindle length, have exclusively fusimotor innervation. They become significantly atrophic after selective de-efferentation performed in adult animals, in contrast to equatorial regions which remain innervated and preserved (Tower, 1932). After neonatal de-efferentation, the development of rat spindles proceeds almost normally. Both nuclear bag and nuclear chain fibers differentiate in de-efferented spindles (Zelená, 1964). One month after de-efferentation, intrafusal fibers become somewhat atrophic, but their ultrastructural fiber type characteristics are comparable to those of normal spindles not only in the innervated equatorial regions (Zelená and Soukup, 1973), but also in the completely denervated polar zones (Zelená and Soukup, 1974).

It thus can be concluded that sensory innervation is essential for the development and differentiation of muscle spindles, whereas fusimotor innervation only has a trophic effect upon polar zones of intrafusal fibers.

## Neural influence

The neural influence of sensory terminals upon specialized cells is assumed to be mediated by a substance produced by the nerve cell body, transported to the periphery and released by the nerve terminals, according to the hypothesis first proposed in order to explain the neural effect upon receptor cells of taste buds and lateral line organs (Olmstead, 1920; May, 1925; Parker, 1932). The possible carriers of an active substance may be dense core vesicles observed in sensory terminals of various receptors. However, there is as yet no convincing evidence of exocytosis and transfer of substances at the sensory junction. Thus, the mechanisms of the neural influence upon peripheral receptors still remains to be elucidated.

## SUMMARY

Sensory nerve terminals apparently induce and maintain the differentiation of non-nervous components of muscle receptors and Pacinian corpuscles of the rat. The development of muscle spindles, Golgi tendon organs and Pacinian corpuscles is arrested after neonatal neurotomy, and the immature receptors disintegrate within 10 days after denervation. On the other hand, rat muscle spindles continue to develop and differentiate ultrastructurally after neonatal de-efferentation, if their sensory innervation remains preserved.

A similar effect of sensory nerve terminals upon the differentiation of receptor cells was previously described in the cases of taste buds and other secondary receptors. The ultrastructural findings appear to support the hypothesis that the neural effect is mediated by substances produced by the sensory neuron and released by its terminals, but direct evidence of this is still lacking.

## REFERENCES

BARKER, D. (1974) Morphology of muscle receptors. In C. C. HUNT (Ed.), *Handbook of Sensory Physiology, Vol. III, Part 2, Muscle Receptors.* Springer-Verlag, Berlin, pp. 1–190.

GUTH, L. (1968) "Trophic" influences of nerve on muscle. *Physiol. Rev.,* **48**, 645–687.

GUTH, L. (1971) Degeneration and regeneration of taste buds. In L. M. BEIDLER (Ed.), *Handbook of Sensory Physiology, Vol. IV, Part 2, Chemical Senses.* Springer-Verlag, Berlin, pp. 63–74.

GUTMANN, E. (1968) Development and maintenance of neurotrophic relations between nerve and muscle. In G. E. M. WOLSTENHOLME AND M. O'CONNOR (Eds.), *Growth of Nervous System.* Churchill, London, pp. 233–243.

GUTMANN, E. AND ZELENÁ, J. (1962) Morphological changes in the denervated muscle. In E. GUTMANN (Ed.), *The Denervated Muscle.* Academia, Prague, pp. 57–102.

HNÍK, P. AND ZELENÁ, J. (1961) Atypical spindles in reinnervated rat muscles. *J. Embryol. exp. Morphol.,* **9**, 456–467.

JACOBSON, M. (1971) Formation of neuronal connections in sensory systems. In W. R. LOEWENSTEIN (Ed.), *Handbook of Sensory Physiology, Vol. I.* Springer-Verlag, Berlin, pp. 166–190.

KALUGINA, M. A. (1956) K voprosu o razvitii proprioceptorov poperechnopolosatykh myshts mlekopytayushchikh. *Arkh. Anat. Gistol. Embriol.,* **33**, 59–63.

LANDON, D. N. (1972) The fine structure of the equatorial regions of developing muscle spindles in the rat. *J. Neurocytol.,* **1**, 189–210.

MATTHEWS, P. B. C. (1972) *Mammalian Muscle Receptors and Their Central Actions.* Edward Arnold, London, 630 pp.

MAY, R. M. (1925) The relation of nerves to degenerating and regenerating taste buds. *J. exp. Zool.,* **42**, 371–410.

MILBURN, A. (1973a) The early development of muscle spindles in the rat. *J. Cell Sci.,* **12**, 175–195.

MILBURN, A. (1973b) *The Development of the Muscle Spindle in the Rat.* Ph.D. Thesis, University of Durham.

OLMSTEAD, J. M. D. (1920) The results of cutting the seventh cranial nerve in *Ameiurus nebulosus*. *J. exp. Zool.*, **31**, 369–401.

PARKER, G. H. (1932) On the trophic impulse, so-called, its rate and nature. *Amer. Naturalist*, **66**, 147–158.

TOWER, S. S. (1932) Atrophy and degeneration in the muscle spindle. *Brain*, **55**, 77–90.

WERNER, J. K. (1973) Mixed intra- and extrafusal muscle fibers produced by temporary denervation in newborn rats. *J. comp. Neurol.*, **150**, 279–301.

ZELENÁ, J. (1957) The morphogenetic influence of innervation on the ontogenetic development of muscle spindles. *J. Embryol. exp. Morphol.*, **5**, 283–292.

ZELENÁ, J. (1962) The effect of denervation on muscle development. In E. GUTMANN (Ed.), *The Denervated Muscle*. Academia, Prague, pp. 103–126.

ZELENÁ, J. (1964) Development, degeneration and regeneration of receptor organs. In M. SINGER AND J. P. SCHADÉ (Eds.), *Mechanisms of Neural Regeneration, Progress Brain Research, Vol. 13*. Elsevier, Amsterdam, pp. 175–213.

ZELENÁ, J. AND HNÍK, P. (1960) Absence of spindles in muscles of rats reinnervated during development. *Physiol. bohemoslov.*, **9**, 373–381.

ZELENÁ, J. AND HNÍK, P. (1963a) Motor and receptor units in the soleus muscle after nerve regeneration in very young rats. *Physiol. bohemoslov.*, **12**, 277–290.

ZELENÁ, J. AND HNÍK, P. (1963b) Effect of innervation on the development of muscle receptors. In E. GUTMANN AND P. HNÍK (Eds.), *The Effect of Use and Disuse on Neuromuscular Functions*. Academia, Prague, pp. 95–105.

ZELENÁ, J. AND SOUKUP, T. (1973) Development of muscle spindles deprived of fusimotor innervation. *Z. Zellforsch.*, **144**, 435–452.

ZELENÁ, J. AND SOUKUP, T. (1974) The differentiation of intrafusal fibre types in rat muscle spindles after motor denervation. *Cell Tissue Res.*, **153**, 115–136.

ZELENÁ, J. AND SOUKUP, T. (1975) Ultrastructural changes of developing muscle spindles after denervation. *Folia morph. (Warszawa)*, 23, in press.

## DISCUSSION

CHOUCHKOV: How long was the peripheral nerve stump below the site of nerve transection performed in newborn rats?

ZELENÁ: The peripheral nerve stump was extirpated, so that the length of the peripheral axons was reduced to about 1 mm. Therefore, the progress of nerve degeneration was very fast.

MAVRINSKAJA: How did the nuclear bag and nuclear chain fibers differentiate in polar regions after neonatal de-efferentation?

ZELENÁ: The contractile polar regions differentiated into distinct fiber types in 70% of de-efferented spindles (Zelená and Soukup, 1974). In contrast to that, extrafusal muscle fibers remained undifferentiated after de-efferentation.

# Vegetative Component of Interoceptors

E. K. PLETCHKOVA AND E. B. KHAISMAN

*The B. I. Lawrentiew Neurohistological Laboratory, Institute of Normal Physiology AMS U.S.S.R., Moscow (U.S.S.R.)*

The problem of the regulative and adaptation-trophic influence of the vegetative nervous system on various neural formations, including the tissue receptors, represents also a morphological problem. The task of morphologists is to study the substrate of these influences; in other words it is necessary to study the interrelationships between the vegetative nerve structures and the terminal sensory endings of spinal and bulbar sensory fibers.

This is a very difficult problem. The difficulties are caused by the structure of the majority of the tissue receptors as well as by the features characterizing the existing methods of their investigation. The major part of neurohistological methods, actually considered as classical, fails to identify simultaneously the sensory and the motor vegetative components in the region of terminals of the receptor fibers, and are characterized by inconstancy of the hoped for results. The method of methylene blue staining identifies more surely than other methods both afferent and efferent conductors and the terminal structures, so that they may be observed in one visual field of the microscope. However, this method also has its disadvantages. What particular features of the morphology of receptor tissue hamper the investigation of the above-mentioned problem? It should be noted that a very large group of the tissue receptors in the connective tissue and muscle structures of the visceral organs represents the so-called "free endings" of sensory cerebrospinal fibers. The terminals of free receptors run over the tissue substrate forming large terminals bushes, and come into immediate contact with the tissue elements.

We know that in smooth muscles of the visceral organs and in their well vascularized connective tissue sheaths another nerve structure is present, a ubiquitous network of the terminal vegetative fibers and their endings. Unfortunately, the sensory and effector components of innervation are extremely rarely observed simultaneously in one preparation. If all fibers were identified in one preparation, we observed a mutual overlapping in the dense network of terminal nerve structures: more or less close contacts of sensory and vegetative terminals. These pictures would permit us to speak of the mediator influences of the vegetative fibers upon the receptors, or to judge their mediatory action on the activity of the tissue receptors through the smooth musculature. However, such judgements are speculative. Thus, we believe that the morphological study of the role of the vegetative innervation in the activity of free tissue receptors, using morphological methods, is actually very difficult.

*References p. 74–75*

In connective tissue sheaths and the layers of connective tissue in the visceral organs, one clearly defined morphological group of the receptors — encapsulated receptors, is observed. Obviously, this group of receptors can be used to ascertain the indicated problem, as shown by the new researches of Santini (1969). It must be recalled that the so-called Timofeyev's apparatus of Vater–Pacinian corpuscles was readily taken for a sympathetic fiber, *i.e.* for the morphologic substrate of sympathetic influences upon the activity of the encapsulated receptor, as first indicated in the work of Juriewa (1927). Later on, however, experimental morphological studies have shown that the Timofeyev's apparatus is formed by the accessory fiber of the same (or the neighboring) cerebrospinal conductor which forms the given receptor (Lawrentiew and Lawrenko, 1933; Lawrenko, 1938; Pletchkova, 1948).

It has been shown that these fibers are always very abundant in the regions of the nodes of Ranvier along the course of sensory fibers. These are thin and unmyelinated along its full length. They may run far away from the site of their origin and intermingle with terminal nerve structures. They are hardly differentiated from the vegetative fibers by usual neurohistological methods of investigations.

In the last decade morphologists have obtained new methods for furthering the studies of vegetative regulation of the receptor structures. These concern the histochemical methods of revealing the vegetative nerve conductors of sympathetic and parasympathetic origin. With the aid of these methods we attempted to find out the interrelationships of vegetative and sensory cerebrospinal fibers in the zone of tissue receptors in the visceral organs and blood vessels. To reveal the parasympathetic fibers we have used the thiocholine method of Koelle–Gomori enabling one to identify the cholinergic nerve fibers by the presence of specific cholinesterase. For the elective identification of sympathetic adrenergic nerve fibers we employed the fluorescent microscopic method of Falck–Hillarp with the modification of Govyrin (1967) or Krokhina (1973).

However, it should be noted that despite their indubitable advantages these methods also have negative qualities. The most essential defect of the luminescent adrenergic method is that the correlation of the adrenergic luminescent fibers and the innervated substrate may only be indicated by various indirect signs. As regards the cholinesterase method it can not safely be said that we are dealing with true cholinergic (*i.e.* parasympathetic) fibers. However, different indirect proofs obtained by us permit us to suggest, like many other authors, that this group of nerve fibers may be considered as fibers of parasympathetic origin.

Since it is often difficult to ascertain the localization of the adrenergic component in the innervated substrate, we tried to choose limited and well outlined reflexogenic zones with a relatively dense arrangement of the interoceptors having definite boundaries and outlines permitting them to be identified even in cases when the nerve component was not revealed by the method used. The reflexogenic zone of the aortic arch and of the carotid sinus and the baroreceptor zones situated in these zones meet the proposed requirements.

The study of the vegetative component of baroreceptors of the vascular reflexogenic zones is of importance because the influence of the tonus of the vegetative nervous system upon the functional activity of these receptors has been the object of physiological observations (Palme, 1944; Anokhin, 1952; Landgren, 1952; Floyd and Neil, 1952; Kezdi, 1954; Diamond, 1955; Navakatikjan, 1956; Eyzaguirre and Levin, 1961; Edmonson and Joels, 1969; Aars, 1971).

To understand and ascertain the interrelationships of the receptor apparatus with the vegetative nerves we have examined the reflexogenic vascular zones of the aortic arch and the carotid sinus by various methods combined with that of experimental morphology, *i.e.* the sectioning of the nerve conductors along with extirpation of nerve ganglia. To examine the structure of baroreceptors we have used the method of silver impregnation after Bielschovsky–Gros or Campos and methylene blue staining after Dogiel with the modification of Shabadash. The histochemical method used was that of Gomori for alkaline and acid phosphomonoesterase and, finally, as mentioned above, the method of Falck–Hillarp was used for investigation of sympathetic adrenergic fibers, and that of Koelle–Gomori for revealing acetylcholinesterase fibers. The subjects of the investigations were young normal dogs. The baroreceptors of the aortic arch and of the carotid sinus in man and in mammals are non-encapsulated, but at the same time non-free receptors. The terminals of the afferent fibers of the baroreceptors are plunged in the sensory sole which consists of syncytium of special cells, derivatives of Schwann glia.

Fig. 1a shows a receptor from the dog's aortic arch obtained with the Campos method. Preterminal fibers forming terminals plunging into the sole of the receptor are visible. Fig. 1b distinctly shows the nuclei of the sole. As already mentioned, the

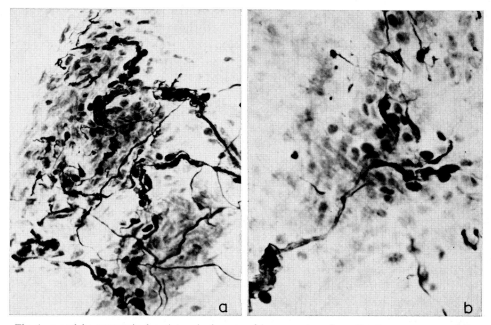

Fig. 1. a and b: preterminal and terminal parts of baroreceptors from the depressor zone of the aortic arch in dog. Nuclei of the soles of receptors are seen. Silver impregantion after Campos. × 150 (a) and × 400 (b).

*References p. 74–75*

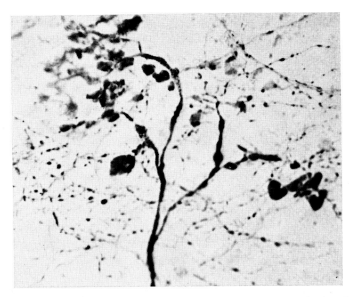

Fig. 2. Baroreceptor apparatus from the depressor zone of the aortic arch in dog. Thin varicose fibers of vegetative origin are seen. Methylene blue staining after Shabadash. × 500.

method of methylene blue staining reveals that in the zone of baroreceptor endings another kind of nerve fiber is found which is considered to be vegetative. Fig. 2 illustrates the baroreceptor of the aortic arch stained with methylene blue. The afferent fiber divides into terminal fibers ending in terminal rings and lattices showing here a homogeneous character. Close to the terminal structures of the baroreceptor, in the zone of their spreading, we see typical thin vegetative fibers which, when stained with methylene blue, look like varicose fibers.

Already in the first work made in our laboratory (Khaisman and Lawrentiewa, 1963) by histochemical methods it became clear that the soles of baroreceptors represent regions of the enzyme activity where different baroreceptors show different degrees of this activity. Fig. 3a shows the baroreceptors of the aortic arch with identified acid phosphatase. The enzyme is seen in the preterminal fibers, in terminal branches and terminal structures and also in the sensory soles of the receptors. The same method allows one to see, in the receptor zones, a dense plexus of thin fibers situated in the region of the sole of the receptor (Fig. 3b), that is the vegetative fibers lying in the plexus of Schwann syncytium.

It is to be noted that this plexus belongs to the baroreceptor zone. Beyond its limits a similar density of arrangement of the vegetative fibers is absent. The experimental morphological investigations (Khaisman and Lawrentiewa, 1964) have shown that the vegetative component of innervation of the depressor zone of the aortic arch is formed by sympathetic and parasympathetic postganglionic nerve fibers. The extirpation of the inferior cervical and stellate sympathetic ganglia was followed by degeneration and a subsequent disappearance of a considerable part of the nerve fibers from the vegetative plexus of the aortic zone.

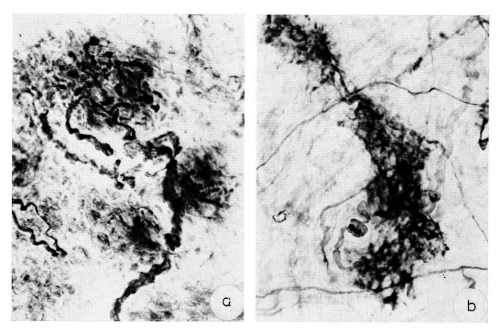

Fig. 3. a and b: baroreceptors from the depressor zone of the aortic arch in dog. Enzyme active elements of the receptor sole are seen. Method of Gomori for acid phosphomonoesterase. × 350 (a) and × 500 (b).

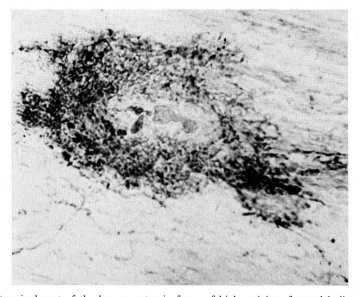

Fig. 4. Preterminal part of the baroreceptor in focus of high activity of acetylcholinesterase. Depressor zone of the aortic arch in dog. Thiocholine method of Koelle–Gomori. × 400.

*References p. 74–75*

It is to be emphasized that in the experiments involving sympathectomy a considerable part of the nerve fibers of the vegetative plexus of the aortic arch remained intact, suggesting that these fibers are of another origin, namely that they are parasympathetic preganglionic fibers. In the territory of depressor zones of the aortic arch and in the sinocarotid zone, parasympathetic neurons with their synaptic apparatuses are found. The conclusion concerning two types of vegetative fibers (sympathetic and parasympathetic) in the baroreceptor zone could be verified by histochemical methods.

As shown in the depressor zone of the aortic arch treated with the cholinesterase method of Koelle–Gomori (Khaisman and Lawrentiewa, 1963), separate areas are revealed which may be regarded as foci of high activity of acetylcholinesterase in the region of endings of the baroreceptor fibers. Fig. 4 shows such an area. The characteristic pattern of the preterminal nerve fiber distinctly shows that this is a baroreceptor. It does not contain active cholinesterase but in virtue of the contrast stain of the sole of the baroreceptor, sinking of this fiber with its terminal branches into the region of the sole is distinctly observed. The terminal branchings of the baroreceptor fibers have no active enzyme and show the appearance of light strands. The study of the depressor zone of the aortic arch and the carotid sinus with the Falck–Hillarp method has shown that, apart from the adrenergic nerve fibers belonging to the sympathetic vascular innervation of vasa vasorum, there are always revealed adrenergic nerve structures in the form of a widely branched net-like system of nerve conductors with dense interlacements characteristic of the vegetative periphery, and representing foci of density of the Schwann syncytium (Borodulja and Pletchkova, 1972; Khaisman, 1974). In their immediate proximity brightly luminescing (with fluorescence of catecholamine type) cellular formations of rounded, ovoid or irregular form are frequently detected.

Their size varied within the limits of 30 and 60 $\mu$m. These cells project small thin, varicose luminescing processes soon entering the adrenergic plexus and being lost among vegetative nerve fibers similar in the appearance and the character of the fluorescence (Fig. 5a, b). The observed morphological features allow one to consider these cellular formations as neurons of adrenergic (sympathetic) origin. These observations agree with the well known facts of location of the adrenergic neurons in the intramural ganglia of the heart and other organs (Hamberger and Norberg, 1965; Furness and Costa, 1971; Krokhina and Pletchkova, 1971; Krokhina, 1973). Along with the adrenergic neurons, the depressor zone of the aortic arch as well as the carotid sinus may contain single chromaffin cells or their small accumulations. They are distinguished from adrenergic neurons by their structural characteristics and by the specific luminescence.

Similar pictures of adrenergic innervation are observed in the sinocarotid reflexogenic zone. Fig. 6a shows fragments of an adrenergic plexus in the adventitial layer of the wall of the carotid sinus in dog. Luminescing nerve fibers with varicosities characteristic of the terminal parts are present. Fig. 6b illustrates the area of adrenergic perivascular plexus innervating the vasa vasorum of the carotid sinus wall. Here, also, are seen brightly luminescing cellular formations similar to those described in the

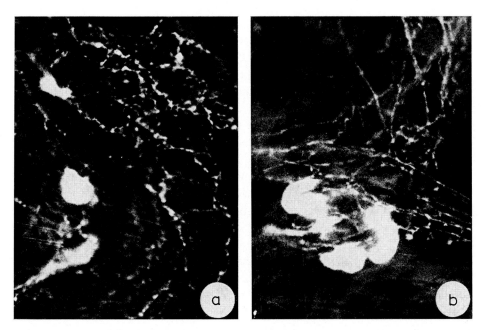

Fig. 5. a and b: fragments of the adrenergic plexus from the depressor zone of the aortic arch in cat. Explanation in the text. Catecholamine method of Falck–Hillarp $\times$ 450 (a) and $\times$ 500 (b).

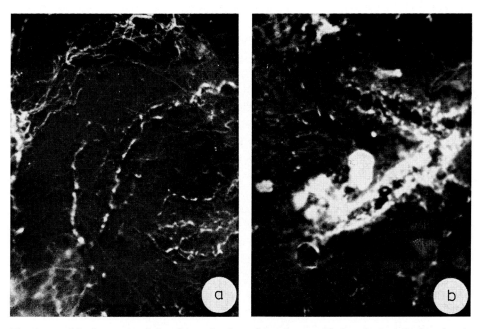

Fig. 6. a. and b: fragments of the adrenergic plexus from the carotid sinus in dog. Explanation in the text. Catecholamine method of Falck–Hillarp. $\times$ 500 (a) and $\times$ 400 (b).

*References p. 74–75*

depressor zone of the aortic arch and, probably, representing adrenergic neurons.

At present many physiological investigations have been accumulated showing the existence of the sympathetic influence of the baroreceptors. This question was most intensely studied in relation to baroreceptors of the carotid sinus (Landgren *et al.*, 1953; Kezdi and Geller, 1968; Koizumi and Sato, 1969; Sampson and Mills, 1970; Bagshaw and Peterson, 1972).

In the works of these authors we find many controversial opinions. However, it is to be emphasized that in the process of the analysis of influences exerted by electrical stimulation of the sympathicus or by the local action of adrenaline, noradrenaline, and other active substances on the vascular wall, the above authors unanimously suggest that the physiological mechanism of the sympathetic influence on the baroreceptors consists of a change in tone activity in the vascular wall. It is only in the work of Koizumi and Sato (1969) that we find an indication that the electrical stimulation of sympathetic fibers in the opossum shows a direct influence of the sympathetic nerve on the receptors of the carotid sinus. However, this opinion is disputed because in these experiments the changes in blood pressure do not occur at once, as expected, but only gradually.

In our opinion there is no doubt that the vegetative influences on the baroreceptors of reflexogenic zones do really exist. There are very few morphological works devoted to the morphological substrate of these influences. We know the works of Rees (1967) and Reis and Fuxe (1968), who investigated the distribution of adrenergic nerve fibers of the carotid zone in normal rabbits, cats and rats and in the same animals after ganglionectomy of the superior cervical ganglion. These authors studied the distribution of sympathetic fibers in the carotid sinus in the electron microscope. A similar study by the fluorescent method with the same results has been made by Reis and Fuxe (1968). In white rats the authors could not find any adrenergic fibers in this region. They also failed to show the presence of sympathetic adrenergic fibers in the area of the baroreceptor endings. They have observed these fibers only in the adventitia of the sinocarotid region in cat and rabbit, and suggest that under the influence of sympathetic impulses there occurs a change in the adventitia as long as there is a small number of muscle cells. Thus, according to these authors the influence on the receptors of the sinocarotid region is effected through the smooth musculature. They remark that the sympathetic fibers can also act immediately on the mechanoreceptors and change their sensitivity. However, the authors do not describe the morphological substrate of these influences.

In this connection we should refer to our previous investigations (Khaisman and Lawrentiewa, 1964; Khaisman, 1967) in which a powerful vegetative innervation of specialized smooth muscle cells on the territory of the depressor zone of the aortic arch was shown. While comparing this innervation system with the above-described adrenergic plexus we came to the conclusion that here we are dealing with the same structural organization of the vegetative component in the depressor zone of the aortic arch. This suggests that adrenergic plexiform structures also effect the effector sympathetic innervation of smooth muscle elements of the depressor zone of the aortic arch.

Thus, our morphological and histochemical investigations, together with the results of Reis and Fuxe (1968), suggest the existence within the aortic and sinocarotid reflexogenic zones of neuromuscular mechanisms able to effect the autonomic regulation of the tissue tone of these zones, and so act upon the functional activity of the baroreceptors. At the same time it is to be emphasized that the existence of intimate topographical interrelationships between the aortic and sinocarotid baroreceptors on the one hand, and the vegetative structures of the sympathetic and parasympathetic origin on the other, suggests the presence of one more mechanism of vegetative influence on the activity of baroreceptors.

There is implied an immediate action of functionally active synaptic structures (of adrenergic or cholinergic origin) on the aortic and sinocarotid baroreceptors by the release of chemical mediators — noradrenaline or acetylcholine — and the associated change in the thresholds of sensory baroreceptors (Anokhin, 1952; Landgren, 1952; Landgren et al., 1953; Navakatikjan, 1956; Aars, 1971).

Probably, a number of other tissue receptors are interrelated with the peripheral vegetative structures and undergo their immediate or indirect influence. Further morphological and histochemical investigations in this direction will contribute to the knowledge of the mechanisms underlying the adaptational-trophic and regulatory influences of the vegetative sympathetic and parasympathetic nervous systems upon the activity of the receptors of visceral organs.

### SUMMARY

The present study is devoted to the morphological and histochemical investigation of the vegetative component of interoreceptors. Attention was paid mainly to baroreceptors of the aortic and sinocarotid reflexogenic zones in dog and cat. The following methods were used: impregnation after Campos and supravital staining with methylene blue after Shabadash; the method of Gomori for acid phosphomonoesterase; the thiocholine method of Koelle–Gomori and the catecholamine method of Falck–Hillarp. To study the sources of innervation the experimental morphological method of nerve sectioning was applied.

The results establish the existence within the limits of the aortic and sinocarotid reflexogenic zones of a specialized vegetative component formed by nerve fibers of sympathetic and parasympathetic origin. There is an intimate interrelationship of the terminal structures of the vegetative component with the baroreceptors. Attention is directed to the part of the vegetative component in the innervation of smooth muscle cells on the area of the aortic and sinocarotid zones.

It is suggested that the vegetative component described may contribute to effecting the adaptational-trophic and regulatory influences of the sympathetic and parasympathetic nervous systems on the functional activity of vascular baroreceptors.

74    E. K. PLETCHKOVA AND E. B. KHAISMAN

REFERENCES

AARS, H. (1971) Effects of noradrenaline on activity in single aortic baroreceptors fibers. *Acta physiol. scand.*, **83**, 335–343.

ANOKCHIN, P. K. (1952) On the two-phase action of adrenaline on the baroreceptors of the aortic nerve. In *Nerve Regulation of Blood Circulation and Respiration*. Medguiz, Moscow, pp. 147–155.

BAGSHAW, R. AND PETERSON, L. (1972) Sympathetic control of the mechanical properties of the canine carotid sinus. *Amer. J. Physiol.*, **222**, 1462–1468.

BORODULJA, A. V. AND PLETCHKOVA, E. K. (1972) Adrenergic innervation of internal carotid arteries. *Dokl. Akad. Nauk SSSR, Otd. Biol.*, **202**, 200–202.

DIAMOND, J. (1955) Observations on the excitation by acetylcholine and by pressure of sensory receptors in the cat's carotid sinus. *J. Physiol. (Lond.)*, **130**, 513–532.

EDMONDSON, P. AND JOELS, N. (1969) Changes in carotid sinus baroreceptor activity induced by angiotensin. *J. Physiol. (Lond.)*, **202**, 82–83.

EYZAGUIRRE, C. AND LEVIN, J. (1961) The effect of sympathetic stimulation on carotid nerve activity. *J. Physiol. (Lond.)*, **159**, 251–267.

FLOYD, F. AND NEIL, E. (1952) The influence of the sympathetic innervation of the carotid bifurcation on chemoceptor and baroceptor activity in the cat. *Arch. int. Pharmacodyn.*, **140**, 230–239.

FURNESS, J. AND COSTA, M. (1971) Morphology and distribution of intrinsic adrenergic neurons in the proximal colon of the guinea pig. *Z. Zellforsch.*, **120**, 346–363.

GOVYRIN, V. A. (1967) *The Trophic Function of the Sympathetic Nerves in the Heart and Skeletal Muscles*. Nauka, Leningrad.

HAMBERGER, B. AND NORBERG, K. (1965) Studies on some systems of adrenergic synaptic terminals in the abdominal ganglia of the cat. *Acta physiol. scand.*, **65**, 235–242.

JURIEWA, E. T. (1927) On the nature of the second thin fibre reaching the encapsulated sensory neural apparatuses. *Russ. Arch. Anat. Histol. Embryol.*, **6**, 209–215.

KEZDI, P. (1954) Control by the superior cervical ganglion of the state of contraction and pulsatile expansion of the carotid sinus arterial wall. *Circulat. Res.*, **2**, 367–371.

KEZDI, P. AND GELLER, E. (1968) Baroreceptor control of postganglionic sympathetic nerve discharge. *Amer. J. Physiol.*, **214**, 427–435.

KHAISMAN, E. B. (1967) *Aortic Baroreceptors*. Medizina, Moscow.

KHAISMAN, E. B. (1974) An adrenergic component of the nervous apparatus of the aortic reflexogenic zone. *Bull. exp. Biol. med.*, **78**, 109–112.

KHAISMAN, E. B. AND LAWRENTIEWA, N. B. (1963) Histochemical studies of the ferment activity of the receptors in the depressor zone of the aortic arch in dog. *Arch. Anat. Histol. Embryol. (Leningrad)*, **44**, 62–68.

KHAISMAN, E. B. AND LAWRENTIEWA, N. B. (1964) The morphology of the vegetative component of depressor zone of the aortic arch. *Dokl. Akad. Nauk SSSR, Otd. Biol.*, **157**, 674–677.

KOIZUMI, K. AND SATO, A. (1969) Influence of sympathetic innervation of carotid sinus baroreceptor activity. *Amer. J. Physiol.*, **216**, 321–329.

KROKHINA, E. M. (1973) *Functional Morphology and Histochemistry of the Vegetative Innervation of the Heart*. Medizina, Moscow.

KROKHINA, E. M. AND PLETCHKOVA, E. K. (1971) Adrenergic neurons in the intramural ganglia of the heart. *Dokl. Akad. Nauk SSSR, Otd. Biol.*, **196**, 211–213.

LANDGREN, S. (1952) The baroreceptor activity in the carotid sinus nerve and the distensibility of the sinus wall. *Acta physiol. scand.*, **26**, 35–56.

LANDGREN, S., SKOUBY, A. AND ZOTTERMAN, Y. (1953) Sensitization of baroreceptors of the carotid sinus by acetylcholine. *Acta physiol. scand.*, **29**, 381–388.

LAWRENKO, V. V. (1938) Participation of sympathetic nerve fibres in the structure of sensory nerve-endings. *Bull. biol. med. exp. (Moscou)*, **5**, 37–38.

LAWRENTIEW, B. I. ET LAWRENKO, V. V. (1933) Les fibres sympathiques participent-elles à la structure des appareils sensitifs périphériques? (De la nature de l'appareil de Timofejew). *Trav. Lab. Rech. Biol. l'Univ. Madrid*, **28**, 187–195.

NAVAKATIKJAN, A. O. (1956) Change in sensitivity of the mechanoreceptors in the aortic reflexogenic zone to adrenaline following bilateral cervicothoracic sympathectomy. *Physiol. J. SSSR*, **42**, 88–95.

PALME, F. (1944) Zur Funktion der brachiogenen Reflexzonen für Chemo- und Pressoreception. *Z. ges. exp. Med.*, **113**, 415–461.

PLETCHKOVA, E. K. (1948) (Ed.) Innervation of the urinary bladder. In *The Morphology of Sensory Innervation of Visceral Organs*. AMS USSR, Moscow, pp. 163–180.

REES, P. (1967) The distribution of biogenic amines in the carotid bifurcation region. *J. Physiol. (Lond.)*, **193**, 245–253.

REIS, D. AND FUXE, K. (1968) Adrenergic innervation of the carotid sinus. *Amer. J. Physiol.*, **215**, 1054–1057.

SAMPSON, S. and MILLS, E. (1970) Effects of sympathetic stimulation on discharges of carotid sinus baroreceptors. *Amer. J. Physiol.*, **218**, 1650–1653.

SANTINI, M. (1969) New fibres of sympathetic nature in the inner core region of Pacinian corpuscles. *Brain Res.*, **16**, 535–538.

## DISCUSSION

WIDDICOMBE: (1) You have shown that there are four ways in which baroreceptor discharge may be modified, by sympathetic and parasympathetic nerves either acting indirectly on the smooth muscle, or directly on the receptor. Do you know the relative functional importance of the four systems? (2) Do your results apply equally to receptors with non-myelinated fibres and those with myelinated fibres? (3) How do you explain the fact that baroreceptors are insensitive to applied acetylcholine?

PLETCHKOVA: (1) Our morphological and histochemical observations suggest that sympathetic and parasympathetic nerve fibers situated in the soles of baroreceptors can, by means of their mediators, change the functional state of the receptive apparatus. Other mechanisms of action of the vegetative nerves on the baroreceptors discussed above are known from the literature and we cannot judge their comparative functional role. (2) The results reported are related only to baroreceptors with thick myelinated fibers and from those of mean caliber, that is to the type II receptors of De Castro. (3) As far as I know from various literature sources acetylcholine does act on the baroreceptors.

# Ultrastructural Differences Between the Preterminal Nerve Fibres and their Endings in the Mechanoreceptors, with Special Reference to their Degeneration and Mode of Uptake of Horseradish Peroxidase

CH. N. CHOUCHKOV

*Department of Anatomy and Histology, Medical Academy, Sofia 31 (Bulgaria)*

Although different views concerning the ultrastructural classification of the receptor organs still exist, the basic principles of their intimate structure are already resolved (Cauna, 1966; Quilliam, 1966; Munger, 1971; Andres and Von Düring, 1973). However, independently of the great advances which electron microscopy and cytochemistry have produced for estimation of the specificity of the capsule cells, Schwann-like cells and of the non-myelinated segments of the myelinated nerve fibres entering the receptor organs, the functional significance of some ultrastructural and cytochemical findings awaits careful evaluation.

No physiological studies appear to have investigated the differences between the non-myelinated segments or preterminals in the sensory receptors and their terminal swellings or so-called nerve endings. The classical neurohistologists attach a valuable importance to the latter structure. Merkel (1875) was the first who found that the naked axon in Grandry corpuscles terminates with a disc ("Scheibe") between two clear cells. Using a combination of acetic acid and gold chloride Ranvier (1889) established that the nerve fibres in the Meissner corpuscle end with flat expanded buttons, while Renaut (1881) considered that these buttons are oval. Krause (1881) brought up for discussion different views concerning the existence of the terminal nerve swellings. He had concluded that all sensory receptors have these structures and they could be demonstrated only in fresh tissue preparations, and that the form of these endings depended on the staining procedure. Using methylene blue, Dogiel (1891) established that the nerve endings in Meissner's corpuscle are more intensively stained than their terminal fibres. After these conclusions the following papers discussed the problem of the nerve endings only with regard to their form and distribution in various organs. Thus Pianese (1891) described 30 different forms of endings in Pacinian corpuscles, while Ruffini (1896) gave various forms of nerve endings in diverse receptor organs.

Ultrastructurally, the nerve endings have been very rarely encountered. Very little is known even in the case of the most investigated Pacinian corpuscle, because of obvious difficulties in the representation of its nerve endings (Chouchkov, 1971; Spencer and Schaumburg, 1973). A precise and clear differentiation between the preterminals and their endings is lacking in the investigations devoted to the mechano-receptor ultrastructure. In addition, the nature of most of the specific organelles in the nerve endings and their functional significance for nerve conduction still require investigation.

The goal of this report is to present the unit design of the terminal nerve swellings or nerve endings in various receptor organs and to clarify the differences between them and the preterminals. At the same time, denervation experiments on the Pacinian corpuscles and the demonstration of horseradish peroxidase uptake by the Herbst and Grandry corpuscles sheds some light on the functional importance of the organelles on both sides of the receptor membrane.

MATERIAL AND METHODS

Three kinds of material were examined. (1) Thin slices of human digital glabrous skin, as well as Pacinian corpuscles from 10 individuals taken at biopsy and processed immediately. (2) The experimental analysis of the effects of denervation was carried out on male cats. The abdominal cavity was opened and nerves going to the Pacinian corpuscles were cut at a distance of 5–8 cm. From 6 hr to 120 days after the operation the receptors were removed and examined electron microscopically. (3) The location of the intravenously injected horseradish peroxidase was visualized from 15 to 60 min after injection in thin slices of duck bill skin from 10 newborn birds. The sections were examined in Hitachi 11A, Jem 100B and Zeiss 9A electron microscopes.

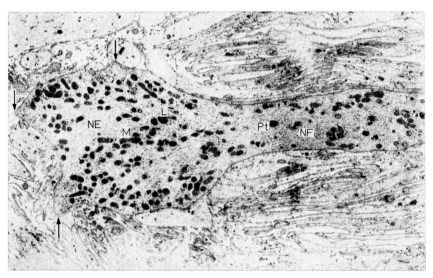

Fig. 1. The nerve preterminal (Pt) and its ending (NE) in Pacinian corpuscle. The nerve ending contains a great accumulation of mitochondria (M), lysosomes (L) and finger-like processes (arrows) Only the neurofilaments predominate in the preterminal (NF). × 35,000.

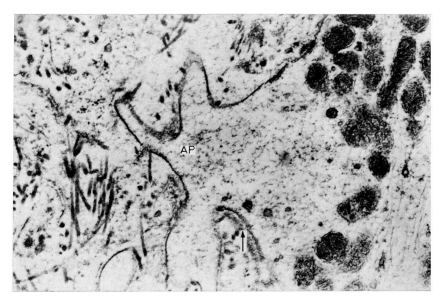

Fig. 2. Finger-like processes (AP) belonging to the terminal portion of the nerve ending. They are surrounded by the intercellular substance. Sometimes the base of the processes is covered by a basement membrane (arrow). × 70,000.

## RESULTS

The Pacinian corpuscle was the receptor in which the differences between the preterminal and its ending could be seen most clearly. In the slices along the corpuscular length, the preterminal contains a peripheral palisade of elongated mitochondria lying parallel to the axonal length. The inside of the axoplasm was predominantly occupied by neurofilaments and neurotubules (Fig. 1). Only in transverse or in oblique sections was it possible to detect lysosomes, clear and coated vesicles, multivesicular bodies and glycogen granules thinly dispersed in the regions adjacent to the cytoplasmic cleft of the inner core cells. In these places the axolemma makes up particular protrusions known as finger-like processes (Figs 1 and 2). This characteristic pattern of the preterminal in Pacinian corpuscles did not differ from the corresponding preterminals in all capsulated mechanoreceptors. The preterminals in non-capsulated receptors, such as free dermal endings, Merkel cell–neurite complexes, intraepidermal and hair nerve endings, do not possess finger-like processes or a considerable vesicular material in adjacent Schwann-like cells.

### Characteristics of terminal regions

The terminal swellings of the preterminals or so-called nerve endings possess specific characteristic patterns of cellular organization which allow their precise definition in both the capsulated and the non-capsulated receptors. The nerve endings contain principally the same organelles mentioned in the preterminals, but their quantity and distribution differ considerably.

*References p. 86–87*

The mitochondria occupy the central part of the nerve endings. They are much more numerous than in the preterminals, and most of them have an oval or spherical form. Many glycogen granules are scattered amongst the mitochondria. One very characteristic feature is the relative accumulation of lysosomes. In most cases they possess a lamellated myelin-like structure (Fig. 3). Their quantity varies in diverse receptor organs, but their presence is an obligatory sign. The most characteristic feature of the ultraterminal sectors of the nerve endings are the so-called "denuded" axoplasm–axolemma complexes. They represent the extensive direct contact of the sensory axoplasm with the surrounding intercellular substance. In some cases they are covered by a basement membrane or they make up finger-like processes partially covered or without a basement membrane. These "denuded" complexes vary in diverse receptor organs. Thus, in the very rapidly adapting mechanoreceptors with a thick lamellated capsule, such as Pacinian, Herbst and Golgi–Mazzoni corpuscles, the finger-like processes show the most extensive growth (Fig. 2), while in the slowly adapting mechanoreceptors, such as Merkel cell–neurite complexes, and also in the intraepidermal and free dermal nerve endings, the "denuded" sectors with a basement membrane predominate. The axoplasm of "denuded" sectors in all mechanoreceptors contains neurofilaments, clear vesicles of various sizes, coated vesicles and multi-vesicular bodies.

Three kinds of vesicles can be distinguished in the nerve endings: clear vesicles, dense core vesicles and coated vesicles (Fig. 3). However, it must be emphasized that the clear and dense core vesicles are not identical with the well known synaptic vesicles proposed to be vesicles of acetylcholine (ACh) and catecholamines (CA) in the other parts of the nervous system. The following indirect arguments can be

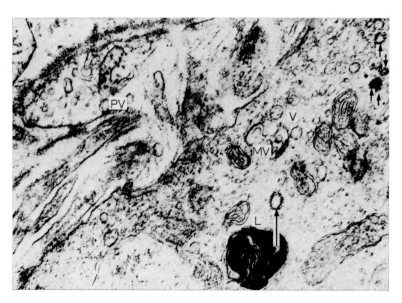

Fig. 3. A part of the nerve ending axoplasm possessing different kinds of vesicles: clear vesicles (V), coated vesicles (arrows), dense core vesicles (double arrow), multivesicular bodies (MV). The surrounding cytoplasm of the inner core lamellae contains numerous pinocytotic vesicles (PV). × 60,000.

presented against the suggestion that the receptor vesicles contain the above-mentioned transmitters. *First*, the vesicle sizes range from 20 to 120 nm, which is not typical for the synaptic vesicles, *Second*, most of the vesicles are scattered in the nerve endings axoplasm and they do not show any clusters characteristic of synaptic vesicles. *Third*, no synaptic differentiation between the adjacent axolemma and plasmalemma near the vesicles can be established. The desmosome-like contacts between the membranes are irregularly distributed and do not possess any reasonable connections with the vesicles. *Fourth*, there is no histochemical evidence for the transmitter role of ACh and CA. The cytochemical reactions for acetylcholinesterase (AChE) normally present in Schwann-like cells in Pacinian corpuscles do not change immediately after denervation of the receptors and persist for up to 14 days, by which time the inner core cells have disappeared (Chouchkov, 1970). Also, the direct cytochemical reaction for CA is negative in the sensory nerve fibres of Pacinian and Herbst corpuscles (Chouchkov, 1968, unpublished data, 1973; Saxod, 1973). The coated vesicles range between 75 and 130 nm and can be found in various degrees of formation. The multivesicular bodies present in very different sizes are invariably present in the nerve ending axoplasm. The highest pinocytotic activity was seen in the cytoplasmic lamellae most closely related to the nerve endings. This process of endocytosis is relatively much more common in the capsulated mechanoreceptors than in the non-capsulated ones.

### Denervation studies

After section of the nerve fibres entering the Pacinian corpuscles, the first changes were seen in the nerve endings, especially in the finger-like processes and vesicular material, after less than 6–12 hr. The differences in time depend on the distance from which the nerve fibres were crushed. These changes were characterized by the appearance of great vacuoles at the bases of the finger-like processes (Fig. 4), accompanied by disintegration and disappearance of both clear and coated vesicles. At the same time the endocytotic activity of the cytoplasmic lamellae increases. *After 12–24 hr* most of the finger-like processes were disrupted and lying isolated among the intercellular substance (Fig. 5). The axonal membrane was fully destroyed. Neurofilaments roughened and changed their orientation. No more vesicles could be seen. The mitochondria lost their characteristic structure and were involved in the process of secondary lysosome formation. Autophagic vacuoles have been observed. The endocytotic activity of the adjacent lamellae diminished abruptly and an increase of lysosomes both in the nerve fibre and the cytoplasmic lamellae were detected. *Between 24 and 48 hr* the non-myelinated nerve fibre and its ending were eliminated. Their places were occupied by degenerated axonal fragments (Fig. 5) filled with destroyed mitochondria and secondary lysosomes. This sequence of events began from the nerve ending and travelled in a proximal direction towards the myelinated nerve segments. At the beginning of the third day conglomerates of denerated bodies replaced the axonal fragments. The process of phagocytosis was observed among the cytoplasmic lamellae followed also by destruction and degeneration. The increase

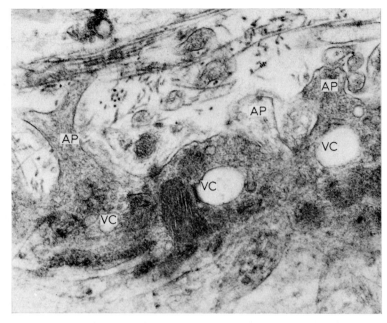

Fig. 4. The nerve ending axoplasm 6 hr after denervation. The vesicular material disintegrates and great vacuoles (VC) appear at the base of the finger-like processes (AP). × 46,000.

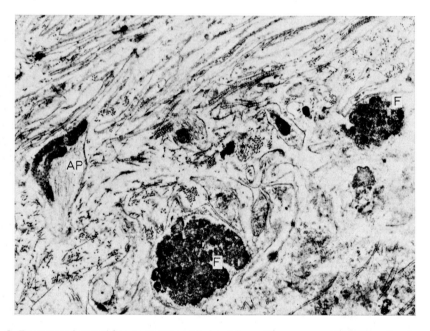

Fig. 5. Degenerated axonal fragments (F) and isolated finger-like processes (AP) 24 hr after denervation of Pacinian corpuscles. × 21,000.

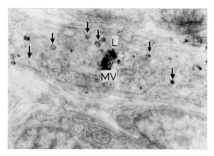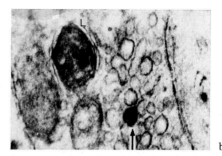

a                                                                          b

Fig. 6. The ultrastructural localization of exogenous peroxidase. a: lamellae of the Herbst corpuscle —
the lysosomes (L), multivesicular bodies (MV) and pinocytotic and coated vesicles (arrows) are
occupied by the electron opaque product. × 5000. b: the nerve ending of Grandry's corpuscle. The
reaction product is localized in some of the nerve ending clear vesicles (arrow) and lysosomes (L).
× 79,000.

of disoriented collagen fibres replaced the destroyed lamellae. The elimination of the
inner core cells began from 7 days and ended at 20 days after denervation. The
analogous process of activation followed by disintegration and degeneration involved the innermost capsule cells. Pacinian corpuscles examined 120 days after
denervation retained their outermost lamellae cells while the places of the inner
core cells and adjacent outer core lamellae were occupied by intensively developed
collagen fibres.

### Peroxidase experiments

The pattern of distribution and the extent of penetration of horseradish peroxidase
into the mechanoreceptors have been examined for the first time. Thirty minutes
after intravenous injection the electron-opaque peroxidase reaction product was
found in all components of Herbst and Grandry corpuscles: capsule cells, Schwann-
like cells, specific sensory cells and nerve fibres and their endings. The ultrastructural
localization was restricted to the pinocytotic vesicles, coated vesicles, multivesicular
bodies and lysosomes of the non-nervous elements (Fig. 6a), and to the vesicular
material and lysosomes of the nerve non-myelinated fibres and their endings (Fig. 6b).

### DISCUSSION

The comparative study of different mechanoreceptors shows that the terminal
swellings of the nerve fibres or the nerve endings have unit ultrastructural patterns
which allows their clear distinction from the preterminals. The specific ultrastructural
signs such as "denuded" axoplasma–axolemma complexes, with or without a basement membrane (finger-like processes), as well as the vesicles (especially coated
vesicles), multivesicular bodies, lysosomes, mitochondria and glycogen granules are
present in greatest quantity in the nerve endings or in the restricted places of the
preterminals situated near to the cytoplasmic cleft of the capsulated mechanoreceptors.

*References p. 86–87*

In brief, the nerve endings and, closely related to them, Schwann-like lamellae give strong morphological evidence as places where the dynamics of the cell processes in the receptors are the most intensive. On the other hand, the denervation experiments show that the nerve endings, especially the finger-like processes and the vesicular material, are the most sensitive parts in the process of degeneration because they first react with disintegration and destruction. Both considerations furnish ground for the suggestion that the nerve endings are the most responsible sites involved in the process of sensory transduction.

In relation to the transducer mechanism employed by the mechanoreceptors, an attempt of following speculations as regards the functional significance of the ultrastructural organelles will be made. The "denuded" axoplasma–axolemma complexes, and especially the finger-like processes, suggest that they are ideally situated to detect mechanical deformations transmitted from the non-neuronal parts. These deformations applied to the surface of the Pacinian corpuscle are selectively transmitted by the elastic elements provided by the lamellae and the intercellular spaces (Hubbard, 1958; Loewenstein and Mendelson, 1965; Loewenstein and Skalak, 1966). Also, some physiological studies have indicated that Pacinian corpuscles possess directional sensitivity to the bilateral arrangement of the inner core in the terminal regions (Ilyinsky, 1964; Nishi and Sato, 1968). However, for such considerations it must be remembered that in physiology electric potentials are never the cause but, on the contrary, the consequence of metabolic activities (Frey-Wyssling, 1973). A simple physical hypothesis of transduction does not take account of the elaborate arrays of organelles present at the nerve endings and so it is not known which biochemical reactions produce the necessary potentials in the receptor sites. It has been proposed that ACh and CA are less acceptable to fulfill a transmission role in the mechanoreceptors. Eccles (1966) suggests that there are specific transmitting mechanisms having a very slow organizational action, such as ribonucleic acids of different kinds. Recently, Hammerschlag and Weinreich (1972) have proposed that glutamic acid plays an important role as the transmitter of primary afferent neurones, but the same physiological effect has not been confirmed for the sensory nerve fibres. Thus it is evident that the question concerning the transmitter substance is open to speculation. On the other hand, it is interesting that at the present time little attention has been paid to one of the most prominent ultrastructural feature in the receptor organs — the vesicular material, especially the pinocytotic vesicles, the coated vesicles and multivesicular bodies. This vesicular material demonstrates the intensive rate of endocytosis on both sides of the receptor membrane. All these types of endocytosis have been shown to constitute a way of transporting extracellular material, especially protein, to lysosomes (Friend and Farquhar, 1967). In the nervous tissue of the adrenal medulla (Holtzmann and Peterson, 1969) uptake of exogenous peroxidase into lysosomes of capsule and Schwann cells is much more extensive than uptake into neurones. Presumably, capsule and Schwann cells act in a kind of "filtering" mechanism controlling access of exogenous material to the neurones. Our results proved that exogenous peroxidase also accumulates in the vesicular material and lysosomes of the receptor organs. Increased catabolism can only occur subsequent to an increased rate of endocytosis. This presumably explains the great occurrence of lysosomes in the sensory nerve endings. Novikoff (1967) has proposed that some lysosomes, especially with tubular shapes, may form outside the Golgi area and that they may arise directly within smooth endoplasmic reticulum by accumulation of dense material and acid hydrolases. Such accumulation of acid phosphatases reaction product was established in Pacinian nerve endings (Chouchkov, 1968). It is very attractive to assume that the main stages of this formation are selective adsorption of certain proteins on the plasma membrane, formation of endocytotic vesicles and transport of these vesicles into the close proximity of primary lysosomes. During the latter process some of the endocytotic vesicles will have fused together so that the final stage of fusion leads to the formation of multivesicular bodies of very different sizes. However, the significance of protein uptake by sensory nerve endings and the sequestration of exogenous protein in lysosomes are open to speculation. The evaluation of the role of lysosomes in processing exogenous material will require a fuller understanding of such transport, and of the sites of synthesis and degradation of neurotransmitters and axoplasmic protein. Independently of these speculations, the ultrastructural evidence presented here suggests that the morphological unit formed by sensory nerve ending constituents is the likely site for the generation of the receptor potential.

SUMMARY

The ultrastructural differences between the preterminals (non-myelinated segments of the sensory nerve fibres) and their terminal swellings, or so-called nerve endings, in different capsulated and non-capsulated mechanoreceptors are described. The nerve ending axoplasm possesses a great accumulation of centrally located mitochondria, much more glycogen granules, lysosomes and multivesicular bodies than the preterminals. Besides that, the nerve endings possess specific signs such as "denuded" axoplasma–axolemma complexes, clear vesicles, dense core vesicles and coated vesicles. The "denuded" complexes, especially the finger-like processes represent the extensive direct contact of the sensory axoplasm with the surrounding intercellular substance. These processes show a different growth in the capsulated and non-capsulated receptors. In connection with the vesicular material, the indirect arguments are presented against the suggestion that ACh and CA fulfill a transmitter role in the mechanoreceptors. The use of the denervated Pacinian corpuscle suggests that the nerve endings, especially the finger-like processes are the most sensitive parts of the receptors because they first react with disintegration and destruction; in other words, they are probably the most responsible sites involved in the process of sensory transduction.

The ultrastructural localization of exogenous peroxidase in the pinocytotic vesicles, coated vesicles, multivesicular bodies and lysosomes of the non-nervous receptor structures, as well as in the vesicular material and lysosomes of the nerve endings are also described. Some speculations as regards the significance of protein uptake by sensory receptors and the sequestration of exogenous protein in lysosomes are discussed.

## REFERENCES

ANDRES, K. H. AND VON DÜRING, M. (1973) Morphology of cutaneous receptors. In A. IGGO (Ed.), *Handbook of Sensory Physiology, Vol. II.* Springer-Verlag, Berlin. pp. 3–28.

CAUNA, N. (1966) Fine structure of the receptor organs and its probable functional significance. In A. V. S. DE REUCK AND J. KNIGHT (Eds.), *Touch, Heat and Pain, Ciba Foundation Symposium.* Churchill, London. pp. 117–136.

CHOUCHKOV, CH. (1968) Histochemical demonstration of primary catecholamines in Pacinian corpuscles of the cat. *Experientia (Basel)*, **24**, 826–827.

CHOUCHKOV, CH. (1970) Experimental histochemical investigation of the cholinesterases and of the primary catecholamines in the Pacinian corpuscles. *C. R. Acad. Bulg. Sci.*, **23**, 863–866.

CHOUCHKOV, CH. (1968) Histochemical demonstration of certain phosphomonoesterases in the Vater-Pacini receptors of the cat. *C.R. Acad. Bulg. Sci.*, **21**, 717–720.

CHOUCHKOV, CH. (1971) Ultrastructure of Pacinian corpuscles in men and cats. *Z. mikr.-anat. Forsch.*, **83**, 17–32.

CHOUCHKOV, CH. (1973) The fine structure of small encapsulated receptors in human digital glabrous skin. *J. Anat. (Lond.)*, **114**, 25–33.

DOGIEL, A. S. (1891) Die Nervenendigungen in Tastkörperchen. *Arch. Anat. Physiol.*, **10**, 182–192.

ECCLES, J. C. (1966) General discussion. In A. V. S. DE REUCK AND J. KNIGHT (Eds.), *Touch, Heat and Pain, Ciba Foundation Symposium.* Churchill, London.

FREY-WYSSLING, A. (1973) *Comparative Organellography of the Cytoplasm.* Springer-Verlag, Berlin.

FRIEND, D. S. AND FARQUHAR, M. G. (1967) Function of coated vesicles during protein absorption in the rat vas deferens. *J. Cell Biol.*, **35**, 357–376.

HAMMERSCHLAG, R. AND WEINREICH, D. (1972) Glutamic acid and primary afferent transmission. In E. COSTA, G. L. GESSA AND M. SANDLER (Eds.), *Advanc. Biochem. Psychopharmacol., Vol. 6.* Raven Press, New York, pp. 165–180.

HOLTZMAN, E. AND PETERSON, E. R. (1969) Uptake of protein by mammalian neurons. *J. Cell Biol.*, **40**, 863–869.

HUBBARD, S. J. (1958) A study of rapid mechanical events in a mechanoreceptor. *J. Physiol. (Lond.)*, **141**, 198–218.

ILYINSKY, O. B. (1964) Process of excitation and inhibition in single mechano-receptors (Pacinian corpuscles). *Nature (Lond.)*, **208**, 351–353.

KRAUSE, W. (1881) Die Nervenendigung in den Tastkörperchen. *Arch. mikr. Anat.* **20**, 212–221.

LOEWENSTEIN, W. R. AND MENDELSON, M. (1965) Components of receptor adaptation in a Pacinian corpuscle. *J. Physiol. (Lond.)*, **177**, 377–397.

LOEWENSTEIN, W. R. AND SKALAK, R. (1966) Mechanical transmission in a Pacinian corpuscle. An analysis and a theory. *J. Physiol. (Lond.)*, **182**, 364–378.

MERKEL, FR. (1875) Tastzellen und Tastkörperchen bei den Haustieren und beim Menschen. *Arch. mikr. Anat.* **11**, 636–652.

MUNGER, B. L. (1971) Patterns of organization of peripheral sensory receptors. In W. R. LOEWENSTEIN (Ed.), *Handbook of Sensory Physiology, Vol. I.* Springer-Verlag, Berlin, pp. 523–556.

NISHI, K. AND SATO, M. (1968) Depolarizing and hyperpolarizing receptor potentials in the non-myelinated nerve terminal in Pacinian corpuscles. *J. Physiol. (Lond.)*, **199**, 383–396.

NOVIKOFF, A. B. (1967) Lysosomes in nerve cells. In H. HYDEN (Ed.), *The Neuron.* Elsevier, Amsterdam, pp. 319–377.

PIANESE, G. (1891) La natura della clava centrale i le diverse forme di terminazione della fibra nervose nel'corpuscoli Pacini-Vater del mesentere dell gatto. E. Detken, Napoli.

QUILLIAM, T. A. (1966) Unit design and array patterns in receptor organs. In A. V. S. DE REUCK AND J. KNIGHT (Eds.), *Touch, Heat and Pain, Ciba Foundation Symposium.* Churchill, London.

RANVIER, L. (1889) *Traité technique d'Histologie.* Savy, Paris.

RENAUT, J. (1881) Sur les terminaisons nerveuses. *Ann. Dermatol.*, **2**, 208–211.

RUFFINI, A. (1896) Sullo strozzamento preterminale nelle diverse forme di terminazioni nervose periferiche. *Mon. Zool. Ital.*, **5**, 1–4.

SAXOD, R. (1973) Organisation ultrastructurale des corpuscules sensoriels cutanés des oiseaux. *Sci. Naturelles*, **1**, 79–98.

SPENCER, P. S. AND SCHAUMBURG, H. H. (1973) An ultrastructural study of the inner core of the Pacinian corpuscle. *J. Neurocytol.*, **2**, 217–235.

## DISCUSSION

KHAJUTIN: In your report you say that no physiological study appears to have investigated the difference between non-myelinated segments of preterminals and their terminal swelling, or so-called nerve endings. What difference might be found by physiologists? The attempt should be made to differentiate these two structures. It is obviously very difficult and is connected with the removal of the inner core. Why do I believe that the difference between these non-myelinated segments and nerve endings exists? Because of the difference in the number of morphological organelles which, however, were also observed in the nerve endings. I should underline again that there is only a quantitative difference. These structures are also observed in the Pacinian corpuscle terminals, but only in the area of the axoplasm protrusion in the inner core. You might see the nerve ending in the axoplasma.

CHOUCHKOV: I do not know whether such differences exist or not, I only suggest it.

# Living Interoceptor Structure

V. N. MAYOROV

*Laboratory of Functional Neuromorphology, I. P. Pavlov Institute of Physiology, Academy of Sciences of the U.S.S.R., Leningrad (U.S.S.R.)*

## INTRODUCTION

Study of the processes taking place in interoceptors is at present being held back due to methodological difficulties. A single living receptor is, in the majority of cases, inaccesible for the investigation. Therefore, it is not at all surprising that its morphology, reactive structural changes and morphophysiology of reactive states have been inadequately studied so far. However, studies of these states are not only of theoretical, but also of clinical significance. For instance, interoceptors located at different distances from ulcerous niches or cancerous tumours respond differently to pathological processes. Structural changes of both a reactive and degenerative nature are certainly taking place in them. Studying reactive phases (states) of interoceptors would be of great significance for correct histological diagnosis, and for revealing the mechanism of the pathological process.

The present report deals with peculiarities of living interoceptor structure. It summarizes results of many years of observation. The investigations have been carried out by the author alone, and also together with Podolskaya and other colleagues from his laboratory (Mayorov, 1957a, b, 1960a, b, 1961, 1965, 1969; Mayorov *et al.*, 1971; Podolskaya, 1972).

## METHODS

The research has been carried out on the living preparations of the grass frog bladder and small intestine of the steppe turtle, rabbit and cat. The preparations were examined with light microscope in light transmitted by means of a special device for living observations (Mayorov, 1969).

Interoceptors have been studied in control preparations and in experiments following the transection of the corresponding sensitive fibres and the exposure of the preparation to ethanol, high temperature (41–44 °C), etc.

For staining living interoceptors a solution of methylene blue (0.01 %) has been used. We considered the above-mentioned solution to be a stain as well as an irritating agent.

Cinemicrographic techniques were used for recording and for investigating structural changes in the interoceptor. The head of the laboratory of scientific cinematography, Y. I. Levkovitch, supervised the process of filming.

## RESULTS

Living interoceptors were found to have a characteristic structure, free of distortions and artifacts of any kind, which generally appeared following fixation and in the course of histological procedures.

Living interoceptors, compared with fixed and coloured ones, are approximately 1.5–2 times greater in size; for instance, if a living interoceptor reaches 478 $\mu$m in length and 443 $\mu$m in width, in the fixed preparation these dimensions are 237 and 161 $\mu$m respectively.

Terminal branches and end-plates of the living interoceptors are revealed in more detail than in *in vitro* surviving and dead preparations. As is known, these highly delicate formations could be lost or subjected to deformation during histological procedures. In the living preparation they are characterized by brighter and more intensive colouration. Following severe irritation, end-plates strongly refract light and can be seen without any staining — this never occurs in the dead preparation. Their dimensions and contours may change, as can distinctly be seen under greater magnification.

On the whole the range of observations is much greater compared with that seen in *in vitro* fixed and stained preparation. The latter reveals only a small part of the changes taking place in a living interoceptor.

The living interoceptor is a dynamic formation. Its structure and its tinctorial features are continuously changing under normal physiological conditions and in the course of experiment. The following phases can be recognized in the process of its reactive changing.

(a) Phase of initial structure. This implies an interoceptor in the unstained, intact preparation. Under these conditions it is not seen all along its length but only partly. Distinctly exposed is the initial thick medullary fibre, medullary preterminals and initial (proximal) parts of terminal branches. Distal parts of these branches, end-plates inclusive, can not be revealed.

(b) Phase of stained structure. (Figs. 1 and 2). This phase begins with the first symptoms of staining of the receptor, and is over at the very beginning of its de-colouring. Usually this phase begins within 14 min after the vital stain has been applied and lasts 11 min. Staining makes earlier invisible details of the interoceptor (terminal branches and end-plates) well defined on the background of colourless and transparent tissues of living preparations. Following the experimental stimulation, changes in the development of the phase can be seen. While thermal stimulation promotes the appearance and development of the given phase, transection of sensory fibres and exposure to alcohol, on the contrary, slow down its development.

(c) Phase of negative response to the stains. The beginning and development of

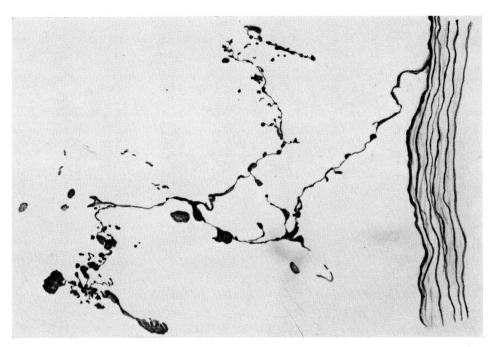

Fig. 1. Living interoceptor in phase of stained structure in the small intestine of the steppe turtle. Staining 2.5 hr after cutting-off of the blood flow (Preparation by V. G. Lucashin.) The figure is prepared from the photomicrograph; Ob. 40, oc. 2.4; nozzle 2.5.

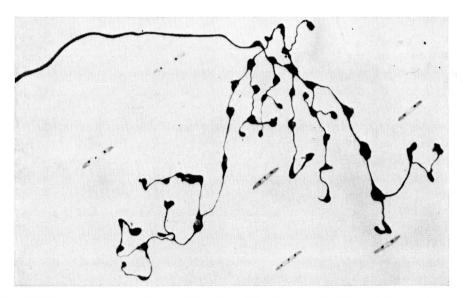

Fig. 2. Living interoceptor in the small intestine of the steppe turtle. Phase of stained structure (preparation by E. K. Morosov); Ob. 20, oc. 10 ×, nozzle 1.6 ×.

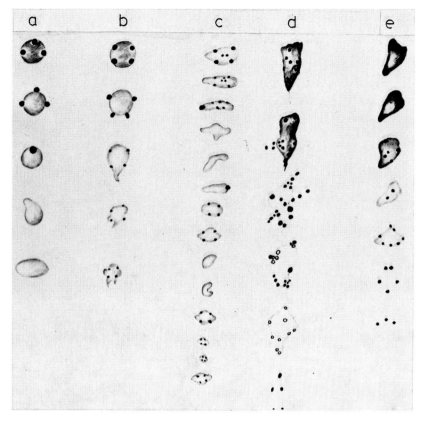

Fig. 3. Irritated end-plates a–e after the cessation of irritation develops to their initial state. Time of observation 30 min (preparation by L. A. Podolskaya). Ob. 20, oc. 10 ×, nozzle 1.6 ×.

this phase is an indication of severe irritation of the nerve terminal (Fig. 3). This phase begins with the first signs of receptor decolouring. Decolouring starts with end-plates and terminal fibres and then spreads onto preterminal medullary branches and further onto initial thick medullary fibres. At last complete structure decolouring sets in. It should be emphasized that during this phase, despite the decolouration, the nerve terminal, contrary to its initial structure phase and due to an increased co-efficient of transmitted light refraction, becomes visible all along its length up to the sensory end-plates. Under experimental conditions this phase varies to a great degree. It is most pronounced in the control preparations stained with methylene blue and in the preparations exposed to high temperature. On the other hand, in the experiments with cutting of nerve fibres and exposure to alcohol, this phase is con-siderably less pronounced.

(d) Reverse development phase. This phase begins with the first signs of a decrease in end-plate sizes. Gradually their contours become weaker and at last invisible. In the long run the interoceptor returns to its initial state, i.e., develops into the phase of initial structure.

These findings suggest that interoceptors respond to any irritation of adequate force by changing their structural and tinctorial characteristics. The dynamics of these changes are of a regular nature; one state of the interoceptor is being replaced by another. There are four phases in this process and each has a characteristic set of structural and tinctorial symptoms.

The end-plate is the most sensitive, most vulnerable and highly plastic structural component of the interoceptor. It is the first to become stained and the first to swell, gelatinize and undergo reverse development. In the phase of stained structure, considerable swelling of end-plates can be seen. During a period of 6 min some of them grew by 20%. Maximal growth takes place in the phase of negative response to the stain. Thus observations of one of the end-plates in this phase has shown that during 13 min it has increased by 34.5%. Some end-plates in this phase reached 13.2 $\mu$m. In the reverse development phase the end-plates shrink. One of the end-plates in this phase had decreased by 40% during 28 min, its size reaching the level characteristic of the stained structure phase. On decreasing in size the end-plates turn from circular and oval formations into polygonal structures. Their shapes are continuously changing; they form bulges which make their movements look more like an amoeba's. Therefore, in a sense, we can speak of mobility of these formations.

How do we estimate the results of studies of living interoceptor structure? We consider these results to be of a certain theoretical significance since they open prospects in the sphere of joint morphological and electrophysiological studies of single receptors. These data supply a reliable methodological basis for morphological studies in the form of anatomohistological preparations, and make the physiological approach more specific. Now, when the phases in the process of interoceptor structural changes have been revealed, it is possible to perform our physiological investigations during the definite phase of the receptor structural changes.

It is obvious that the development of generator potentials in the interoceptor does depend upon a given phase state. Evidently, during each phase of interoceptor structural change, generation of excitation impulse develops differently. Further experiments are necessary to confirm this assumption.

SUMMARY

Studies of interoceptor structure in living preparations reveals sensitive end-plates and terminal branches in more detail. As is known, these end-plates and terminal branches can be lost or considerably deformed in fixed and stained preparations. In the living preparation the receptor is much larger in size and much more brightly coloured. The interoceptor is not a static formation, its structure is continuously changing under experimental and normal conditions in response to any stimulation. During this process the following phases can be seen: phase of initial structure, phase of stained structure, phase of negative response to the stains and phase of reverse development of irritation symptoms. After the cessation of stimulation gradual restoration of the initial state can be observed. In the fixed and stained preparations interoceptors can be seen only in the phase of stained structure. Fixation and histological procedures result in shortening and disappearance of all other phases. End-plates are the most sensitive, most vulnerable and highly plastic structural components of the interoceptor. Their forms and dimensions are continuously changing in the course of structural changes of the receptor. Therefore, in a sense, one can speak of mobility of these formations.

## REFERENCES

MAYOROV, V. N. (1957a) Lebendbeobachtung der interneuronalen Verbindungen und Rezeptoren in der Harnblase. *Z. mikr.-anat. Forsch.*, **63**, 442–449.

MAYOROV, V. N. (1957b) On living observation of interneuronal relations and receptors in the bladder of grass frog. *Dokl. Akad. Nauk SSSR, otd. Biol.*, **115**, 826–828 (in Russian).

MAYOROV, V. N. (1960a) On living observation of sensory nerve endings. *Arch. Anat., Histol Embryol.*, **38**, 31–34 (in Russian).

MAYOROV, V. N. (1960b) On living observations of nerve cells, synapses and receptors. *Leningrad Soc. nat. Sci.*, **71**, 69–70 (in Russian).

MAYOROV, V. N. (1961) On living observation in the transmitted light of pericellular apparatus and sensory terminations. In *Proc. VIth All-Union Congr. Anat., Histol. Embryol., Kharkov, Vol. 1.* pp. 834–836 (in Russian).

MAYOROV, V. N. (1965) On structural and functional shifts in the living interneuronal synapses on staining it with methylene blue. In *Morphology of Ways and Relations of the Central Nervous System.* Nauka, Moscow, pp. 87–97 (in Russian).

MAYOROV, V. N. (1969) *Morphology of Reactive States of Vegetative Interneuronal Synapses.* Nauka, Leningrad (in Russian).

MAYOROV, V. N., MOROZOV, E. K., PODOLSKAYA, L. A. AND LEVKOVITCH, Y. I. (1971) Living observations of interoceptors. In *Proc. IIIrd All-Union Conf. Physiol. Vegetative Nervous System, Erevan.* p. 132 (in Russian).

PODOLSKAYA, L. A. (1972) On reverse phenomena in the receptor on the basis of living studies of its fine structure. In *Proc. IInd Symp. Local and Spreading Excitation, 120th Anniversary of N. E. Vvedensky,* Leningrad University Press, Leningrad. pp. 84–85 (in Russian).

# Morphometric Study of Fine Structure of Living Receptor by Cinemicroscopic Technique

Yu. I. LEVKOVICH AND L. A. PODOLJSKAYA

*Laboratory of Scientific Cinematography, Laboratory of Functional Neuromorphology, I. P. Pavlov Institute of Physiology, Academy of Sciences of the U.S.S.R., Leningrad (U.S.S.R.)*

## INTRODUCTION

At present only a few morphological papers in which a quantitative approach was used for the investigation of the nerve structures on the living and surviving preparations are available. We were not able to find any papers dealing with the morphometric study of the fine structure of living receptors. This may probably be explained by the technical difficulties which have been met. We made an attempt to overcome these difficulties by using the cinemicrographic technique. This method makes it possible to observe the living structures of the mobile preparation through its whole depth and to record a picture during a fraction of a second with the subsequent quantification of the recorded pictures.

## METHOD

Free bush-like sensory nerve endings were studied on the histological preparation made from the bladder of *Rana temporaria* (Mayorov, 1957). Vessels and nerve connections of the organ remained intact. Nerve endings were revealed by staining with vital dye, methylene blue (concentration 0.013%).

A morphometric technique was used for the processing of the obtained material. The cinemicrographic data were correlated with the results of microscopic examination and photography. At microscopic examination it was necessary to sum up the data of several experiments on various animals, because it does not seem possible to evaluate simultaneously all the details of the receptor structure during one experiment, due to the object mobility and small dimensions of the receptor terminal structures. (Fig. 1).

Photomicrography was used as an objective method of structure recording. Photographs were taken with a special apparatus for vital studies on line with a camera (Mayorov, 1969) on RF-3 film with exposure times of 1/500 and 1/250 sec. However, only a limited area of a structure and in a single plane might be photographed.

Cinemicroscopy proved to be the most objective and complete method for re-

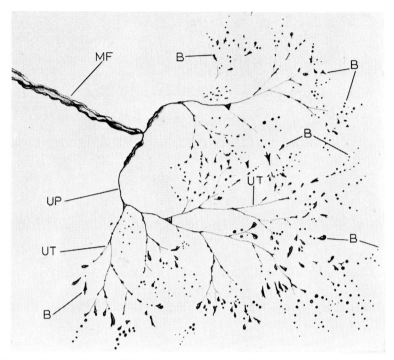

Fig. 1. Composite general view of the living receptor in the bladder of *Rana temporaria*. Methylene blue staining. MF, myelinated fibre; UP, unmyelinated preterminal; UT, unmyelinated terminal; B, terminal sensory boutons. Magnification: ($\times$ 350, $\times$ 1050) 20 $\times$ objective lens; 60 $\times$ water-immersion objective lens; 7 $\times$ ocular; 2.5 $\times$ attachment. The final receptor picture obtained from several experiments on various animals. The figure is subjective and is not suitable for quantitative analysis.

cording the structures. Vertical panning permits observation of a structure in several planes in less than a second. Mobility of the object did not affect the image quality and the stained structure did not fade in the intensive light.

Microfilms were made with 'Rodina' and 'Convas-1' cameras on colour LN-6 and LN-7 films at a rate of 24 pictures per second and exposure time in the range of 1/260–1/50 sec (Levkovich, 1971). The cinemicrographic negative was developed up to the contrast factor values in the range of 0.65–0.90. Positives were printed on TsR-8 films. The cinemicrographic material was analysed frame-by-frame and projected on to a screen, and the contours of all necessary details of the receptor were traced. Their shape was not distorted and the scale was the same. Several pictures were then super-imposed (Fig. 2). To match the images of the same receptor, the basic detail, common for all the pictures was used (*e.g.* characteristic bending of a vessel, part of the nerve fibre, etc.). These details were matched every time, and thus the repeated counting of the same bouton was excluded. Therefore, in the final picture the details of the receptor located at various depths may be observed.

The maximum "diameter" of the terminal boutons was measured. The obtained data were classified into the groups including the boutons of various dimensions.

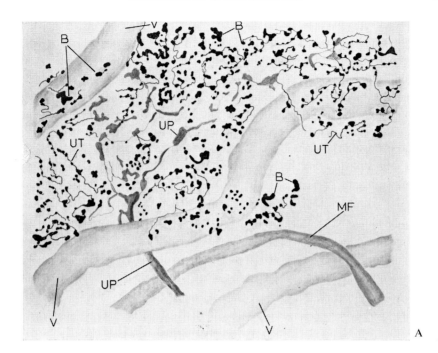

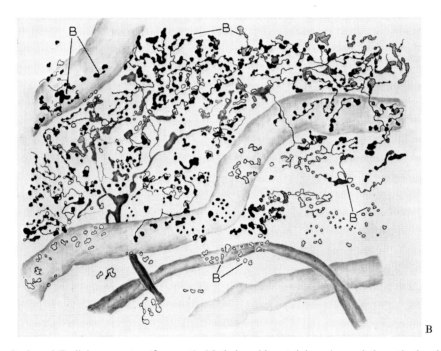

Fig. 2. A and B: living receptor (fragment). Methylene blue staining. A: semischematic drawing derived from a film picture. B: semischematic drawing derive from four film pictures Vertical panning. ■, first picture; □, second picture; hatched, third picture; cross-hatched, fourth picture; MF, myelinated fibre; UP, unmyelinated preterminal; UT, unmyelinated terminal; B, terminal sensory boutons; V, vessel. Magnification ($\times$ 220) 20 $\times$ objective lens; 10 $\times$ ocular; 1.1 $\times$ attachment.

Optic section area of the terminal structures in a receptor has been also measured and the number of boutons of a various size per 1000 sq.$\mu$m of the receptor area was evaluated.

At microscopic examination the bouton "diameter", measured on the scale of an ocular micrometer and the scale ruler, was used for measurement of the bouton size on the recorded pictures. Only in the film pictures can the bouton area be evaluated by the weight method because mathematical evaluation is difficult due to irregular shapes of boutons (Fig. 3) (Roskin and Levinson, 1957). In microscopic observations the terminal bouton distribution was determined by means of an ocular grid.

The number of boutons was counted per square of the projected pictures. The results were recounted per 1000 sq.$\mu$m of the receptor area.


RESULTS


Absolute dimensions of the receptor terminal structures are presented in Table I. The data obtained in cinemicrographic and microscopic examinations appeared to be identical. "Diameter" of one bouton was 6.1–6.2 $\mu$m on average, with minimal and maximal values of 0.6 $\mu$m and 11.9–12.1 $\mu$m.

As seen from Table II the boutons of 1–9 $\mu$m in "diameter" are widely spread, whereas the boutons of smaller size (up to 1 $\mu$m) and larger size (from 9 $\mu$m and above) occur comparatively rarely. Thus, small forms makes up 13.3% and large ones 2.7% of the total 150 boutons of the same receptor studied (high magnification), while the boutons of 1–6 $\mu$m in "diameter" constitute 75.3%.

At the same magnification visual observations showed 84% boutons of 1–6 $\mu$m


TABLE I

SIZES OF THE RECEPTOR TERMINAL BOUTONS IN $\mu$m (MAXIMAL "DIAMETER"). (AVERAGE DATA)

| Groups (in $\mu$m) | Average "diameters" of terminal boutons | | |
| --- | --- | --- | --- |
| | Cinemicroscopic method | Microscopic examinations | |
| | Objective lens 60 × Ocular 10 × Attachment 1.1 × | Objective lens 60 × Ocular 7 × Attachment 2.5 × | Objective lens 20 × Ocular 7 × Attachment 2.5 × |
| (1)  Less than 1 | 0.60 ± 0.01 | 0.55 ± 0.00 | |
| (2)  From 1 to 3 | 1.55 ± 0.02 | 1.80 ± 0.20 | |
| (3)  From 3 to 6 | 3.89 ± 0.03 | 4.00 ± 0.03 | |
| (4)  From 6 to 9 | 6.83 ± 0.04 | 7.10 ± 0.06 | |
| (5)  From 9 and above | 11.90 ± 0.50 | 12.10 ± 0.31 | |
| Total number of measured boutons | 747 | 334 | |

NOTE: These measurements were not performed in the case of photography.

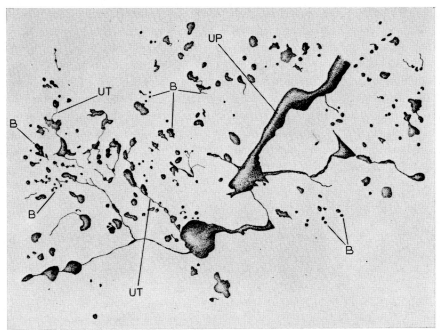

Fig. 3. Living receptor (fragment). Methylene blue staining. UP, unmyelinated preterminal; UT, unmyelinated terminal; B, sensory terminal boutons. Magnification: ($\times$ 660) 60 $\times$ water-immersion objective lens; 10 $\times$ ocular; 1.1 $\times$ attachment. Figure is derived from a transformed film picture.

## TABLE II

DISTRIBUTION OF THE RECEPTOR TERMINAL BOUTONS OF VARIOUS SIZES
(AVERAGE DATA)

| Groups (in μm) | Cinemicrographic method 60 ×, 10 ×, 1.1 ×, | 20 ×, 10 ×, 1.1 × | Microscopic studies 20 ×, 7 ×, 2.5 × | 20 ×, 7 ×, 2.5 × | Photography 20 ×, 7 ×, 1.6 × |
|---|---|---|---|---|---|
| (1) Less than 1 | 20 13.3% | — | — | — | — |
| (2) From 1 to 3 | 67 44.7% | 43 5.9% | 7 28 % | 6 20.7% | — |
| (3) From 3 to 6 | 46 30.6% | 328 44.9% | 14 56 % | 14 48.3% | — |
| (4) From 6 to 9 | 13 8.7% | 354 48.4% | 3 12 % | 7 24.1% | — |
| (5) From 9 and above | 4 2.7% | 6 0.8% | 1 4.0% | 2 6.9% | — |
| Average number in one film picture or experiment | 150 100 % | 731 100 % | 25 100 % | 29 100 % | 89 100% |

size and only 4% boutons of larger size of the total 25 registered in one experiment.

A correlation was made between the total numbers of boutons determined with different methods. The cinemicrographic method appeared to be the best: we were able to register 731 boutons, on average, for one receptor studied, 89 in the photograph and 29 in one microscopic examination at average magnification.

*References p. 102*

In Table III the area dimensions of the receptor terminal structures are presented. These measurements could be made only by the cinemicroscopic method. A single bouton area was 5.8 sq.$\mu$m on average, with minimal and maximal values being 0.3 and 39 sq.$\mu$m, respectively. In some cases the value might even reach 62.7 sq.$\mu$m. The total area of 146 boutons measured in one receptor studied was 855.8 sq.$\mu$m.

Terminal boutons of the sensory bush in the bladder of *Rana temporaria* are rather densely distributed (Figs. 1–3). To make it more evident, the density of boutons distribution per 1000 sq.$\mu$m of the receptor area was evaluated. On average magnification 28 boutons were registered visually; 10 and 5 boutons in the film picture and photograph, respectively.

TABLE III

AREA OF THE RECEPTOR TERMINAL BOUTONS IN sq.$\mu$m
(AVERAGE VALUES DERIVED FROM 5 FILM PICTURES)

| Item number | Number of boutons in one film picture | Total area of all the boutons in one film picture | Area of one bouton in one film picture | Area of the largest bouton | Area of the smallest bouton | Magnification |
|---|---|---|---|---|---|---|
| (1) | 154 | 911.3 | 5.9 | 55.7 | 0.4 | Objective lens 60 × Ocular 10 × Attachment 1.1 × |
| (2) | 205 | 555.9 | 2.7 | 24.4 | 0.4 | Same |
| (3) | 133 | 872.4 | 5.6 | 62.7 | 0.3 | Same |
| (4) | 131 | 1410.8 | 10.8 | 33.1 | 0.3 | Same |
| (5) | 107 | 528.5 | 4.9 | 23.0 | 0.2 | Same |
| On average | 146 | 855.8 | 5.8 | 39.8 | 0.3 | |

TABLE IV

DENSITY OF DISTRIBUTION OF TERMINAL BOUTONS PER 1000 sq.$\mu$m OF THE RECEPTOR AREA

| Method | Number of boutons | Magnification |
|---|---|---|
| Visual observations | 28 | Objective lens 20 × Ocular 7 × Attachment 2.5 × |
| Cinemicrography | 10 | Objective lens 20 × Ocular 10 × Attachment 1.1 × |
| Photomicrography | 5 | Objective lens 20 × Ocular 7 × Attachment 1.6 × |

A correlation between the results obtained by the three different methods showed that the cinemicrographic method had evident advantages over microscopic and microphotographic techniques. It takes less than 1 sec to film the living structure, with subsequent quantification of a recorded picture. By its use at average magnification it is possible to detect 731 boutons in a single picture as compared to 29 boutons during one microscopic examination. Analysis of a recorded image permits simultaneous evaluation of a greater number of the receptor terminal structures, their topography, dimensions, number, area, distribution density, etc., in the same animal. The scale is not distorted. Visual observation permits the collection of data only by stages through different experiments performed on various animals. Therefore, such presentation of a receptor structure proves to be schematic and subjective (compare Fig. 1 with Figs. 2 and 3). Besides, some parameters can be measured only by the cinemicrographic method. For instance, it is impossible to measure the area of some small details of irregular shape in the living mobile object during visual observation.

The microphotographic method proved to be time-consuming and unsuitable for our purposes because a structure may be photographed only in one plane.

Good agreement between the cinemicrographic and microscopic values of the receptor terminal boutons areas confirms the accuracy of the data obtained. Quantitative analysis showed that terminal boutons of 1–9 $\mu$m in diameter were most commonly found, the incidence of smaller and larger forms being lower. The significance of these findings remains somewhat unclear. Whether the smaller forms are less mature than the larger ones is not known. The increased number of the terminal boutons with diameters in the range of 1–9 $\mu$m might be related to neuroplasma mobility or could be explained by their different functions. Further studies are needed to clarify these assumptions and to investigate the relationship between the function and the dimensions of the boutons.

The same may be said of the terminal structures area. We do not know what is the role of the smallest and the largest boutons. Only the area of a number of boutons which acquire the information from the environment can be determined. Thus, the total area of 146 boutons measures 855.8 sq.$\mu$m. A correlation between this value and the value of the receptive field of one receptor, which measures 478 sq.$\mu$m × 443 sq.$\mu$m on average, may give some idea on the receptor function. We did not determine the total number of boutons in one receptor.

The number of boutons per 1000 sq.$\mu$m of the receptor area was used as a measure of density. We consider that this parameter might be accepted as a morphologic criterion of sensitivity of free bush-like receptors.

SUMMARY

Morphometric studies of free bush-like sensory nerve endings were carried out on the living mobile preparation from the bladder of *Rana temporaria*, with special emphasis on terminal boutons (end-plates) as the most sensitive and labile part of a receptor. A correlation was made between the data obtained by microscopic, cinemicrographic and photomicrographic techniques. The cinemicrographic technique was found to be the most suitable for quantitative assessments in vital microscopic studies. Good agreement was found between the geometrical dimensions of the boutons obtained with microscopic and cinemicrographic techniques. Mean diameter (the longest axis) of a single bouton was 6.1–6.2 $\mu$m, range 0.6–12.1 $\mu$m. Terminal boutons of 1–9 $\mu$m in diameter were most commonly found, whereas small (up to 1 $\mu$m) and large sized (from 9 $\mu$m and above) boutons occurred much more rarely. The mean area of a single terminal bouton measured with the cinemicrographic technique was 5.8 sq.$\mu$m, the smallest and largest boutons had the area of 0.3 and 39.8 sq.$\mu$m, respectively. The density of terminal boutons distribution, *i.e.* the number of boutons per 1000 sq.$\mu$m of the receptor area was 28 in microscopic examination; cinemicrographic and photomicrographic methods revealed 10 and 5 boutons, respectively.

## REFERENCES

LEVKOVICH, YU. I. (1971) A device for cinemicrography of the living objects. *Cinema and Television Technique*, N **2**, 74–77 (in Russian).

MAYOROV, V. N. (1957) On the vital study of interneural connections and receptors in the bladder of *Rana temporaria*. *Rep. Acad. Sci., U.S.S.R.*, **115**, 826–828 (in Russian).

MAYOROV, V. N. (1969) *Morphology of the Reactive States of Vegetative Interneural Synapse*. Nauka, Leningrad (in Russian).

ROSKIN, G. I. AND LEVINSON, L. B. (1957) *Microscopic Method*. Sovietskaya. Nauka, Moscow (in Russian).

SESSION III


# THERMORECEPTOR MECHANISMS

# Functional and Structural Basis of Thermoreception

HERBERT HENSEL

*Institute of Physiology, University of Marburg/Lahn, Marburg/Lahn (G.F.R.)*

Physiology of thermoreception includes various experimental approaches: (1) the phenomenological analysis of temperature sensations, (2) the recording of neural events, mainly by electrophysiological methods and (3) the investigation of physiological and behavioral responses to thermal stimuli (Hensel, 1973a and 1974a). All three approaches have led to substantial results but when trying to connect the findings, we are still at the beginning.

In a number of homoiothermic and some poikilothermic species, populations of warm and cold receptors have been identified. The specificity of thermoreceptors can be defined in man by warm or cold sensations related to the excitation of the sensory nerve endings in question, or, in man and animals, by the specific response of these endings to thermal stimuli, as assessed by electrophysiological methods. In the first case we speak of "sensory specificity", in the second case of "biophysical specificity".

A warm receptor is characterized by a dynamic overshoot in frequency on sudden warming and a transient inhibition on sudden cooling, whereas a cold receptor responds in the opposite way, namely, with an overshoot on cooling and an inhibition on warming. Furthermore, these receptors are insensitive to mechanical stimulation in the physiological range. When a rectangular temperature step is applied to the skin, the frequency will show an overshoot after which a static level of activity is attained. The new level can be reached either asymptotically, or, as was found recently, in the form of a damped oscillation. An example are the warm receptors in *Boa constrictor* (Hensel, 1974b). This snake, like other members of the snake family Boidae, possesses highly sensitive warm receptors in the upper and lower lip, their functional significance being the detection of infrared radiation from warm-blooded prey. These receptors are insensitive to mechanical stimulation, and no cold receptors have been found in this region. A quantitative single-fiber analysis has revealed a high overshoot in frequency on rectangular warming with a subsequent depression, after which a new static level is reached (Fig. 1).

Besides their dynamic response, all thermoreceptors show a more or less regular static discharge at constant temperature. The static frequency has a maximum at a certain temperature and decreases at higher and lower temperatures. Fig. 2 shows average static and dynamic frequencies for various populations of single warm and cold fibers. As can be seen, the static maxima for warm receptor populations in the

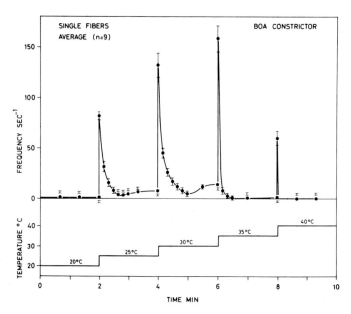

Fig. 1. Average impulse frequency of single warm fibers in the trigeminal nerve of *Boa constrictor* when applying temperature steps to the upper labial region. Bars show standard error of mean. (From Hensel, 1974b).

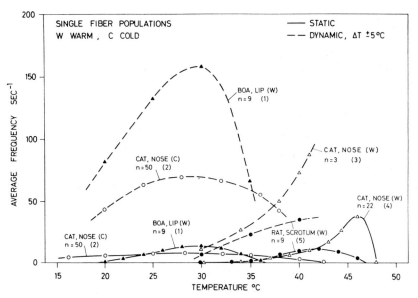

Fig. 2. Average static and dynamic impulse frequency of various populations of warm and cold fibers. Dynamic curves show the maximum overshoot on temperature changes of $\Delta T = +5\,°C$ for warm fibers and $-5\,°C$ for cold fibers as a function of adapting temperature. (1) From Hensel (1974b); (2) from Hensel and Schöner (unpublished); (3) from Hensel and Huopaniemi (1969); (4) from Hensel and Kenshalo (1969); (5) from Hellon *et al.*, (1975).

TABLE I

AVERAGE OVERSHOOT FOLLOWING IDENTICAL DYNAMIC STIMULI OF $\Delta T = +5\,°C$ FOR VARIOUS POPULA-
TIONS OF SINGLE WARM FIBERS AND OF $\Delta T = -5\,°C$ FOR A POPULATION OF SINGLE COLD FIBERS. THE
ADAPTING TEMPERATURES PREVIOUS TO THE STIMULUS ARE $5\,°C$ LOWER THAN THE TEMPERATURES OF
THE STATIC MAXIMUM

| Species Region | Receptor | n | Adapting temperature °C | Average overshoot sec⁻¹ |
|---|---|---|---|---|
| Rat[1] Scrotal | Warm | 9 | 37 | 29 ± 3 |
| Cat[2] Nasal | Cold | 50 | 23 | 56 ± 3 |
| Cat[3] Nasal | Warm | 3 | 41 | 88 ± 11 |
| Boa[4] Labial | Warm | 9 | 25 | 132 ± 11 |

(1) From Hellon et al. (1974): (2) from Hensel and Schöner (unpublished); (3) from Hensel and
Huopaniemi (1969); (4) from Hensel (1974).

rat's scrotum and in the cat's nose are at $42\,°C$ and $46\,°C$, respectively, whereas the
warm receptors in the boa have their maximum at $30\,°C$ which is very close to the
maximum of $28\,°C$ for the cold receptors in the cat's nose. This demonstrates clearly
that the static discharge is not sufficient to define a cold or warm receptor.

The magnitude of the dynamic overshoot on sudden warming or cooling, respectively, is a function of the adapting temperature and follows the general shape of the
static frequency curve. Thus the cold and warm receptors are most sensitive to
temperature changes in the range of their static maximum. The higher the dynamic
response to a given temperature change, the higher is the dynamic differential sensitivity
of a particular thermoreceptor. In Fig. 2 the dynamic values can immediately be
compared since thermal stimuli of similar shape and magnitude ($+5\,°C$ or $-5\,°C$)
have been used for all receptor populations. The ratio between dynamic and static
response increases in the sequence: warm receptors in the rat's scrotum, cold receptors
in the cat's nose, warm receptors in the cat's nose and warm receptors in the lip of
the boa (Table I).

A particular feature of cold receptors in the trigeminal region of cats (Hensel,
1973b) and in the skin of monkeys (Iggo, 1969; Hensel and Iggo, 1971; Iggo and
Iggo, 1971) and rats (Hellon et al., 1975) is the occurrence of periodic bursts of
impulses, separated by silent intervals (Fig. 3). An analysis of this pattern has shown
that, in contrast to the bell-shaped curve of mean frequency versus temperature,
several parameters of the burst discharge are related to temperature in a monotonic
way over a large range. For example, in monkeys the number of impulses per burst
increased when the temperatures fell slowly from about $33\,°C$ to $24\,°C$ (Fig. 4),
whereas the mean frequency decreased below $27\,°C$ (Iggo and Iggo, 1971). A similar
pattern was found in the cat, where the average static frequency of nasal cold re-

## a) CAT, SINGLE COLD FIBRE, INFRAORBITAL NERVE

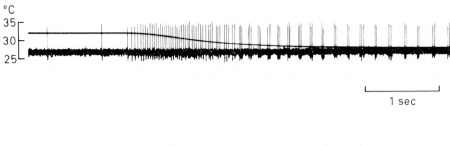

1 sec

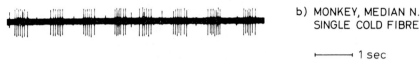

## b) MONKEY, MEDIAN N.
## SINGLE COLD FIBRE

1 sec

## c) RAT, SINGLE COLD FIBRE, SCROTAL NERVE

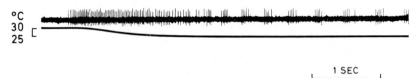

1 SEC

Fig. 3. Burst discharge of single cutaneous cold fibers. a: dynamic discharge of a fiber from the cat's infraorbital nerve and temperature of the thermode when cooling the nose from 32 °C to 27 °C. At constant temperatures the discharge was regular. From Hensel and Wurster (1970). b: static discharge of a fiber from the median nerve in the monkey at constant temperature of the hairy skin in the forearm. From Iggo (1969). c: dynamic discharge of a fiber from the scrotal nerve of the rat. From Hellon *et al.*, (1975).

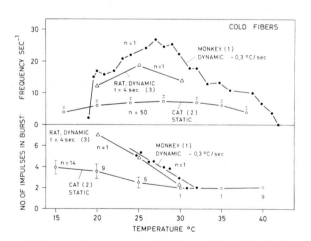

Fig. 4. Average frequency and number of impulses in bursts of single cutaneous cold fibers from monkey, cat and rat as a function of temperature. The curves for the monkey are obtained from a single fiber during slow dynamic cooling, the curves for the cat are average values of a cold fiber population under static conditions, the curves for the rat are obtained at t = 4 sec after the onset of a cold step of $\Delta T = -5\,°C$ to the final temperature indicated on the abscissa. Bars show standard error of mean. (1) From Iggo and Iggo (1971); (2) from Hensel and Schöner (unpublished); (3) from Hellon *et al.*, (1975).

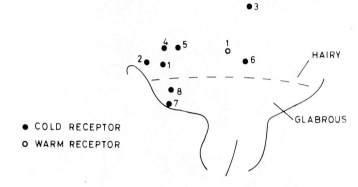

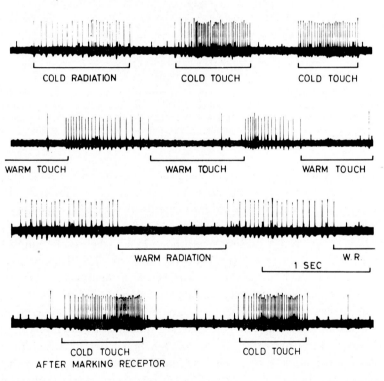

Fig. 5. Functional identification of a cold receptor in the cat's nose. Above: schematic diagram of cat's nose showing receptive fields of single cold and warm fibers. Below: afferent impulses from the single fiber serving cold spot 7 in the above diagram. Cold and warm touch was applied by a copper thermode of 60 μm diameter. (From Hensel *et al.*, 1974).

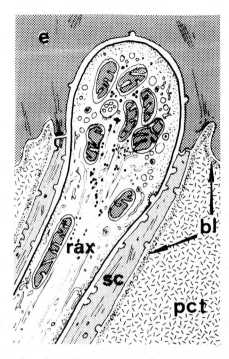

Fig. 6. Schematic representation of a cold receptor axon from the cat's nose. The terminal protrudes into a basal epidermal cell. The Schwann cell cover and basal lamina fuse with the epidermis. The typical structures of the receptor matrix are present below the receptor membrane. Receptor axon (rax), Schwann cell (sc), epidermis (e), papillary connective tissue (pct), basal lamina (bl). From Hensel *et al.*, (1974).

ceptors decreased at temperatures below 28 °C, whereas the average number of impulses per burst increased in the range from 35 °C to 15 °C. However, in contrast to the monkey, only about 20 % of the cat's cold fibers showed a static burst pattern. In the rat, the average dynamic frequency of cold fibers 4 sec after the onset of a cold step of $\Delta T = -5$ °C had a maximum at about 25 °C, whereas the number of impulses in the burst increased in the range from 30 °C to 20 °C (Hellon *et al.*, 1975). It is not yet known which of the various parameters of the discharge are significant. But theoretically the burst discharge would considerably reduce the ambiguity of information carried by the mean frequency above and below the static maximum.

The existence of highly specific cold and warm cutaneous thermoreceptors completely refutes earlier claims that neither on functional nor on structural grounds could cutaneous receptors be regarded as modality specific. Furthermore, the specific morphological substrate of two types of cutaneous thermoreceptors has now been identified: that of cold receptors in the cat's nose (Kenshalo *et al.*, 1971; Hensel, 1973b; Hensel *et al.*, 1974) and that of warm receptors in the skin of various species of snakes (Barrett *et al.*, 1970), most recently in *Boa constrictor* (Andres and v. Düring, unpublished).

The identification of specific cold receptors in the cat's nose was possible by a direct combination of electrophysiological and electron microscopical methods

(Fig. 5). In the hairy skin of the nose the receptive structures at the site of cold spots are served by thin myelinated axons dividing into several non-myelinated terminals within the stratum papillare (Fig. 6). The terminal axons are accompanied by un-myelinated Schwann cells as far as the epidermal basal lamina. A continuous connection between the basal lamina of the epidermis and that of the nerve terminals is seen. The receptive endings which penetrate a few microns deep into the basal epidermal cells contain numerous mitochondria as well as an axoplasmic matrix with fine filaments and microvesicles.

Various hypotheses have been put forward about the underlying processes occurring in a thermoreceptor, but no direct evidence is available so far (for references see Hensel, 1973b). Any satisfactory theory should at least account for (1) the specificity of cold and warm receptors, (2) the static discharge and (3) the dynamic response. There are, however, a few findings which may be pertinent to the question of the receptive process.

The ampullae of Lorenzini in sharks and rays show properties similar to the cold receptors in homoiotherms, although the ampullary receptors may serve as electro-receptors rather than as thermoreceptors (Kalmijn, 1971; Bromm et al., 1974). Nevertheless, they offer a unique possibility of studying thermoreceptive processes, the more so as they are functioning as an isolated preparation. Normally dynamic cooling causes an overshoot in frequency, whereas dynamic warming leads to a transient inhibition. It has been found, however, that one and the same single fiber can spontaneously change its response into an inversed pattern, i.e. an overshoot on warming and a transient inhibition on cooling, its other properties being practically unchanged (Hensel, 1974c; Nier and Hensel, 1974). The cause of this spontaneous

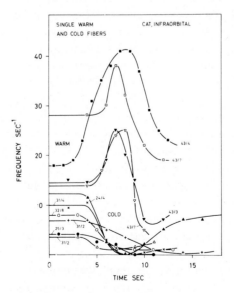

Fig. 7. Impulse frequency of single warm fibers (4 upper curves) and cold fibers (6 lower curves) from the nasal area of cats following intravenous injection of calcium gluconate. At each curve the skin temperature and the intravenous dose of calcium ions per kg body weight is indicated.

References p. 116–117

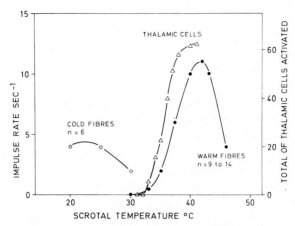

Fig. 8. Average static frequency of single cold and warm fibers from the rat scrotal nerve and number of activated cells in the thalamus as a function of scrotal temperature. From Hellon *et al.*, (1975).

change from cold-receptive to warm-receptive behavior is not yet known. From these findings we may conclude that cold and warm sensitivity may be based on the same fundamental processes, the difference being a quantitative shift in some unknown parameters.

Among ionic components involved in neural activity, calcium deserves particular interest. It is well known that an intravenous injection of calcium causes warm sensations in man and that local injection of calcium lowers the threshold for warm stimuli and raises that for cold stimuli. Electrophysiological investigations have shown that calcium inhibits the discharge of cold receptors in the cat's nose, whereas it increases the spontaneous discharge frequency of warm receptors at a given temperature and causes a discharge of warm impulses at temperatures at which no spontaneous warm fiber activity is present (Fig. 7). The effect is not caused by changes in skin temperature. This shows that there must be some specific action of calcium on thermoreceptors which is not identical with its well known inhibitory action on various cutaneous receptors (for references see Nier and Hensel, 1973; Nier, 1974).

Recently a direct electrophysiological comparison has been made between peripheral and central neural events following the stimulation of a well defined population of warm receptors in the rat scrotum (Hellon *et al.*, 1975). Fig. 8 shows the average static frequency of populations of warm and cold fibers as a function of scrotal temperature. In the same diagram the response of a population of thalamic cells to various constant temperatures of the scrotum is depicted. As shown by Hellon and Misra (1973), single thalamic neurons start firing at various levels of skin temperature, increase their frequency very steeply with rising temperature and then reach a constant level which is maintained throughout the higher temperature range. These neurons thus show a kind of "all or nothing response", the number of simultaneously activated units being a function of scrotal temperature. As can be seen, the average frequency of peripheral warm receptors and the number of thalamic units activated are surprisingly similar.

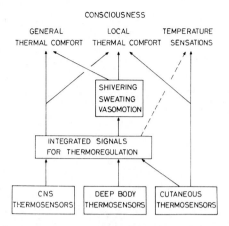

Fig. 9. Sensory inputs of temperature sensation, thermal comfort and temperature regulation. From Hensel (1973c).

Cutaneous thermoreceptors play an important role in conscious temperature sensations, for thermal comfort and behavior as well as for physiological temperature regulation (Fig. 9). In the present state of investigation it is difficult to arrive at a synopsis of experiments dealing with sensory, neurophysiological, behavioral and thermoregulatory aspects of peripheral thermoreceptors. A direct connection seems to exist between cutaneous thermoreceptors and the central structures involved in temperature sensation, whereas the emotional feeling of thermal comfort or discomfort reflects the general state of the thermoregulatory system (Hardy, 1970; Cabanac, 1972; Hensel, 1973c).

At a skin temperature of 33 °C, a number of human cold receptors are continuously firing (Hensel and Boman, 1960) but no conscious temperature sensation is observed. The latter begins only when a relative high number of thermal impulses per unit of time reaches the central nervous system. Attempts have been made to determine this "central threshold" for single cold spots in human subjects (Järvilehto, 1973). We can assume that normally a cold spot is served by a single fiber. After having measured the threshold of sensation by means of a micro-thermode, the same stimulus was applied to single cold receptors in the cat's nose, and the activity of the single fiber serving the receptor was recorded. From the results of direct recording of human cold fiber activity as well as of measurements of the thickness of the epidermis, the assumption is justified that the events in man and cat are comparable.

Fig. 10 shows the relation between the average reaction in man and the average single fiber activity in the cat to a cold stimulus of $\Delta T = -5.9\,°C$. The threshold frequency is reached rather early, when the temperature has dropped by about 2 °C. Such a stimulus, however, does not yet elicit a reaction in man. This reaction occurs more than 1 sec later. On the other hand, the cold sensation persists even if the peripheral frequency adapts to a value considerably below the maximum. This shows that the neural correlate of the "central threshold" is not simply a certain frequency of peripheral impulses. It seems that the frequency has to be maintained

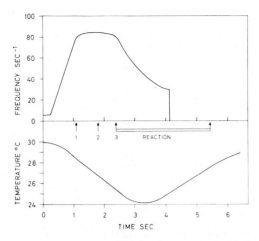

Fig. 10. Comparison between average changes in firing frequency of cold fibers in the cat's nose and reaction in man to a temperature stimulus of $\Delta T = -5.9\,°C$. Arrows: (1) instant of exceeding the threshold frequency in periphery; (2) instant of exceeding "central threshold" and (3) instant of reaction in man. From Järvilehto (1973).

for some time, *i.e.* that the absolute number of impulses arriving into the CNS may also be significant. Furthermore, if there were a critical threshold frequency, then the cold sensation should disappear during the first period of adaptation. However, this is not the case in human experiments. According to Järvilehto (1973), the results in man are much better explained if it is assumed that the "central threshold" is not a threshold in the strict sense, but presents only some kind of limit for the decision process which disappears, once exceeded, and thereafter all impulses arriving into the CNS contribute to the sensation.

A few direct measurements of afferent impulses from cutaneous thermoreceptors in human subjects (Hensel and Boman, 1960) prove the existence of specific cold receptors but do not allow quantitative correlation of the properties of thermo-receptor populations with the data of temperature sensation. In a series of indirect experiments the activity of cold fiber populations in monkeys was compared with cold sensation in human subjects (Darian-Smith *et al.*, 1973; Johnson *et al.*, 1973). The difference limen of sensation for two cooling pulses was found to be a linear function of intensity. Under the assumption that the neural correlate of the difference limen is a certain statistical difference between the average activities of a cold receptor population, the experimental values imply that only cold receptors, but neither warm receptors nor slowly adapting mechanoreceptors can account for human cold discrimination. On the other hand, warmth discrimination cannot be explained on the basis of cold fiber inhibition alone but requires an additional receptor population sensitive to warming.

The theory that the sensory qualities of cold and warmth can be ascribed to a dual set of receptors is further supported by the existence of separate cold and warm spots and by recent experiments with nerve blocking in which selective inhibition of either cold or warm sensation was achieved (Torebjörk and Hállin, 1972; Fruhstorfer, *et al.*, 1974). By injection of mepivacaine into the region of the ulnar nerve in 39 subjects it was possible in 22 subjects to block warm sensibility significantly earlier (average 12.8 min) than cold sensibility (average 16.3 min) (Fruhstorfer *et al.*, 1974). During the differential block of warm sensibility, no decrease in cold sensation was observed. The present findings support the hypothesis that, in man, warm and cold sensations are mediated by two different groups of receptor neurons. The results further indicate that thermal indifference cannot be achieved by simply combining the information delivered by warm and by cold receptors, as in this case the block of one group of thermal afferents should lead to a persisting thermal sensation.

## SUMMARY

Cutaneous warm and cold receptors have been identified in various homoiotherms and poikilotherms. In biophysical terms, warm (cold) receptors are defined by an overshoot (transient inhibition) on dynamic warming and a transient inhibition (overshoot) on dynamic cooling. At constant temperatures thermoreceptors show a static discharge with a bell-shaped temperature frequency curve. The static discharge does not allow an unequivocal discrimination between warm and cold receptors. Specific thermoreceptors are insensitive to mechanical stimulation.

The dynamic overshoot is up to 30 times higher than the static discharge. For a given temperature change, the dynamic response is relatively small for warm receptors in the rat's scrotum, medium for the cold receptors in the cat's nose and large for warm receptors in the cat's nose and in the labial region of *Boa constrictor*.

In certain single fibers from the ampullae of Lorenzini in the dogfish, a spontaneous inversion from cold to warm sensitivity of unknown origin has been observed. Ionized calcium inhibits cold receptor activity but enhances the activity of warm receptors.

Direct comparisons have been made between peripheral and central neural events following thermal stimulation of the rat scrotum. The average static discharge frequency of a population of scrotal warm fibers was closely correlated with the number of activated neurons in the thalamus as a function of scrotal temperature.

Temperature sensation is more directly related to peripheral thermoreceptor discharge than is thermal comfort, which reflects an integrative state of the thermoregulatory system. When stimulating a single cold receptor in man, the threshold of conscious sensation corresponds to an average impulse frequency of about 80/sec in the single cold fiber but some cumulative effects also seem to be involved. Comparisons between the discharge of cutaneous thermoreceptor populations in monkeys and temperature sensation in man suggest a dual set of receptors as a basis for cold and warm sensations. This view is further supported by differential nerve block in human subjects where warm sensations can be abolished while cold sensations persist.

## ACKNOWLEDGEMENT

Supported by the Deutsche Forschungsgemeinschaft.

*References p. 116–117*

## REFERENCES

BARRETT, R., MADERSON, P. F. A. AND MESZLER, R. M. (1970) The pit organs of snakes. In C. GANS AND TH. S. PARSONS (Eds.), *Biology of the Reptilia, Vol. II, Morphology B*. Academic Press, London. pp. 277–314.

BROMM, B., HENSEL, H. AND NIER, K. (1974) Effects of combined electrical and thermal stimulation on steady state response frequency in Lorenzinian ampullae. *Pflügers Arch. ges. Physiol.*, **347**, R 28.

CABANAC, M. (1972) Thermoregulatory behavior. In J. BLIGH AND R. E. MOORE (Eds.), *Essays on Temperature Regulation*. North-Holland Publ., Amsterdam. pp. 19–32.

DARIAN-SMITH, I., JOHNSON, K. O. AND DYKES, R. (1973) "Cold" fiber population innervating palmar and digital skin of the monkey: responses to cooling pulses. *J. Neurophysiol.*, **36**, 325–346.

FRUHSTORFER, H., ZENZ, M., NOLTE, H. AND HENSEL, H. (1974) Dissociated loss of cold and warm sensibility during regional anaesthesia. *Pflügers Arch. ges. Physiol.*, **349**, 73–82.

HARDY, J. D. (1970) Thermal comfort: skin temperature and physiological thermoregulation. In J. D. HARDY, A. P. GAGGE AND J. A. J. STOLWIJK (Eds.), *Physiological and Behavioral Temperature Regulation*. Thomas, Springfield, Ill. pp. 856–873.

HELLON, R. F., HENSEL, H. AND SCHÄFER, K. (1975) Thermal receptors in the scrotum of the rat. *J. Physiol. (Lond.)*, **248**, 349–357.

HELLON, R. F. AND MISRA, N. (1973) Neurones in the ventrobasal complex of the rat responding to scrotal skin temperature changes. *J. Physiol. (Lond.)*, **232**, 389–399.

HENSEL, H. (1973a) Zur Electrophysiologie der Hautsinnessysteme unter Berücksichtigung informationstheoretischer Betrachtungen. *Nova Acta Leopoldina, N.F.*, **37**, 211–222.

HENSEL, H, (1973b) Cutaneous thermoreceptors. In A. IGGO (Ed.), *Handbook of Sensory Physiology*, Vol. II. Springer, Berlin, pp. 75–106.

HENSEL, H. (1973c) Thermoreception and thermal comfort. *Arch. Sci. physiol.*, 27, A359–370.

HENSEL, H. (1974a) Thermoreceptors. *Ann. Rev. Physiol.*, **36**, 233–250.

HENSEL, H. (1974b) Properties of warm receptors in *Boa constrictor. Naturwissenschaften*, **61**, 369.

HENSEL, H. (1974c) Effect of temporal and spatial temperature gradients on the ampullae of Lorenzini. *Pflügers Arch. ges. Physiol.*, **347**, 89–100.

HENSEL, H., ANDRES, K. H. AND V. DÜRING, M. (1974) Structure and function of cold receptors. *Pflügers Arch. ges. Physiol.*, **352**, 1–10.

HENSEL, H. AND BOMAN, K. (1960) Afferent impulses in cutaneous sensory nerves in human subjects. *J. Neurophysiol.*, **23**, 564–578.

HENSEL, H. AND HUOPANIEMI, T. (1969) Static and dynamic properties of warm fibres in the infra-orbital nerve. *Pflügers Arch. ges. Physiol.*, **309**, 1–10.

HENSEL, H. AND IGGO, A. (1971) Analysis of cutaneous warm and cold fibres in primates. *Pflügers Arch. ges. Physiol.*, **329**, 1–8.

HENSEL, H. AND KENSHALO, D. R. (1969) Warm receptors in the nasal region of cats. *J. Physiol. (Lond.)*, **204**, 99–112.

HENSEL, H. AND WURSTER, R. D. (1970) Static properties of cold receptors in nasal area of cats. *J. Neurophysiol.*, **33**, 271–275.

IGGO, A. (1969) Cutaneous thermoreceptors in primates and subprimates. *J. Physiol. (Lond.)*, **200**, 403–430.

IGGO, A. AND IGGO, B. J. (1971) Impulse coding in primate cutaneous thermoreceptors in dynamic thermal conditions. *J. Physiol. (Paris)*, **63**, 287–290.

JÄRVILEHTO, T. (1973) Neural coding in the temperature sense. *Ann. Acad. Sci. fenn. B*, **184**, 1–71.

JOHNSON, K. O., DARIAN-SMITH, I. AND LAMOTTE, C. (1973) Peripheral neural determinants of temperature discrimination in man: a correlative study of responses to cooling skin. *J. Neurophysiol.*, **36**, 347–370.

KALMIJN, A. J. (1971) The electric sense of sharks and rays. *J. exp. Biol.*, **55**, 371–383.

KENSHALO, D. R., HENSEL, H., GRAZIADEI, P. AND FRUHSTORFER, H. (1971) On the anatomy, physiology and psychophysics of the cat's temperature sensing system. In R. DUBNER AND Y. KAWAMURA (Eds.), *Oral-facial Sensory and Motor Mechanisms*. Appleton-Century-Crofts, New York, pp. 23–45.

NIER, K. (1974) Effects of different ionic components on afferent responses to vibrissa receptors. *Pflügers Arch. ges. Physiol.*, **347**, 27–38.

NIER, K. AND HENSEL, H. (1973) Effects of calcium on afferent responses of the ampullae of Lorenzini. *Pflügers Arch. ges. Physiol.*, **338**, 281–287.

NIER, K. AND HENSEL, H. (1974) Special dynamic characteristics of thermosensitive afferents from the ampullae of Lorenzini. *J. comp. Physiol.*, **91**, 241–246.

TOREBJÖRK, H. E. AND HÁLLIN, R. G. (1972) Activity in C fibres correlated to perception in man. In C. HIRSCH AND Y. ZOTTERMAN (Eds.), *Cervical Pain*. Pergamon Press, Oxford. pp. 171–178.

## DISCUSSION

BURGESS: I would like to make a comment and then ask a question. If you electrically stimulate a single cold spot you do not feel any cold sensation until the frequency reaches 50, 60, or 70 impulses. The result of this experiment fits very well with the deductions that you mentioned based on recordings from cold fibers. If you are interested you might try it on yourself and, perhaps, have already done so.

HENSEL: We must do more experiments in this direction and I am very happy that you already have some results of this kind.

BURGESS: Under normal circumstances when you cool the skin you not only excite the cold receptors but you inhibit the warm receptors. Am I to understand from your nerve blocking experiments that the inhibition of warm receptors does not contribute anything to the cold sensation?

HENSEL: At the normal skin temperature, say, 32–33 °C there is only a very low steady discharge of warm receptors, so if you start at the usual ambient temperature, you would have only a very low discharge of warm receptors. The experiment you mentioned should be made with warm skin and a temperature of 40 °C. This we have not done yet.

LINDBLOM: I would like first to make a comment. As a clinical neurologist I have had the opportunity of observing conditions which may be interesting to the question of the separation of warm and cold sensations. In certain cases of neuropathy, that is a lesion which affects certain peripheral nerve fibers but which may leave other nerve fibers intact, you may find that the threshold for cold sensation is increased while the warm sensation is retained. My first question is: was your observation of the fibers which changed from cold fibers to warm fibers a frequent one or a rare one? My second question is: have you observed thalamic cold cells as well as warm cells?

HENSEL: To your first question: the change was only in the ampullae of Lorenzini and not in warm or cold fibers in humans, nor in warm-blooded animals. All our observations as yet show that these receptors keep that property as warm or as cold receptors. As to the ampullae of Lorenzini, it is only about 10 % of the whole population that showed this change, but no such change was observed in the population of homoiothermic thermoreceptors. As to the second question: in this experiment we have only observations when we started with a warm site which is, I think, particularly important. We have found cold fibers in the cat's tongue but we have no information as yet of the higher levels: spinal or thalamic or cortical levels. We should have more experiments on this side.

IGGO: I think I would like to interpolate a warning remark on this point, about trying to correlate too exactly the behavior of the peripheral receptors with the activity of the central thermosensory pathways. There is not very much information about the central thermosensory pathways and in some recent experiments on monkeys, it has become clear in the spinothalamic tract cells that there is no exact correspondence between the activity of the peripheral fibers and the activity of the central cells, and I think we would need a lot more detailed information about the behavior of the central cells before we can start making hypotheses about how the central thermosensory systems work.

HENSEL: I can only agree, and as you saw there seem to be different types of correlations. The usual correlation which has been known before this experiment was an analog correlation and now this other type, and I think we must be very careful in making premature assumption and hypothesis.

TAPPER: I recently finished the study on mechanoreceptors in the skin of the birds in the same region in which you found your thermoreceptors' activity, and I was interested whether you might have observations on the other end organs in the skin that might be related to either slowly adapting or rapidly adapting mechanoreceptor activity.

HENSEL: We have seen some mechanoreceptive activity. This comes regularly in touch of the skin. We have not yet performed any detailed investigations of the mechanoreceptors, we focussed interest on the warm receptors, but when stimulating the warm receptors mechanically there was no response. So, they are rather specific to warming, but I can give you no more quantitative information on mechanoreceptors, although we have found mechanoreceptors in the same area.

MINUT-SOROKHTINA: How can you explain the reactions and the generation of excitation in those touch-cold receptors that you found with Dr. Zotterman in the cat's tongue and that Dr. Iggo has investigated as slowly adapting mechanoreceptors. Do you think the primary processes lie in those reactions to mechanical or to cold stimulation?

HENSEL: That is a very difficult question. I think, speaking of slowly adapting receptors, some receptors might respond to cooling, as it was shown by Dr. Iggo and others. But I think the properties of these receptors are rather different as compared with a specific receptor. So, I think I cannot answer whether it is generally an analog process.

# On the Vascular Component of the Peripheral Cold Reception

O. P. MINUT-SOROKHTINA AND N. F. GLEBOVA

*O. V. Kuusinen State University, Petrozavodsk (U.S.S.R.)*

The recent reviews and monographs (Hensel, 1973; Minut-Sorokhtina, 1972) show that the impulse activity in the finest sensory fibres (myelinated and unmyelinated) in response to thermal stimulation of the skin has been studied in detail. It was established that such stimuli excite not only the specific cold and warm receptors, but the slowly adapting mechanoreceptors of the skin as well. The stable temperature of the skin modifies the rate of tonic (static) activity of the specific cold receptors, while step-changes of the temperature stimulate their phasic (dynamic) responses. The inflow of information to the central nervous system during the skin cooling creates a pattern including tonic discharges from cold receptors, reaching a maximal frequency at 20–30 °C and diminishing outside of this zone, and phasic reactions to sudden cooling of the skin. Simultaneously the tonic activity of warm receptors is reduced.

The touch-cold or mechano-cold receptors belong to the slowly adapting type of receptors which produce rhythmical impulses during the persistent mechanical stimulation of the skin. The frequency of discharges of the static activity depends on the stable level of skin temperature and increases with warming of the skin. In other words, warming increases the reactivity of mechanoreceptors to tactile stimulation. This dependence was first established in experiments carried out on cats (Witt and Hensel, 1959) was confirmed in our experiments on rabbits (Minut-Sorokhtina, 1959) and investigated in detail in recent works of Iggo and Muir (1969) and Duclaux and Kenshalo (1972). As far as the static activity of the slowly adapting mechanoreceptors is concerned, they might be classified as warm receptors. But electrophysiologically they are designated as touch-cold receptors due to their dynamic properties. The step-cooling of the skin elicits such phasic responses in these receptors that cannot be distinguished from the responses of the specific cold receptors. They produce a series of impulses when the skin is cooled and reduce their activity or cease firing if the skin is warmed.

The understanding of the functional properties of receptors and the primary processes which underlie the initiation of nerve impulses greatly depends on the knowledge of the receptors micromorphology. The use of electron microscopy and of histochemical techniques have enabled investigators to reveal morphologic details in cutaneous receptors which could not be discovered using ordinary methods of histology and optic microscopy. In the skin of man and animals, including the

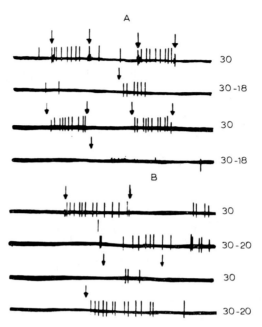

Fig. 1. Isolated skin–nerve preparation (rabbit). Reactions of touch-cold receptors to standard mechanical and cold stimulation of the skin before and after the subcutaneous application of adrenaline (A) and carbachol (B). Beginning and end of stimulation marked by arrows. Numbers on right show temperature of thermode in °C.

epidermis, various structures of encapsulated nerve terminals along with non-encapsulated, so called "free", terminals were found. The recent articles of Cauna (1968); Winkelmann (1968); Iggo and Muir (1969) and Duclaux and Kenshalo (1972) contain the detailed description of touch corpuscles which functionally represent the slowly adapting mechano-cold receptors. These receptors (type I according to Iggo) were subjected to a most thorough investigation which permits an understanding of their reactions to the mechanical deformation of the skin. But the question of how the receptors of this type are stimulated by cooling remains obscure.

Experiments carried out in our laboratory by Olimpienko (1969) showed the possibility of a selective blockade of the reactions of touch-cold receptors to one of the two kinds of stimuli. In a preparation consisting of a strip of cat's or rabbit's skin isolated along with a branch of cutaneous nerve the impulse activity in single nerve fibres was registered during standard stimulation of the skin. Application of adrenaline in doses which caused a spasm of the vessels abolished the response to cooling in 17 trials and reduced it in 5 trials, at the same time the reactions to standard mechanical stimuli remained unchanged. Contrary to this effect, when carbachol ($10^{-3}$–$10^{-4}$ $M$) was applied the reactions to mechanical stimuli were significantly reduced, but the reactions to cooling the skin strip remained nearly unchanged (Fig. 1). The possibility of a selective depression of one of the two components of the touch-cold receptor responses suggests that a single sensory axon can supply by its terminals the touch corpuscle and some other structure responding to cooling.

As to the specific cold (and warm) receptors, it is widely assumed that many of them are represented by the "free" nerve terminals. The old controversy about the question why some nerve terminals are depolarized and produce action potentials during cooling, while others are excited by warming, still remains unresolved. The ramification of the sensory axons with their terminals ending among relatively dense tissues of the skin does not permit the dissection and investigation of a single receptor as is possible, for example, with the Pacinian corpuscle. The absence of specialized cellular structures suggests that in the tissue surrounding the free sensory terminals some kind of transducer may transform the thermal stimuli into chemical or mechanical processes exciting the terminals.

In search of a chemical mediator of the thermal activation of the receptors several hypotheses have been advanced, but none of them brought experimental evidence in favour of such a substance. The presence of a mechanical transducer could be admitted if, among the skin tissues, structures were found which change their physical properties according to temperature changes and cause a deformation (stretching, flexing etc.) of the free sensory terminals. This role can be ascribed to the smooth muscle cells of the cutaneous and subcutaneous vessels with their pronounced basal tone and exclusively high reactivity.

The possibility of evoking the reactions of thermoregulation by local thermal stimulation of the animals' subcutaneous veins (Minut-Sorokhtina, 1950) brought us, some twenty years ago, to a deeper investigation of the vascular receptors function. The subsequent experiments (Minut-Sorokhtina, 1953, 1968, 1970 and 1972) were carried out on humorally isolated segments of cutaneous veins of cats and rabbits using the registration of electrical activity in the afferent nerve fibres supplying this vessel. Most suitable for such a kind of experiment is the external thoracic vein innervated by the lateral cutaneous branches of the intercostal nerves. The segmentary distribution of the nerves permits the dissection of nerve bundles and the recording of receptor activity during the perfusion of the vein *in situ* and in a completely isolated vessel–nerve preparation as well. Another object of the experiments in our laboratory is an isolated and perfused rabbit ear. After the removal of the skin the preparation consists of the auricular cartilage with the epichondrium and a network of subcutaneous vessels and nerves.

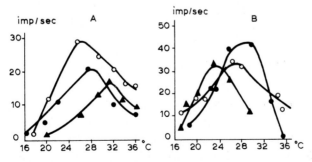

Fig. 2. A: spike activity of smooth muscles of the vessels of rabbit ear. B: tonic activity of three single receptors of a subcutaneous vein in rabbit ear as a function of stable temperature. Abscissa, temperature of the preparation; ordinate, impulse frequency per sec.

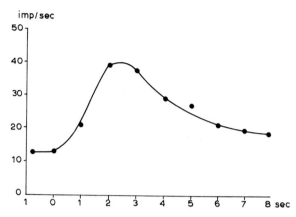

Fig. 3. Frequency of impulses of single receptors of auricular vessels during cooling of thermode from 30 °C to 17 °C. Mean of 40 measurements. The beginning of cooling is at zero time.

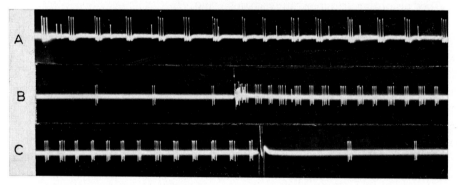

Fig. 4. Activity of single receptors of rabbit's auricular vein, with grouping of impulses. A: perfusion with a solution with a lowered $Ca^{2+}$ concentration. B and C: beginning and end of DC depolarization of the receptive zone.

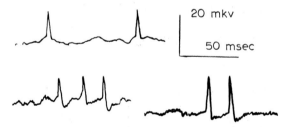

Fig. 5. Prepotentials and spike potentials of single vascular receptors.

The dissection of the auricular nerve into fine filaments allowed us to reveal the impulse activity of single receptors of the subcutaneous vessels. It was ascertained that the functional properties of these receptors correspond, in all details, to those of the specific cold receptors. They are insensitive to touch and produce steady tonic discharges of impulses with a rate according to the temperature. The maximal frequency of impulses corresponds to the temperature in the range of 20 °C to 30 °C and decreases outside this zone. In single units the firing rate usually does not exceed 30 impulses/sec, but occasionally it could be as high as 50–60 impulses/sec (Fig. 2B). With more severe cooling the activity of receptors diminishes and they stop firing at 17–14 °C, but the blockade is completely reversible and when warmed the receptors resume their impulse activity.

The phasic reactions of vascular receptors are revealed by fast cooling, to 10–12 °C, of the thermode placed on the surface of the preparation, as seen in Fig. 3. Warming of the thermode, to 38–40 °C, involved a phasic depression or cessation of impulses. Even such a peculiarity as the grouping of impulses of single units in short bursts of 3–6 potentials in each, which has been described for the specific cold receptors by Iggo (1969) and Hensel and Wurster (1970) can be regularly observed in the activity of vascular receptors. The appearance of such bursts is facilitated by lowering the concentration of calcium in the perfusate or by DC depolarization of the receptive zone (Fig. 4). The method of DC depolarization allows a precise localization of the receptive zone of a single sensory fibre, which occupies an area 3–4 to 12–15 mm along the vascular wall (Minut-Sorokhtina, 1968). In this zone the prepotentials preceding the action potentials in the nerve fibre were registered (Fig. 5). All the units studied belonged to the A-delta medullated fibres with a conduction velocity of 4–15 m/sec.

Are the receptors of the vascular wall directly excited by cooling, or does the origin of their excitation lie in the myogenic reactions of the smooth muscle cells to this stimulus? A series of investigations in our laboratory was carried out to provide an answer to this question. The presence of a basal tone and spontaneous contractions in isolated segments of dog's subcutaneous vessels and in the vessels of denervated bat's wing were described by Johansson and Bohr (1966) and by Wiedeman (1957 and 1966). The high reactivity of cutaneous vessels to various stimuli, including thermal, is well known. The majority of investigators (Folkow, 1964; Webb-Peploe and Shepherd, 1968; Vanhoutte and Shepherd, 1971) believe that the reactions of vessels to thermal stimuli depend not only upon nervous mechanisms, but on a myogenic component as well.

We investigated the myogenic component of vascular reactions on isolated sub-cutaneous vessels of cattle and human subcutaneous veins (Belsky, 1974). The recording of the smooth muscle tone with a mechanoelectrical transducer revealed some differences in the responses of circular and longitudinal strips cut out of various vessels. Lowering the temperature of the perfusate from 40 °C to 12 °C induced first some decrease and then a marked increase of the tone of circular arterial strips, which reached a maximum at 28–19 °C and then fell again. The circular strips of animal veins showed a maximal tone at 30–18 °C, and of human veins at 32–26 °C. The spontaneous contractions were more pronounced in arterial strips and to a lesser extent in the venous ones. The automaticity appeared to be at its maximum at a temperature of 36–37 °C, it lessened with cooling and completely ceased at 20–25 °C in the arteries and at 15–20 °C in the veins.

The thermal reactivity of smooth muscles was also studied in our laboratory by electrophysiological techniques (Kokarev, 1969 and 1970) on arteries and veins of the isolated rabbit ear. The measuring of membrane potential showed that in single smooth muscle cells its average amplitude was $38.2 \pm 1.2$ mV, reaching 56 mV in some cases. The membrane potential of the smooth muscle cells is unstable and a wave of depolarization, when reaching a critical level, is usually accompanied by action potentials with an amplitude of about 5 mV lasting for 20–60 msec. These findings concerning the properties of single smooth muscle cells of the subcutaneous vessels are in accordance with data of several authors describing the properties of smooth muscles of other vessels. The extracellular recording of impulse activity of smooth muscle cells with a tungsten microelectrode showed its dependence on thermal conditions. In 86 experiments the mean firing rate was $13.7 \pm 1.0$ impulses/sec at a temperature of 36 °C; in the range 26–31 °C it increased to $27.7 \pm 1.7$ impulses/sec and decreased to $3.2 \pm 0.5$ impulses/sec at 20–23 °C. There is a great similarity in impulse activity of smooth muscle cells and single receptors of the same vessels, as seen in Fig. 2A and B.

All the data obtained show a close relation between the vascular receptors' activity and the myogenic activity, as revealed by electrical and contractile responses of the vascular muscles. Evidently the mediation of the excitation of receptors during thermal stimuli can be ascribed to myogenic reactions of the smooth muscle which mechanically stimulate the sensory nerve terminals.

But this raises the next question, namely, what kind of primary process takes place in the smooth muscles during cooling? According to investigations summarized in the article of Vanhoutte and Shepherd (1971) temperature exerts a direct non-specific effect on the muscle cells of subcutaneous veins. A moderate cooling enhances the sensitivity of smooth muscles to the vasoconstrictive influence of the catecholamines and of electrical stimulation and when a deeper cooling is applied, then the reactivity of the vessels decreases. Such changes of reactivity were found not only in the inner-vated veins, but also in veins sympathectomized several weeks before the experiment and in isolated segments of subcutaneous veins. In our laboratory similar results were obtained in experiments on isolated strips of subcutaneous arteries of cattle (Belsky, 1974). The constrictive reactions to a standard dose of noradrenaline rose during cooling from 40 °C to about 25 °C and then diminished, finally ceasing at 15 °C.

Thus one can suggest that under physiological conditions local myogenic reactions of subcutaneous vessels are accompanied by an increased sensitivity to endogenous catecholamines. The evoked contraction of the smooth muscles, acting on the vascular receptors, induces the appearance of "cold" impulses in the sensory nerve terminals.

The conduction of impulses from thermoreceptors was traced all along the 3-neurone pathway to the somatosensory area of the cortex in several investigations (Landgren, 1957 and 1959; Poulos and Lende, 1970a and b). It is worth mentioning that in thalamic neurones the pattern of impulse activity during the thermal stimula-tion of the tongue receptors remained essentially unchanged, preserving the main features of the peripheral receptors' firing. The afferent pathways connecting the peripheral receptors with the thermoregulatory centres are hardly known, since for a long time the principal attention of physiologists was directed to the central thermo-sensitivity of the hypothalamic neurones. However, many attempts were made to

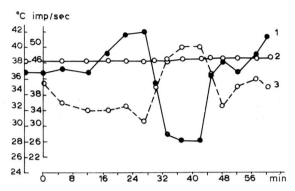

Fig. 6. Impulse activity of a single neurone of the medial preoptic area of hypothalamus during perfusion of the vena thoracica externa of the rabbit. Open circles, impulse frequency/sec; filled circles, temperature of perfusion.

assess quantitatively the relative role of the central and the peripheral stimulations in the induction of various reactions of thermoregulation. But the investigation of hypothalamic neuronal reactions to peripheral receptors' stimulation has begun only recently. One of the first articles on the subject belongs to Wit and Wang (1968). Amongst the single hypothalamic neurones studied, only 15% reacted to thermal stimuli. A detailed investigation of the rabbit hypothalamic neurones' reactions to cutaneous thermal stimulation was carried out in the laboratory of Ivanov (Dymni- kova et al., 1973) and it was found that in physiological conditions about 23–29% of neurones react to thermal stimulation of the skin.

In our laboratory the reactions of single hypothalamic neurones were studied with special attention being paid to peripheral cooling. In the medial preoptic area of the rabbit hypothalamus a relatively high percentage of neurones were found which were excited by skin cooling. But most relevant were the experiments with cold stimuli applied not to the skin surface, but to humorally isolated subcutaneous veins of the rabbits. The cooling of perfusate from 28 °C to 30 °C induced an increase of firing rate in 10 out of 34 neurones of the medial preoptic area. An example of such a reaction is given in Fig. 6.

All the considerations mentioned here suggest that in the formation of well localized discrete cold sensations the activity of mechano-cold receptors takes part. As to the role of the receptors of cutaneous and subcutaneous vessels, this component of the peripheral thermal reception is associated with the thermoregulatory reactions and with more generalized sensations of thermal comfort or discomfort.

## SUMMARY

The functional properties of receptors located in the subcutaneous veins and cutaneous vessels of rabbits and cats are described. Functionally these receptors closely resemble the specific cold receptors of the skin. They display static activity, reaching a maximal firing rate in the temperature zone of 20–30 °C, and a dynamic activity in response to sudden cooling. Evidence is presented that a vascular component takes part in the reactions of the touch-cold receptors of the skin. The activity of single neurones of the hypothalamic medial preoptic area was registered during cold stimuli applied to the skin and to humorally isolated subcutaneous veins of rabbits. Ten out of 34 neurones studied showed increased firing rate during cooling of the vein. It is suggested that the activity of mechano-cold receptors takes part in the formation of well localized discrete thermal sensations, whereas the vascular component of peripheral thermal reception is associated with the thermoregulatory reactions and a more generalized sensation of thermal comfort or discomfort.

## REFERENCES

BELSKY, E. D. (1974) *Mechanisms of Cold Vasodilatation*. Dissertation Thesis. Petrozavodsk.

BROWN, A. G. AND IGGO, A. (1967) A quantitative study of cutaneous receptors and afferent fibres in the cat and rabbit. *J. Physiol. (Lond.)*, **193**, 707–733.

CAUNA, N. (1968) Light and electron microscopical structure of sensory end-organs in human skin. In D. R. KENSHALO (Ed.), *The Skin Senses*. Thomas, Springfield, Ill. pp. 15–37.

DUCLAUX, R. AND KENSHALO, D. R. (1972) The temperature sensitivity of the type I slowly adapting mechanoreceptors in cats and monkeys. *J. Physiol. (Lond.)*, **224**, 647–664.

DYMNIKOVA, L. P., SAKHARJEVSKAJA, N. P. AND IVANOV, K. P. (1973) On afferent projections of the thermoregulation center. *Fiziol. Zh. (Leningr.)*, **59**, 156–163.

FOLKOW, B. (1964) Description of the myogenic hypothesis. *Circulat. Res.*, **15**, Suppl. 1, 14–15.

HENSEL, H. (1973) Neural processes in thermoregulation. *Physiol. Rev.*, **53**, 948–1017.

HENSEL, H. AND WURSTER, R. D. (1970) Static properties of cold receptors in nasal area of cats. *J. Neurophysiol.*, **33**, 271–275.

IGGO, A. (1969) Cutaneous thermoreceptors in primates and sub-primates. *J. Physiol. (Lond.)*, **200**, 403–430.

IGGO, A. AND MUIR, A. R. (1969) The structure and function of a slowly adapting touch corpuscle in hairy skin. *J. Physiol. (Lond.)*, **200**, 763–796.

JOHANSSON, B. AND BOHR, D. F. (1966) Rhythmic activity in smooth muscle from small subcutaneous arteries. *Amer. J. Physiol.*, **210**, 801–806.

KOKAREV, A. A. (1969) Electrophysiological properties of smooth muscles of subcutaneous vessels. In *The Temperature Reception*. Nauka, Leningrad. pp. 10–12.

KOKAREV, A. A. (1970) Intracellular studies of smooth muscles of subcutaneous vessels. *Fiziol. Zh. (Leningr.)*, **56**, 1233–1236.

LANDGREN, S. (1957) Convergence of tactile, thermal and gustatory impulses on single cortical cells. *Acta physiol. scand.*, **40**, 210–221.

LANDGREN, S. (1959) Thalamic units responding to cooling of the cat's tongue. *J. Physiol. (Lond.)*, **147**, 12P.

MINUT-SOROKHTINA, O. P. (1950) On the role of vascular receptors in thermoregulation. *Bull. exp. Biol. Med.*, **29**, 422–425.

MINUT-SOROKHTINA, O. P. (1953) Electrophysiological properties of the venous thermoreceptors. *Fiziol. Zh (Leningr.)*, **39**, 210–217.

MINUT-SOROKHTINA, O. P. (1959) Comparative properties of cutaneous and venous thermoreception. *Trans. Khabarovsk med. inst.*, **17**, 39–48.

MINUT-SOROKHTINA, O. P. (1968) Nature of rhythmic activity of cold receptors. *Fiziol. Zh. (Leningr.)*, **51**, 413–420. (*Neuroscience Translations*, 1968–69, **6**, 615–622).

MINUT-SOROKHTINA, O. P. (1970) The dual character of peripheral cold reception. *Fiziol. Zh. (Leningr.)*, **56**, 886–894. (*Neuroscience Translations*, 1970–71, **16**, 39–46).

MINUT-SOROKHTINA, O. P. (1972) *Physiology of Thermoreception*. Meditsina, Moskow.

OLIMPIENKO, T. S. (1969) On the mechanisms of activation of mechano-cold receptors. In *The Temperature Reception*. Nauka, Leningrad. pp. 17–18.

POULOS, D. A. AND LENDE, R. A. (1970a) Response of trigeminal ganglion neurons to thermal stimulation of oral–facial regions. I. Steady state response. *J. Neurophysiol.*, **33**, 508–517.

POULOS, D. A. AND LENDE, R. A. (1970b) Response of trigeminal ganglion neurons to thermal stimulation of oral–facial regions. II. Temperature change response. *J. Neurophysiol.*, **33**, 518–526.

VANHOUTTE, P. M. AND SHEPHERD, J. T. (1971) Thermosensitivity and veins. *J. Physiol. (Paris)*, **63**, 449–451.

WEBB-PEPLOE, M. M. AND SHEPHERD, J. T. (1968) Responses of the superficial limb veins of the dog to changes in temperature. *Circulat. Res.*, **22**, 737–746.

WIEDEMAN, M. P. (1957) Effect of venous flow on frequency of vasomotion in the bat wing. *Circulat. Res.*, **5**, 641–647.

WIEDEMAN, M. P. (1966) Contractile activity of arterioles in the bat wing during intraluminal pressure changes. *Circulat. Res.*, **19**, 559–563.

WINKELMANN, R. K. (1968) New methods for the study of nerve endings. In D. R. KENSHALO (Ed.), *The Skin Senses*. Thomas, Springfield, Ill. pp. 38–56.

WIT, A. AND WANG, S. C. (1968) Temperature-sensitive neurons in preoptic/anterior hypothalamic region; effects of increasing ambient temperature. *Amer. J. Physiol.* **215**, 1151–1159.

WITT, I. UND HENSEL, H. (1959) Afferente Impulse aus der Extremitätenhaut der Katze bei thermischer und mechanischer Reizung. *Pflügers Arch. ges. Physiol.*, **268**, 582–596.

## DISCUSSION

IGGO: Are you sure that the impulse activity you are recording is propagated by the sensory fibres of the nerve, and not by the efferent ones?

MINUT-SOROKHTINA: We record the impulse activity not only in the nerve filaments supplying the vessel *in situ*, but in completely isolated vessel–nerve preparations as well. Besides, the conduction velocity of 4–15 m/sec indicates that the fibres belong to the A-delta sensory group, but not to unmyelinated efferents.

BURGESS: Do the vascular receptors respond to cold stimuli applied on the surface of the skin?

MINUT-SOROKHTINA: Surely they do, because the temperature of the blood in the capillaries and subcutaneous veins decreases during the skin cooling. But the latencies in this case are longer.

KONRADI: How do the vascular receptors respond to pharmacologically induced vasomotion?

MINUT-SOROKHTINA: Our experiments in this field are not completed yet, but I can say that moderate vasoconstriction stimulates the receptors' firing.

# Some Response Properties of Cold Fibers to Cooling

DAN R. KENSHALO, DENNY CORMIER AND MIKE MELLOS

*Dept. of Psychology and the Psychobiology Research Center, Florida State University, Tallahassee, Fla.*
*(U.S.A.)*

## INTRODUCTION

Application of the methods of systems analysis to biological systems, in order to express more concisely stimulus–response relationships, is not new. Our aim here is to describe the dimensions of a model that account for the averaged responses of a small population of cold receptors to mathematically describable cool stimuli.

The receptive fields of 112 specific cold receptors were identified by extracellular records of the neural activity from the vicinity of the primary axon cell bodies in the trigeminal ganglion of cats. The electrodes were electropolished, insulated tungsten wire. Each unit was identified as a specific cold receptor by the following criteria: (1) each exhibited a steady-state response whose frequency was a function of the static skin temperature; (2) each failed to have its neural activity altered by moderate or even strong mechanical stimulation applied to the receptive field; (3) each showed a phasic increase in neural activity when its receptive field was cooled and (4) each showed a phasic decrease in activity when its receptive field was warmed.

Of the 112 specific cold receptors, 20 were located in areas of skin accessible to the thermal stimulator and were held long enough (about 2.5 hr) to permit records of the responses to the complete series of thermal stimulations. The stimulus series consisted of four intensities of cooling, 0.5, 1.0, 2.5 and 5 °C presented at a rate of 0.4 °C/sec. These intensities of cooling were presented after the receptive fields had been adapted to each of six adapting temperatures, 20, 25, 30, 35, 40 and 45 °C. In addition, the 5 °C cool intensity was presented at rates of 0.3 and 0.2 °C/sec from the 30 °C adapting temperature.

The 20 cold receptors varied considerably, one from another, in their steady-state and dynamic responses. Hence, any attempt to fit a system equation to the responses of individual cold receptors would result in a bewildering number of constants none of which could be thought of as representative of cold receptors in general. An alternative, not without faults, however, is to use simple averages of the responses of the cold receptors to each condition of stimulation. One difficulty with averaging the responses of cold receptors is that there may be several types. Some cold receptors yield spike trains in which the interspike intervals vary independently in length while others show interspike intervals that are highly dependent upon previous interspike

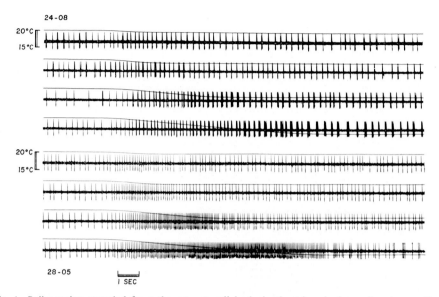

Fig. 1. Spike trains recorded from the neuron cell body in the trigeminal ganglion innervating a bursting cold receptor (24-08) and a non-bursting cold receptor (28-05).

intervals (Kenshalo *et al.*, 1975). It is not known if this represents a fundamental difference in the receptor mechanism or if, from the standpoint of systems analysis, they can be grouped together. For the present, however, they will be averaged together.

Fig. 1 shows examples of the spike trains of two of the 20 cold receptors in response to cool stimuli of 0.5, 1.0, 2.5 and 5 °C intensity from the 20 °C adapting temperature. The bursting discharge, seen in receptor 24-08 was first described by Hensel and Zotterman (1951) in lingual cold receptors of the cat, and is a characteristic of 80 % of the cold receptors in this sample. Bursts of impulses during the steady-state response first appeared at an adapting temperature of about 30 °C and the amount of bursting increased linearly as the adapting temperature decreased to 20 °C (Kenshalo *et al.*, 1975). Measurements of bursting were not made at lower adapting temperatures. Cold receptor 28-05 is an example of the 20 % that did not discharge in bursts under any of the conditions of stimulation.

The steady-state response of cat cold receptors is a function of the temperature to which they are adapted. The mean steady-state response of the 20 cold receptors reached a maximum frequency at an adapting temperature of about 27 °C, and the mean frequency declined at both higher and lower adapting temperatures.

The dynamic responses of the 20 cold receptors to 0.5, 1.0, 2.5 and 5 °C intensities of cooling from the several adapting temperatures were represented by mean post-stimulus time (PST) histograms. These were smoothed and variations in the bin to bin content were filtered out, leaving relatively smooth curves that estimate the main trends of the responses, as seen in Fig. 2.

The form of the model was first proposed by Sand (1938) to account for the responses of the ampullae of Lorenzini to thermal stimulation. It was later elaborated by Hensel (1952 and 1953) as a model for cold receptors found in the tongue of the cat.

### Dynamic responses

The dynamic responses of cold receptors can be considered to be the result of the interaction of at least two processes, an excitatory process (E) and an inhibitory process (I). Thus, the change in frequency of activity ($\Delta F$) of cold receptors should be equal to the difference between the E and I process

$$\Delta F = E - I \tag{1}$$

During the dynamic response to cooling E and I change and their interaction governs the frequency of the response. These changes take time and can be described as exponential functions. It is further assumed that E and I have rate constants such that it takes longer to establish the end value of $E_2$ than $I_2$. Expressed algebraically,

$$E = ae^{-t/k_E}$$

$$I = ae^{-t/k_I} \tag{2}$$

$$\Delta F = a[e^{-t/k_E} - e^{-t/k_I}] \tag{3}$$

where $k_E$ and $k_I$ are the rate constants for E and I, t is the time following the stimulus onset, and a is a scaling constant that is a function of the adapting temperature.

Equation (3) represents the change in frequency to a step stimulus. However, we have used ramp stimuli, hence, over time

$$\frac{d(\Delta F)}{dt} = a \left[ \frac{e^{-t/k_I}}{k_I} - \frac{e^{-t/k_E}}{k_E} \right] \tag{4}$$

and for a ramp stimulus, S, the frequency at any time t, is the following convolution expression:

$$F(t) = S * \frac{d(\Delta F)}{dt} \tag{5}$$

### Steady-state responses

When equal temperature changes are applied at different adapting temperatures the amplitude of the peak dynamic response varies approximately as the steady-state response (Hensel and Zotterman, 1951; Iggo, 1969; Kenshalo et al., 1971). In spite of this correspondence, which suggests that the same processes are involved, the systems analysis suggested that different processes give rise to the steady-state and the

*References p. 139*

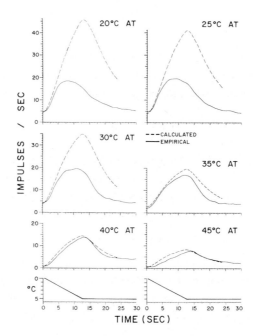

Fig. 2. The empirical and calculated dynamic responses to 5 °C cooling from each of the adapting temperatures (AT). In these calculated response curves linearity was assumed between the stimuli and the responses.

dynamic responses. It further suggested that the steady-state process continued during the dynamic response, modulating the frequency of the dynamic response to some extent, and manifests itself by the appearance of bursts during the dynamic response. Further evidence that separate processes are antecedent to the steady-state and the dynamic responses is provided by the report that the steady-state response frequency declined while the dynamic response to a standard cool stimulus increased with increasing concentrations of potassium ions in the external medium bathing frog cold receptors (Spray, 1974).

If the steady-state response is of a different source than the dynamic response, we have not yet been able to formulate a meaningful steady-state system equation. The steady-state response is likely the result of several unknown processes whose interactions we have not yet been able to specify. In these calculations inclusion of the steady-state response was based upon the empirical data.

In order to determine if equation (5), with proper constants, can satisfy the requirements of the empirical data, mean PST histograms of the dynamic responses to 5 °C cooling from each of six adapting temperatures were used for curve fitting. Rate constants, $k_E$ and $k_I$, and the scaling constant a were assumed for equation (5) and convolved with ramp-shaped stimuli of 5 °C intensity. The constants were adjusted, following the method of successive approximations, until the best fits were obtained between the calculated and the empirical PST histograms at the 35, 40 and 45 °C adapting temperatures. The empirical and calculated PST histograms are compared in Fig. 2. The agreement of the PST histograms at the 40 °C and 45 °C adapting

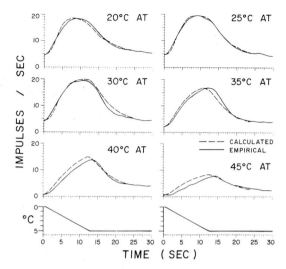

Fig. 3. The empirical and calculated dynamic responses to 5°C cooling from each of the adapting temperatures (AT). Here the obvious non-linearity between stimuli and responses, so prominent in Fig. 2, has been corrected by a term for depletion.

temperatures is good. Quasi-linear correspondence exists between the cool stimuli and the empirical responses at these adapting temperatures. At the 20, 25, 30 and 35 °C adapting temperatures non-linearity between the stimuli and the responses is manifest in two ways. First, the peak of the dynamic responses occurred well before the end of the stimulus and, second, the response to 5 °C cooling was scarcely larger than that to 2.5 °C cooling. Adjustments in the constants to accommodate this non-linearity caused them to assume illogical values and failed to produce satisfactory fits.

The shapes of the empirical PST histograms at the 20, 25, 30 and 35 °C adapting temperatures suggest that one or several of the processes antecedent to the occurrence of action potentials in the axon became depleted before the end of the cooling stimulus. A term for this "depletion" (D)§ has been added to equation (5) so

$$F_D(t) = S^* \frac{d(\Delta F)}{dt} \times D \tag{6}$$

The fit of the empirical PST histograms and the calculated PST histograms adjusted for depletion at the six adapting temperatures are shown in Fig. 3. The inclusion of D in the system equation had little effect upon the calculated PST histograms at the 40 °C and 45 °C adapting temperatures.

The values for the rate constants increased from 4.3 to 5.5 sec for $k_E$ and from 2.3 to 3.3 sec for $k_I$ as the adapting temperature decreased from 45 °C to 20 °C. Evaluated in terms of their half-life, at the 30 °C adapting temperature, $t_{0.5_E}$ = 3.4 sec and $t_{0.5_I}$ = 2.0 sec. The constant $k_E$ is of the same order of magnitude as that reported by Hensel (1953) while $k_I$ is considerably longer. The constant a = $a_0$

---

§ The expanded equation for D appears in Appendix A.

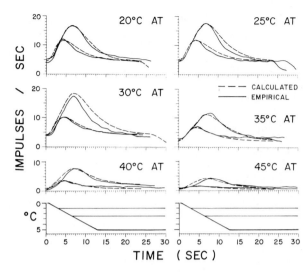

Fig. 4. The empirical and calculated response curves to 1.0 °C and 2.5 °C cooling from each adapting temperature (AT).

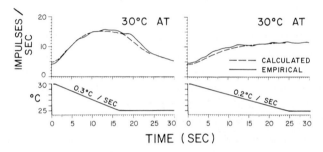

Fig. 5. The empirical and calculated response curves to cooling by 5 °C from a 30 °C adapting temperature at rates of 0.3 and 0.2 °C/sec.

the steady-state frequency ($a_0 \approx 3.5$). Since the steady-state response represents modulations of the impulse generation, a is the link between the steady-state and the dynamic responses.

We have shown that with certain values for $k_E$, $k_I$, a, and D the model will account for changes in the configuration of the dynamic responses to 5 °C cooling from adapting temperatures between 20 °C and 45 °C. Since the model is concerned with only the dynamic responses of the cold receptors, it need not account for the steady-state phenomena of the bursting discharge at low adapting temperatures nor the "paradoxical" response at high adapting temperatures.

If equation (6) is adequate it should also predict changes in the dynamic response to stimuli of different intensities and rates of stimulation. The calculated and empirical PST histograms for the 1.0 °C and 2.5 °C intensities of cooling are shown in Fig. 4. Fig. 5 shows the empirical and calculated PST histograms for 5 °C cool stimuli presented at rates of 0.2 and 0.3 °C/sec. The agreement is considered acceptable.

SOME POSSIBLE PHYSIOLOGICAL CORRELATES

A model based on Hensel's assumption of an inhibitory and an excitatory process, and whose rate constants change slightly with adapting temperature can account for the empirical responses of cold receptors. The assumption of just two processes is the limiting case. Each may be the product of several physiological processes. At this point only suggestions can be made of physiological processes that are represented by these excitatory and inhibitory processes, although some have an empirical basis.

The cold receptor is a tonic receptor. Thus, its frequency of discharge may be expected to be proportional to the degree of the receptor depolarization as in the crayfish stretch receptor (Eyzaguirre and Kuffler, 1955).

The steady-state response of cold receptors occurs without an energy transfer between the environment and the receptor since cold receptors show a continuous discharge even when the temporal and spatial temperature gradients are zero. The sustained discharge requires energy but the energy is derived from the receptor. Temperature merely modulates this discharge, apparently by controlling the metabolic processes of the receptor (Hensel, 1973).

The general morphology of a cold receptor has been described by Andres, von Düring, and Hensel (Hensel, 1973). There appear to be no accessory or special structures such as arterioles, venules, or cells that contain vesicles systematically associated with the receptor, although small vesicles can be seen within the receptive structure. This implies that the unique properties of cold receptors depend upon the morphology of the nerve terminal itself and upon the ionic transport characteristics of its terminal membrane.

The small size of the cold receptor terminals, and hence the large surface area–volume ratio, increases the probability that significant membrane depolarization can result from the exchange of only a few ions across the membrane. Thus, small temperature-induced changes in the ion permeability of the receptor membrane may be expected to produce sufficient changes in membrane potential to result in action potentials. However, the small diameter of the receptor alone does not endow cold receptors with their unique properties. Receptors with axons of the C fiber diameter may be as small in diameter as cold receptors yet they show differential sensitivities to mechanical and noxious stimulation (Burgess and Perl, 1973).

The small size and inability to localize cold receptors beneath the skin make observations difficult on changes in membrane potential associated with stimulation. An alternate approach is to identify, as models, systems that exhibit at least some of the functional properties of cold receptors and that provide greater accessibility to their membranes. The models suggested here are, by no means, the only ones. They represent examples. Others are possible and may better fulfill the requirements as models of cold receptors.

*Steady-state responses*

The origin of the steady-state response to static temperatures is the cold receptor itself. This predicts that large but relatively slow oscillations in the cold receptor membrane potential should occur. The depolarizing phase of the wave should initiate bursts of impulses and the repolarization of the membrane should create interburst intervals.

A model for the proposed oscillating potential in cold receptors comes from the recent work on the bursting neurons in the visceral ganglion of the sea hare *Aplysia*. Here, oscillations in membrane potential result from the interplay of two current components; first, a regenerative inward current drives the membrane potential toward one well beyond the depolarized peak and, second, an outward current, activated by the regenerative depolarization, temporarily overwhelms the negative membrane resistance and drives the membrane potential in the hyperpolarized direction (Carnevale and Wachtel, 1974).

*Dynamic responses*

Modulation of the steady-state discharge by temperature is to be expected considering the known temperature dependency of ionic permeabilities of receptor membranes. However, the transduction of a change in temperature to a receptor depolarization is not known. Some mechanoreceptors, like the Pacinian corpuscle, have a fairly high temperature sensitivity (Ishiko and Loewenstein, 1961). Type I slowly adapting mechanoreceptors, likewise, show a higher discharge rate to maintained pressure at high than at low adapting temperatures (Iggo and Muir, 1969; Duclaux and Kenshalo, 1972). A discharge can be initiated in the cat muscle spindle by cooling alone and it is presumed to be due to the depolarizing effect of the low temperature ($<32°C$) at the receptor terminals (Lippold *et al.*, 1960). But, none of these provide an understanding of the mechanism of membrane depolarization to sudden cooling in specific or even non-specific temperature sensitive receptors.

Mechanisms that have been demonstrated in *Aplysia* neurons and in the spinal motoneurons of cats may account for the temperature sensitivity of specific thermo-receptors. The neurons of *Aplysia* have a ouabain-sensitive active transport process, the sodium–potassium pump, that contributes to the membrane potential. An increased excitability of the *Aplysia* neurons is observed on cooling because of the high temperature dependence of the sodium–potassium pump. Depolarization due to cooling is opposed, however, because these neurons have a higher temperature coefficient for sodium than for potassium permeability (Carpenter, 1970). In the spinal motoneurons of the cat, however, a greater temperature coefficient for potassium than for sodium permeability is linked with depolarization during cooling (Klee *et al.*, 1974).

These results have led Pierau *et al.* (1974) to propose two possible mechanisms for cold transduction and one for warm transduction. Cold transduction may be accomplished by slowing the highly temperature dependent sodium–potassium pump (see also Sperelakis, 1970; Spray, 1974) or, as in the cat motoneuron, depolarization by cooling may occur because of a greater temperature dependency for potassium than for sodium permeability. Warm transduction may occur in membranes that exhibit a greater temperature dependency for sodium than potassium permeability.

Experiments with ouabain, a metabolic inhibitor, on the possible role of the sodium–potassium pump as a cold transducer have yielded apparently conflicting results. Spray (1974) found that the application of ouabain produced an initial discharge in frog cold receptors in the absence of cooling and rendered them less sensitive to cooling by 20 °C from a 30 °C adapting temperature. Pierau *et al.* have reported, however, that ouabain infiltrated into the scrotal skin of rats produced a steady-state response at a 38 °C adapting temperature, when there had been none prior to ouabain, and an increased dynamic response to cooling by 15 °C in specific cold receptors. The differences in these reports may have resulted from differences in the concentration of ouabain reaching the cold receptors, membrane differences in the cold receptors of amphibia and mammals, or, more likely, differences in the temperature ranges of cool stimulation. They both show, however, that metabolic processes in the receptor membrane are somehow involved in the transduction of cold stimuli. Temperature dependent changes in ionic permeability of the cold receptor membrane to active transport, passive transport, or, more likely, a combination of the two appear to be likely candidates to account for cold transduction.

Sufficient information is lacking to permit suggestions of the physiological analogs for E and I or the origins of their rate constants in dynamic responses. However, an unequally coupled active sodium efflux and potassium influx, suggested by Pierau *et al.* may account for the decreasing sensitivity of cold receptors with increasing adapting temperatures, as is apparent in Fig. 3. At high static temperatures ($>30\,°C$) the larger sodium efflux than potassium influx tends to hyperpolarize the terminal and thereby decrease its excitability to cooling. The increased activity of cold receptors at high adapting temperatures (38 °C) after ouabain may be explained by a reduction in hyperpolarization that resulted from inhibition of the sodium–potassium pump. Sodium–potassium pump activity is highly temperature dependent and so the lack of an effect of ouabain on cold fiber activity at low adapting temperatures (24 °C) may be explained by a very low rate of pumping. This leaves the membrane potential, determined at low temperatures largely by passive transport mechanisms, less polarized than it was at higher adapting temperatures and more subject to depletion of its ionic reservoir. As the adapting temperature is decreased further, the membrane may even become partially depolarized to make it even more sensitive to sudden cooling. This increased sensitivity at lower adapting temperatures is limited, however, by the positive temperature coefficient of ion permeabilities.

The hypothesis of Pierau *et al.* (1974) accounts for the bell-shaped steady-state response curves of cold receptors. The gradual slowing ionic movement at low adapting temperatures ($<25\,°C$) and hyperpolarization of the receptor membrane due to the increased activity of the temperature dependent sodium–potassium pump at high adapting temperatures ($>30\,°C$) would be expected to produce a steady-state response maximum in the mid-temperature range. As the adapting temperature is

138 D. R. KENSHALO *et al.*

lowered from 30°C the membrane becomes less polarized, and hence closer to the threshold of action potential production. Oscillations in membrane potential may be more likely to exceed the action potential threshold and thereby produce bursts of impulses that are a characteristic of the cold receptor spike train at low adapting temperatures. Finally, as the adapting temperature is lowered still further cold blocks further action potential generation at temperatures of 10°C to 15°C.

In the same way the slower rate of increase in the frequency of the discharge upon cool stimulation (see Fig. 3) at the 35, 40 and 45°C adapting temperatures, than at lower adapting temperatures, is explained by the hyperpolarized condition of the cold receptor membrane that is produced by increased activity of the unequally coupled sodium–potassium pump.

At low adapting temperatures the dynamic response is a non-linear function of the stimulus. The systems analysis suggests that this is due to a depletion or at least an imbalance in the ion pool responsible for maintaining the membrane potential or the generation of action potentials. This may well depend on the ionic content of the cells, especially in terminals of small diameter (high surface area–volume ratios), where there is a greater effect of interferences with ion diffusion due to connective tissue, Schwann cells and so forth between them and the external volume or a sluggish to inoperative sodium–potassium pump to restore the internal ionic concentrations (Katz, 1966).

SUMMARY

The methods of systems analysis have been employed to describe the responses of feline facial cold receptors to ramp-shaped cool stimuli that varied in rate, intensity, and the temperature to which the skin was preadapted. It was assumed that two processes, an excitatory and an inhibitory process, interact to produce a change in the frequency of cold receptor activity upon cool stimulation.

Linear and non-linear components of the responses to 5°C cool stimuli have been identified. The linear components, which occurred at the 40°C and 45°C adapting temperatures, can be described as exponential functions with rate constants that increased by about 25% as the adapting temperatures decreased from 45°C to 20°C. Non-linearity of the responses to 5°C cool stimuli increased as the adapting temperature decreased from 35°C to 20°C. This non-linearity can be described as an exponential function whose rate constant was a function of the adapting temperature. This component of the system equation might be due to depletion of the ionic reservoir responsible for restoring the receptor membrane polarization or action potential generation.

The second major outcome of the system analysis indicated that the steady-state and dynamic responses of cold receptors arose from different processes, although they may be loosely coupled.

Some possible physiological mechanism underlying the steady-state response and cool stimulus transduction are considered along with some possible physiological correlates for the excitatory and inhibitory processes of the system equation.

ACKNOWLEDGEMENT

This research was supported by USPHS Grant NB-02992. Assistance of the Psychobiology Research Center of Florida State University, through USPHS Grant NB-7468 and NSF Grant GU-2612 is also acknowledged.

REFERENCES

BURGESS, P. R. AND PERL, E. R. (1973) Cutaneous mechanoreceptors and nociceptors. In A. IGGO (Ed.), *Handbook of Sensory Physiology, Vol. II, Somatosensory System*. Springer, Berlin. pp. 30–78.

CARNEVALE, N. T. AND WACHTEL, H. (1974) Slow oscillations in *Aplysia* bursting neurons are produced by the interaction of two currents. *Physiologist*, **17**, 193.

CARPENTER, D. O. (1970) Membrane potential produced directly by the $Na^+$ pump in *Aplysia* neurons. *Comp. Biochem. Physiol.*, **35**, 371–385.

DUCLAUX, R. AND KENSHALO, D. R. (1972) The temperature sensitivity of the type I slowly adapting mechanoreceptors in cats and monkeys. *J. Physiol. (Lond.)*, **224**, 647–664.

EYZAGUIRRE, C. AND KUFFLER, S. W. (1955) Processes of excitation in the soma of single isolated sensory nerve cells of the lobster and crayfish. *J. gen. Physiol.*, **39**, 87–119.

HENSEL, H. (1952) Physiologie der Thermoreception. *Ergebn. Physiol.*, **47**, 166–368.

HENSEL, H. (1953) The time factor in thermoreceptor excitation. *Acta physiol. scand.*, **29**, 109–116.

HENSEL, H. (1973) Cutaneous thermoreceptors. In A. IGGO (Ed.), *Handbook of Sensory Physiology, Vol. II, Somatosensory System*. Springer, Berlin. pp. 79–110.

HENSEL, H. AND ZOTTERMAN, Y. (1951) Quantitative beziehungen swischen der Entladung einzelner Kaltfasern der Temperatur. *Acta physiol. scand.*, **23**, 291–319.

IGGO, A. (1969) Cutaneous thermoreceptors in primates and sub-primates. *J. Physiol. (Lond.)*, **200**, 403–430.

IGGO, A. AND MUIR, A. R. (1969) The structure and function of a slowly adapting touch corpuscle in hairy skin. *J. Physiol. (Lond.)*, **200**, 763–796.

ISHIKO, N. AND LOEWENSTEIN, W. R. (1961) Effects of temperature on the generator and action potentials of sense organ. *J. gen. Physiol.*, **45**, 105–124.

KATZ, B. (1966) *Nerve, Muscle, and Synapse*. McGraw-Hill, New York.

KENSHALO, D. R., HENSEL, H., GRAZIADEI, P. AND FRUHSTORFER, H. (1971) On the anatomy, physiology, and psychophysics of the cat's temperature-sensing system. In R. DUBNER (Ed.), *Oral–Facial Sensory and Motor Mechanisms*. Appleton-Century-Crofts, New York. pp. 23–44.

KENSHALO, D. R., FRUHSTORFER, H. AND HENSEL, H. (1975) Steady state and dynamic responses of cat's cold receptors to temperature and temperature changes, in preparation.

KLEE, M. R., PIERAU, F. K. AND FABER, D. S. (1974) Temperature effects on resting potential and spike parameters of cat motoneurones. *Exp. Brain Res.*, **19**, 478–492.

LIPPOLD, O. C. J., NICHOLLS, J. G. AND REDFEARN, J. W. T. (1960) A study of the afferent discharge produced by cooling a mammalian muscle spindle. *J. Physiol. (Lond.)*, **153**, 218–231.

PIERAU, F. K., TORREY, P. AND CARPENTER, D. O. (1974) Mammalian cold receptor afferents: role of an electrogenic sodium pump in sensory transduction. *Brain Res.*, **73**, 156–160.

SAND, A. (1938) The function of the ampullae of Lorenzini, with some observations of the effect of temperature on sensory rhythms. *Proc. roy. Soc. B*, **125**, 524–553.

SPERELAKIS, N. (1970) Effects of temperature on membrane potentials of excitable cells. In J. D. HARDY, A. P. GAGGE AND J. A. J. STOLWIJK (Eds.), *Physiological and Behavioral Temperature Regulation*. Thomas, Springfield, Ill. pp. 408–441.

SPRAY, D. (1974) Metabolic dependence of frog cold receptor sensitivity. *Brain Res.*, **72**, 354–359.

APPENDIX A

IONIC DEPLETION THEORY

DENNY CORMIER

An intense study of the cold receptor PST histograms has shown definite stimulus–response activity. As a receptor mechanism this activity is to be expected. However, when analyzing the specific nature of the histogram in light of a "systems approach", linear and non-linear components of the cold receptor response must be differentiated. The linear interaction has already been outlined in equations (4) and (5) of the preceding discussion. Yet, as can be seen from Fig. 2, there is obviously a significant non-linear interaction involved within the receptor response. The following "Ionic Depletion Theory" has been offered as an explanation for the non-linear character of the cold receptor dynamic response.

No nerve fiber or receptor commands access to an infinite ionic reservoir for production of resting and action potentials. More specifically, for any closed electrolytic system there are associated ionic mobilities which limit the membrane charge transport; in the receptor system sodium and potassium play the most important roles regarding charge transport. In addition, there are active transport systems (sodium–potassium pump) which require energy to repolarize the membrane. For smaller receptor diameters, the recovery or refractory period associated with action potential generation becomes increasingly important. The net contribution of these considerations upon the receptor membrane is simply that continued or prolonged discharge activity results in a gradual decrease of its ability to recover electrical polarization. In effect, its available charge reservoir has been "depleted". If the assumption is then made that the active transport mechanisms exert greater energy toward an equilibrium state when the resting potential has been upset, as during the action potential, it follows that

$$k_D \frac{dD}{dt} = - D(t) \tag{1a}$$

where $k_D$ is a proportionality constant $>0$, $D(t)$ is the driving ionic concentration as a function of time and $dD/dt$ its respective return rate to an equilibrium condition. Equation (2a) is the solution to equation (1a):

$$D(t) = A_0 e^{-t/k_D} \tag{2a}$$

$$A_0 = \text{constant of integration}$$

Since $D(t)$ determine the recovery state within the nerve fiber away from an equilibrium condition, $D_0$, such that $D(t) = D_0$ during periods when no excitation occurs, equation (2a) becomes:

$$D(t)_J = A_0 e^{-t/k_D} + D_0 \tag{3a}$$

For a "discrete" case whereby the action potential is the sole source of ionic depletion

$$D(t) = \left[ \left( A_0 \sum_{i=1}^{n} e^{-(t-t_i)/k_D} \, u_{-1}(t-t_i) \right) + D_0 \right] \qquad (4a)$$

For n action potentials occurring at respective times, $t_i$, and $u_{-1}(t - t_i)$ is the unit step function defined as 0 for $t < t_i$ and 1 for $t > t_i$.

Since the average interspike frequency is approximately the reciprocal of the average interspike interval, a simple expression for depletion in $\Delta F(t)$ resulting from a step input would be:

$$F_D(t) = \frac{\Delta F(t)}{D(t)} \qquad (5a)$$

where $F_D$ and $\Delta F$ are defined in the main text. Equation (5a) demonstrates the relationship of D(t) to the system equation; in other words, D(t) acts directly upon the generator potential to lengthen the effective refractory period.

When large numbers of action potentials are involved, Equations (4) and (5) from the main text and equation (5a) may be combined into a general expression in terms of the convolution integral:

$$F_D(t) = \frac{a}{D_0} \frac{\displaystyle\int_0^t S(t-\tau)\,[E(\tau) - I(\tau)]_h \, d\tau}{1 + \dfrac{a}{D_0} \left[ \displaystyle\int_0^t D(t-\tau)\,F(\tau)\,d\tau \right]} \qquad (6a)$$

Where a, E, I, F, and S are as previously defined in the paper, and $\tau$ is the dummy time variable of the convolution integral. Equation (6a) applies equally well for a continuous F(t).

## DISCUSSION

KHAJUTIN: What can you tell of physical mechanisms in this set of calculations you have described?

KENSHALO: We can only speculate because it is very dark inside the skin and microelectrodes do not probe it very well. But we do speculate on possible models for the ion E–I processes. And the model is taken from the different visceral ganglia and neurons of *Aplysia*. In the first place at high adapting temperatures, as Pierau and his colleagues suggested, the membrane becomes hyperpolarized because of the high temperature dependency of the sodium pump. At the low-adapting temperature the pump is no longer operative or is sluggish and the ionic mobility is also sluggish. We can only expect that to have a steady-state bell-shaped curve. Now the transduction of a change in temperatures is quite another matter. The model here is the cat motoneuron. I do not know if anybody has investigated the temperature changes in a cat motoneuron. At any rate they can be excited by cooling and the reason for their being excitable by cooling is thought to be that they have a higher temperature coefficient for potassium permeability than for sodium permeability. They propose that warm receptors show just the opposite temperature coefficients. They have a higher temperature coefficient for sodium permeability than for potassium permeability.

HENSEL: I would like to make two brief comments. One point is that we should bear in mind that we have cold and warm receptors. And I think it is very attractive to arrive at a theory that we have both, so we should not focus attention too much on cold receptors. Another question is that I think there are more complicated processes in terms of the damped oscillation and I believe that this type of response is only a special case of a more general type of response.

IGGO: I think in addition that it is necessary that your equation should also account for the paradoxical response of some of the cold receptors, because in your slide where you compared the smoothed curve, some of the receptors showed a paradoxical discharge, that is a rise in activity with the higher temperature in cold receptors. Did your equation account for that?

KENSHALO: No, it excludes paradoxical responses, it does include bursting, however. One comment I should make about Dr. Hensel's remark. Our first approximation of this gave us, assuming the different constants, less than critically damped oscillations in the response. However, it was not shown in the system we were working with. If we pursue this line of investigations it should be tried out not only on the cold receptors from the face of cat but also on cold receptors from monkeys. Perhaps, the same equation can account for warm receptors' activity. We do not have data available on warm receptors.

# Physiological Mechanisms of Skin Thermosensitivity

K. IVANOV, V. KONSTANTINOV, N. MALOVICHKO, N. DANILOVA AND V. TRUSOVA

*I. P. Pavlov Institute of Physiology, Academy of Sciences of the U.S.S.R., Leningrad (U.S.S.R.)*

In the present work a careful study was made of the regularities of skin thermo-receptors' firing rate changes in the strictly physiological limits of skin temperature changes. The temperature was changed at constant rates to which the animals are normally exposed.

The thermoreceptors of skin of the dorsal surface of the nose of a rabbit (nose back skin) were examined. This region of skin has a large number of thermoreceptors and plays an important role in thermoregulation. Biopotentials were registered from the thin (100–200 $\mu$V) twigs of nervus infraorbitalis. With the help of the thermodes, or environmental temperature changes, the nose skin temperature was shifted within 22–37 °C with the rate of 0.3 or 0.8 °C/min.

The succession of the experiment was as follows. First, the skin temperature was increased to 36–37 °C, then it was decreased immediately to 22 °C, then again increased to 36–37 °C. In every experiment several successive skin temperature changes were carried out in such a way. Nerve biopotentials were summed up automatically every 15 sec. For more detailed analysis the biopotentials were registered on photographic film. The skin surface temperature was measured by a thermocouple. The rabbit was under light anaesthesia.

The firing rate of the impulses, with an amplitude no more than 50 $\mu$V, changed in response to the skin temperature change and was unaffected by mechanical stimulation of the skin. We attributed these impulses to thermoreceptor functions. In all the experiments we studied only the nerve twigs with the impulses that did not exceed this amplitude.

In the thermoneutral zone (24–26 °C environmental) the nose skin temperature was 28–30 °C. The frequency of impulses under these conditions depended on the number of active afferent fibres in a nervous twig. Frequency was 250–100 impulses/sec with large numbers of active fibres. In individual experiments we were able to register the impulses from only three, two or even from one active unit. In such a case the frequency was equal to from 3 to 20–25 impulses/sec. An increase of the skin temperature to 36–37 °C was always followed by a decrease of the firing rate. A decrease of nose skin temperature in all the experiments gave rise to an increase of the firing rate. As can be seen in Fig. 1, an increase of skin temperature from 25 to 33 °C was followed by a distinct decrease of summary firing rate. Consequently, in the nose

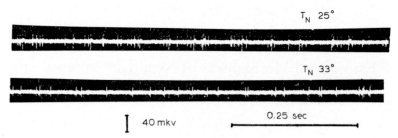

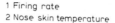

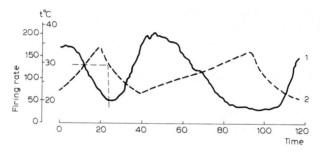

Fig. 1. The firing rate of cold thermoreceptors. The upper line: that at the nose back skin temperature of 25 °C; the lower line: that at 33 °C.

Fig. 2. The cold thermoreceptors' firing rate changes in dependence on the nose back skin temperature. The continuous line shows the thermoreceptors firing rate and the dotted line the nose back skin temperature. x-axis: the time in minutes; y-axis: the firing rate in impulses/sec and temperature in °C.

back skin of the rabbit, the cold thermoreceptors were registered in our experiments, rather than warm thermoreceptors.

Trying to determine the maximum of the summed thermoreceptors' firing rate, we managed to establish some special, unknown till now, functional properties of thermoreceptors that could be found only at the physiological fluctuations of temperature and with continuous registration of the firing rate. In Fig. 2 such a registration of the firing rate during one continuous experiment is shown. With an increase of the skin temperature the firing rate decreased gradually. Further, under the decrease of skin temperature the summed firing rate is distinctly increased. The special features of this process are that the firing rate does not reach the minimum at the highest skin temperature, 37 °C, but continues to fall for some time, in spite of the skin temperature beginning to decrease. On the contrary, the summed firing rate of the thermoreceptors does not reach a maximum at 22 °C, the minimal skin temperature. It continues to increase for some time in spite of the skin beginning to get warm. A regular delay of the changes of thermoreceptors' firing rate takes place with respect to the skin surface temperature changes. This, in its turn, results in a striking phenomenon. As can be seen from Fig. 2, at the same temperature of the skin surface the firing rate depends on the direction of the temperature shifts. The role of the dynamics of the temperature changes appears most distinctly under the statistical treatment

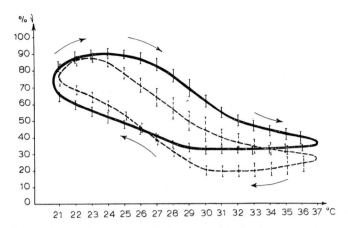

Fig. 3. The thermoreceptors' firing rate change under the velocity of skin temperature changes equal to 0.8 °C/min (the continuous line) and 0.3 °C/min (the dotted line). x-axis: the skin temperature (°C); y-axis: the firing rate change (%).

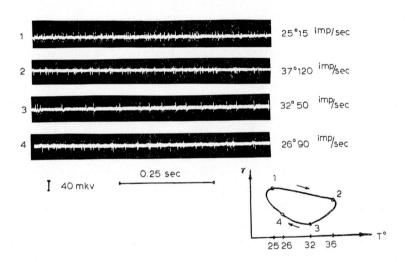

Fig. 4. The firing rate of the cold thermoreceptors at different nose back skin temperature. 1: temperature at 25 °C; the firing rate is 155 impulses/min; 2: temperature at 37 °C; the firing rate is 120 impulses/min; 3: temperature at 32 °C; the firing rate is 50 impulses/min; 4: temperature at 26 °C; the firing rate is 90 impulses/min. At the foot of the figure is shown the scheme of the cold thermo- receptors' firing rate changes in dependence on the direction of nose back skin temperature changes.

of all the experiments, when the continuous firing rate changes in dependence on the skin temperature are expressed as a continuous loop. This is shown on Fig. 3.

These figures show quite distinctly that during continuous temperature changes of skin the firing rate of cold thermoreceptors is different at the same temperature of skin surface. Let us consider, for instance, the firing rate at 26 °C. It can be seen from the figure that during heating at this temperature of skin surface, the firing rate is considerably higher than at the same temperature of skin surface when reached under cooling.

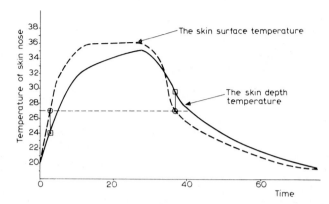

Fig. 5. The skin temperature changes on the surface (continuous line) and at the depth of 2 mm (dotted line) under increase and decrease of environmental temperature. x-axis: time (min); y-axis: temperature (°C). The thin horizontal line unites the points with the same temperature of the skin surface.

This phenomenon is illustrated in Fig. 4. Attention should be given to the first and the fourth firing rate record recorded at the same skin temperature. However, the first line is recorded under heating and the firing rate is 155 impulses/sec. The fourth is recorded at practically the same skin temperature, but under cooling, and has a firing rate of only 90 impulses/sec.

What is the cause of this delay? It can be accounted for by the inertia of temperature changes. Our special measurements have shown that at the depth of about 2 mm from the skin surface, the temperature shifts are delayed with respect to the skin surface under the given experimental conditions, as is shown in Fig. 5. During heating of the skin at the rate of 0.8 °C/min, the skin surface temperature was 3 °C higher (27 °C) than it was at the depth of 2 mm. Conversely, with skin cooling at the same rate, when the skin surface temperature was 27 °C the temperature at the depth of 2 mm was equal to 29 °C, *i.e.* it was 2 °C higher than at the surface. If one assumes that cold thermoreceptors of the skin are situated at different levels, and even in the deepest ones, then the phenomenon of the firing rate delay can be explained. Indeed, during heating of the skin the temperature of its deeper levels will be lower than on the surface. If the deep thermoreceptors do participate in the summed firing rate changes, then their firing rate will be higher. During cooling at the same temperature of the skin surface, temperature of deep skin level will be higher. Consequently, the summed firing rate of cold thermoreceptors will be lower.

If the presence of cold thermoreceptors in different levels of the skin is accepted, then an important conclusion follows that the skin thermoreceptors can determine the temperature gradients of skin, their value and direction. But value and direction of the temperature gradients depend on those of the heat flow. There follows one more conclusion: that skin thermoreceptors can measure the intensity and the direction of the heat flow.

This is a very important function from the point of view of organism thermoregulation. But is it true in reality?

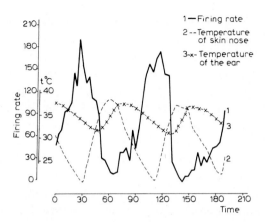

Fig. 6. The vasomotor thermoregulatory reaction of the rabbit's ear and its correlation with the cold thermoreceptors firing rate. Continuous line shows the cold thermoreceptors firing rate; dotted line the nose back skin temperature and the dotted line with crosses the temperature of the ear. x-axis: time (min); y-axis, firing rate (impulses/min) and the temperature (°C).

Recently in our laboratory a special technique has been elaborated for the registration of the potentials from very thin twigs of nervus infraorbitalis in an unanaesthetized rabbit. Thanks to this method, we were able to carry out the simultaneous observations of the skin thermoreceptors' firing rate changes and of appearance, development and disappearance of the specific thermoregulatory reactions. The reaction observed was that of the vessels of the rabbit's ear. The ear is known to be a specific organ of heat loss in these animals.

In Fig. 6 the results of one of these experiments are presented. The reaction of strict dilatation of ear vessels and, consequently, the increase of heat loss appear when the temperature of the nose skin is about 31 °C. The cold thermoreceptors' firing rate is at a minimum under these conditions. We believe this to be the cause of vessel dilatation and of the increase of heat loss.

During the further course of the experiment, when the environmental temperature decreased, which leads to a decrease of the nose skin temperature, the ear vessels remain dilated for a long time. However, of utmost importance is the fact that the cold thermoreceptors' firing rate also remains at a very low level. In other words, if the increase of the cold thermoreceptors' firing rate is delayed, then the appearance of the ear vessels' reaction is also delayed. The vessels remain dilated and the heat loss continues at a high level. Only when the cold thermoreceptors' firing rate begins to grow quickly does narrowing of the ear vessels occur and the heat loss decrease. This allows us to postulate that cold thermoreceptors play a very important role in the regulation of the vessel's thermoregulatory reactions. What is the physiological meaning of this phenomenon?

Consider Fig. 5, when the temperature of the skin surface is 27°C; it is near the temperature of the skin surface in the thermoneutral zone. However, in the thermoneutral zone the temperature of the deep levels of the skin at a depth of 2 mm is only 0.3–0.4°C higher than that at the surface. This is normal. In our case, when we deal with the gradual cooling of the skin after heating, the temperature of the deep levels of the skin is 2 °C higher than at the surface, that is to say, much greater. This tells us that in the deep levels of the skin there is a surplus of heat. Until this surplus is removed from the organism, the temperature of the deep levels will be high, and, until the temperature falls, the cold thermoreceptors will have a low firing rate. Until they have a low firing rate the ear vessels will remain dilated and the heat loss will be on a high level. This is a supposed physiological meaning of these phenomena. It gives rise to the supposition that skin thermoreceptors, being situated in different levels, can provide the information into the central nervous system not only about the temperature of the skin surface, but about the value and direction of the heat flow inside the skin. This supposition is of interest for the common theory of thermoregulation. It also widens our knowledge about the mechanisms of skin thermosensitivity.

### SUMMARY

The firing rate changes of the rabbit's nose back skin thermoreceptors were studied under physiological fluctuations of the environmental temperature. The observed delaying of thermoreceptor firing rate changes with respect to the skin temperature can be explained by the temperature shifts in its deep levels. The thermoreceptors, situated in different levels of the skin, are supposed to be able to register the value and direction of the temperature gradients.

The simultaneous registration of skin thermoreceptors' firing rate changes and of the development of a specific thermoregulatory vasomotor reaction have shown that the strict dilatation of the ear vessels and, consequently, the increase of the heat loss of an organism, appears when the cold thermoreceptors' firing rate decreases to a minimum. The vessels remain dilated until the firing rate has a low value. With a decrease of the environmental temperature, the cold thermoreceptors' firing rate begins to increase quickly. At the same time the narrowing of the ear vessels occurs and the heat loss decreases. Consequently, the skin cold thermoreceptors can play an important role in the regulation of the thermoregulatory vasomotor reactions.

### DISCUSSION

HENSEL: Do you not think that the hysteresis that you have found is the dynamic reorganization of a receptor—that the delaying is natural?

IVANOV: The dynamic properties of the thermoreceptors can be found only under very quick changes of the skin temperature (0.3–0.5 °C, and even more, per sec). In our experiments the skin temperature was changed very slowly. That is why there is no reason to attribute the hysteresis phenomena to the dynamic properties of the receptors.

HENSEL: The cold thermoreceptors are known to be situated on the very surface of the skin. What significance has the gradient that you have measured for them?

IVANOV: The cold thermoreceptors are considered to be situated only in the surface level of the skin. Our data have shown that they can be situated even in the deep levels of the skin. The data of Minut-Sorokhtina confirm our hypothesis.

BURGESS: It is interesting that the hysteresis described in this report, which is caused by the thermal inertia of the skin, is reversed when compared with that shown by mechanoreceptors and that would be predicted from the dynamic responses of cold receptors. Would the hysteresis you describe not cause a problem for the animal in determining the temperature of an object touching the skin because the same discharge frequency occurs at different temperatures, depending on the rate and direction of the temperature change?

IVANOV: Our investigation has shown that at the same temperature of the skin surface, its deep levels can have different temperatures. The hysteresis reflects this fact. The nervous pathways from the thermoreceptors of different skin levels to the central nervous system may end at the specific groups of neurones. Such neurones may have different situations. This is one of the possible ways of the estimation of the value and direction of skin temperature gradients that is of utmost importance for thermoregulation.

TSYRULNIKOV: Is it possible that you have studied not only cold receptors, but the warm ones?

IVANOV: The hysteresis concerns mainly the cold thermoreceptors. Warm thermoreceptors change the course of the hysteresis loop a little, but only in the region of high temperature, where the difference between the firing rates at the same skin surface temperature is minimal.

# Analysis of Activity in A and C Fibres Under Mechanical and Thermal Stimulation of the Skin Receptor Field

A. V. ZEVEKE, E. D. EFES, G. I. MALYSHEVA AND V. L. SHAPOSHNIKOV

*Department of Biocybernetics of the Institute of Applied Mathematics and Cybernetics, N. I. Lobachevsky State University, Gorky (U.S.S.R.)*

In beginning this report we should like to cite Academician Chernigovsky (1970) who wrote: "How, from the collossal flow of 'depersonalized' spikes rushing along nerve fibres and on the whole creating a fairly depressing picture of monotony, do the nerve centres choose the necessary information? What combinations of spikes transfer information on certain peripheral events and what combinations of spikes signalize about others? How does this monotony convert into the splendour of the reflectory activity of a living organism?".

It is these questions that lured us into work the aim of which was to disclose the mystery of the peripheral nerve system code.

An important contribution to the investigation of skin receptors was made by Adrian (Adrian and Bronk, 1928) whose method permitted the qualitative and quantitative characteristics of various receptor units to be determined. The works of Zotterman (1939), Maruhashi *et al.* (1952), Iggo (1966 and 1969), Hensel (1966), Minut-Sorokhtina (1972), Burgess *et al.* (1968) and Kenshalo and Nafe (1962, 1963a and b) are relevant.

It is known that under natural conditions external stimulation causes excitation of a great number of receptors of various kinds. The impulse flow from receptors should vary on various stimuli affecting the skin. This difference is perhaps the reason for the determination of sensation modality by the central nervous system.

For determination of quantitative characteristics of the total afferent flow under various externally applied stimuli one should use methods that permit quantitative analysis of afferent impulses in all nerve fibres simultaneously.

For this purpose we employed the modified method of colliding impulses of Douglas and Ritchie (1957), which permitted the determination of not only the relative number of active fibres but the frequency spectrum of orthodromic flow in these fibres as well (Zeveke and Khayutin, 1966; Zeveke and Gladysheva, 1969). The principle of modification lies in a gradual increase of antidromic stimulation frequency which results in ortho- and antidromic impulse collisions being forced out from the interelectrode section of the nerve in the fibres where orthodromic frequency is less than the antidromic one. The recorded antidromic potential increases. There have been established certain limitations of the modifications and discrepancies in

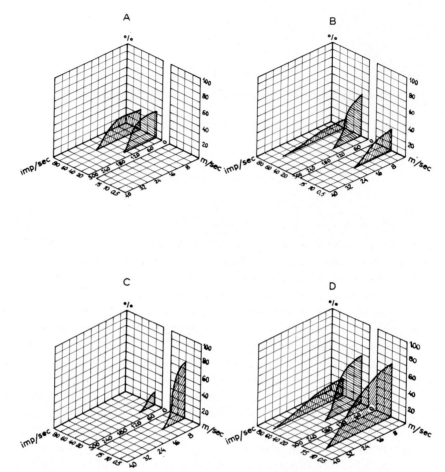

Fig. 1. Cumulative curves for impulse activity of cat. Each point of the curve reflects the number of active fibres whose impulse frequency exceeds a given frequency of antidromic stimulation. Axis "x" is for the relative number of fibres where ortho- and antidromic impulses have collided; axis "y" is for the impulse conduction velocity (m/sec), and axis "z" is for the frequency of antidromic stimulation (impulses/sec). Skin receptors were stimulated A: by the air flow with pressure of 20 mg/sq.cm; B: by pins with pressure of 0.5 g/pin, pin distribution density being 5 pins/sq.cm; C: by cooling the skin from 27°C to 17°C at a rate of 1°C/sec; D: by needles with pressure of 10 g/needle, needle distribution density being 5 needles/sq.cm.

absolute values of afferent frequencies in comparison with the results obtained by recording the potentials from a single fibre. However, irrespective of these limitations, the modification which we suggest gives rather good results when determinating the afferent flow pattern which in the modal groups of fibres can be characterized by a relative number of conductive fibres, by impulse frequency therein and by the conduction velocity. Fig. 1A shows the results of afferent flow analysis during peak activity in the skin nerve fibres when the medial part of the cat's paw is exposed to an air stream at a pressure of 20 mg/sq.cm during 1 sec.

Axis "z" is for the relative number of fibres involved in impulse conductance, axis "x" is for conduction velocity in the fibre group investigated and axis "y" is for impulse conductance frequency. At the given stimulation intensity the impulse activity was observed in modal fibres Aβ and δ with maximal frequencies of 180 and 135 impulses/sec. The relative number of these fibres involved in conductance was 25% and 32% respectively.

The increase of the air flow pressure up to 40 mg/sq.cm leads to an increase in the number of fibres involved in conductance, to an increase of frequency of afferent impulses, and to the appearance of activity in non-myelinated fibres with a frequency of 9 impulses/sec. The relative number of C fibres involved in conductance was less than 10%.

The afferent flow pattern changed when blunt pins were placed on the skin surface with a force of 0.5 g/pin and with a density of distribution of 5 pins/sq.cm (Fig. 1B). In this case the activity of Aβ fibres was less and the activity of C fibres was much greater than when affecting the skin receptors with a stream of air. When stimulating the skin with sharp needles with the same density but with a pressure of 10 g/needle the afferent flow pattern changed as a result of the increasing number of active fibres and the increasing frequency of afferent impulses in all the modal groups of nerve fibres. Particularly large changes were found in non-myelinated fibres, (Fig. 1D). On stimulation with needles there was always a nociceptive reaction, which was never present when stimulating the skin with pins.

No activity was observed in Aβ fibres during cooling of the skin from 37°C down to 17°C at the rate of 1°C/sec. The number of excited Aδ fibres was small and their frequencies were insignificant. The number of excited C fibres in some experiments reached 70%, and peak frequencies did not exceed 12 impulses/sec (Fig. 1C).

On comparing the afferent flow patterns during peak activity of the receptors, it is possible to see clearly the difference between them and get some idea about the code which enters the central nervous system and calls forth a certain modality of sensations (Fig. 1). It would be wrong to think that stimulation coding is carried out only by modal groups of Aβ, Aδ and C fibres. Shunting of the input signal by nerve tissue and the electronic equipment noise does not permit reliable recording of small potentials of non-modal fibre groups in the evoked response of the entire nerve trunk. For picking the low-amplitude potentials out of equipment noise on electrical stimulation of the nerve we employed the method of coherent accumulation of signals with subsequent averaging by the computer (Zeveke et al., 1973a and b). When stimulating the nerve with an intensity several times exceeding the threshold for the group of Aδ fibres, we picked out potentials of nerve fibres with conduction velocities from 2 to 14 m/sec. Potentials with conduction velocities from 0.8 to 0.15 m/sec were registered on supramaximal stimulation of C fibres.

For determining the presence of afferent fibres in non-modal groups we employed the method of colliding impulses. The results showed that after ortho- and antidromic impulse collision the potentials of fibres with low conduction velocities in myelinated as well as in non-myelinated fibres were drastically reduced (Fig. 2). It can be supposed that the activity in these fibres supplements in a certain way the activity of modal groups.

It is known that a great number of slowly adapting mechanoreceptors respond by

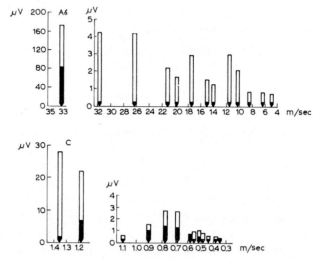

Fig. 2. Nervus saphenus antidromic potentials amplitudes. The potential value after collision of ortho- and antidromic impulses is marked with black colour. Skin receptors were stimulated by scratching with a soft brush. Abscissa axis is for fibre conduction velocity, ordinate axis is for potential amplitudes, mV.

excitation to thermal stimulation (Hunt and McIntyre, 1960; Iggo, 1968 and 1969; Perl, 1968; Chambers *et al.*, 1972). This permitted Kenshalo and Nafe (1962, 1963a and b) to adopt the hypothesis of a common excitation mechanism for thermo- and mechanoreceptors. According to this hypothesis, the main part in stimulation perception is played by the tissues surrounding the receptors and, particularly, by skin smooth muscles. This hypothesis was confirmed by Minut-Sorokhtina's (1972) experiments on subcutaneous vessels' thermoreceptors. Studying the afferent flow in A$\delta$ and C fibres in response to variation of skin temperature we registered contraction of the skin. The experiments showed that under the conditions of isometry and cooling the intact and isolated skin of various animals and of man contracts mainly along Langer's lines. The observation of hair behaviour during skin cooling revealed no change in the hairs' inclination to the skin surface.

Experiments with the skin of various hairless animals (fish, frog, bird, dolphin) were carried out to check the role of pilomotors in the thermal deformation of skin. Contraction of skin during cooling and its relaxation during heating were registered in all cases but skin contraction intensity of different animals was not equal. This permitted us to suppose that skin deformation can depend on collagen contraction. To verify this supposition, similar experiments were carried out in different animals on the tendon fascia which do not contain smooth muscles. It was found that tendon fascia, consisting mostly of collagen bundles, had a contraction intensity much greater than that of other tissues.

However, all these experiments do not exclude the possibility of smooth muscles not connected with hair follicles participating in the thermal deformation of skin. Besides, it can be supposed that during cooling skin collagen becomes such a rigid substance that pilomotors cannot change the hairs' inclination during contraction.

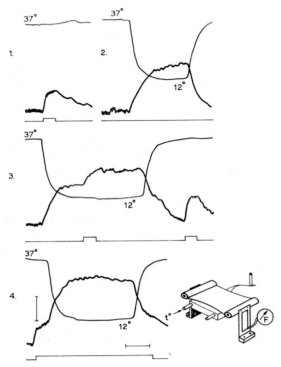

Fig. 3. Cat's skin deformation under: 1: contraction of pilomotors due to the stimulation of C-efferents of skin nerve; 2: cooling the skin, 3: cooling the skin and contraction of pilomotors, and 4: contraction of pilomotors and cooling the skin. From top to bottom: temperature registration, skin deformation force, mark of cutaneous nerve stimulation. Calibration is 10 g and 40 sec. To the right is shown the experiment scheme.

Cat's skin deformation was registered under the common action of these stimuli, skin cooling and pilomotors' efferent stimulation, to verify this supposition (Fig. 3). As can be seen, stimulation of skin nerve efferents caused additional skin contraction on a background of skin contraction, caused by cooling. If the nerve was stimulated before cooling, then skin contraction in response to cooling was observed on a background of skin deformation due to contraction of pilomotors. The total value of skin deformation intensity due to cooling and contraction of pilomotors was always greater than the contraction intensity caused by only one of these factors.

Thus, the results of experiments showed that collagen contracts with lowering of skin temperature. Skin elastin and reticulin fibres cannot, perhaps, participate substantially in the contraction because their number is small (Sokolov, 1973). It can be supposed that collagen is the thermosensitive element in the skin thermoreceptive system. Its deformation excites mechanoreceptors the location of which on collagen bundles has been confirmed histologically by Zazybin (1951) and Semenov (1965). The supposition about the thermoreceptor function of collagen is confirmed by the work on the histology and physiology of Ruffini's body by Chambers et al. (1972). The authors proved that Ruffini's receptor responds to thermal as well as mechanical stimulation. It was found that inside this receptor capsule there are collagen bundles on which the afferent fibre terminals end.

This does not mean that pilomotor contraction during reflex action cannot cause excitation in slowly adapting mechanoreceptors with low excitation threshold. We showed that during contraction of skin pilomotors due to C efferents, stimulation excitation appears in mechanoreceptors innervated by A$\delta$ and C fibres. Twenty per cent of A$\delta$ fibres and from 75 to 95% of C fibres were active. This correlation of activity in fibres is very similar to the pattern of the flow appearing on skin cooling. Perhaps the cat should feel cold during pilomotors' contraction in analogy with the sensation of man at the appearance of "goose-skin" during emotions.

Thus we showed that cat's skin receptors are mechanoreceptors and that they respond to various mechanical stimulations by certain afferent flow patterns. Thermal stimulation causes collagen deformation which is the cause of low threshold mechano-receptor excitation.

## SUMMARY

A conduction velocity spectrum in nerve fibres of 0.15 to 90 m/sec was found by means of electrophysiological methods of analysis and computer-aided processing of experimental data. A greater portion of the non-myelinated fibres in the cutaneous nerve proved to be afferent. Patterns of afferent impulse flows entering the central nervous system are determined under various mechanical and thermal stimulations of cat's cutaneous receptive field. Differences of these flows are considered to be the reasons for various sensation modalities.

The mechanism of cutaneous mechanoreceptor excitation under temperature stimuli is discussed. Special attention is paid to the contraction of cutaneous collagen under cooling. Experimental data on the change of cutaneous mechanical properties and the electrophysiological changes corroborating the thermomechanical hypothesis of receptor excitation are given.

## REFERENCES

ADRIAN, E. D. AND BRONK, D. W. (1928) The discharge of impulses in motor fibres. Part 1. Impulses in single fibres of the phrenic nerve. *J. Physiol. (Lond.)*, **66**, 81–101.

BURGESS, P. R., PETIT, D. AND WARREN, R. M. (1968) Receptor types in cat hairy skin supplied by myelinated fibres. *J. Neurophysiol.*, **31**, 833–848.

CHAMBERS, M. R., ANDRES, K. H., VON DUERING, N. AND IGGO, A. (1972) The structure and function of slowly adapting type II mechanoreceptor in hairy skin. *Quart. J. exp. Physiol.*, **57**, 417–445.

CHERNYGOVSKY, V. N. (1970) *Problems of Physiology of Man and Animals*. Nauka, Leningrad. 239 pp. (in Russian).

DOUGLAS, W. W. AND RITCHIE, J. M. (1957) A technique for recording functional activity in specific groups of myelinated and non-myelinated fibres in whole nerve trunks. *J. Physiol. (Lond.)*, **138**, 19–30.

HENSEL, H. (1966) Classes of receptor units predominantly related to thermal stimuli. In *Touch, Heat and Pain*. Churchill, London. pp. 275–291.

HUNT, C. C. AND MCINTYRE, A. K. (1960) An analysis of fibre diameter and receptor characteristics of myelinated cutaneous afferent fibres in cat. *J. Physiol. (Lond.)*, **153**, 99–112.

IGGO, A. (1966) Cutaneous receptors with a high sensitivity to mechanical displacement. In *Touch, Heat and Pain*. Churchill, London. pp. 237–260.

IGGO, A. (1968) Electrophysiological and histological study of cutaneous mechanoreceptors. In *The Skin Senses*. Thomas, Springfield, Ill. pp. 84–105.

IGOO, A. (1969) Cutaneous thermoreceptors in primates and sub-primates. *J. Physiol. (Lond.)*, **200**, 403–430.

KENSHALO, D. AND NAFE, J. (1962) A quantitative theory of feeling. *Physiol. Rev.*, **62**, 17–33.

KENSHALO, D. AND NAFE, J. (1963a) The peripheral basis of temperature sensitivity in man. *Science and Industry*, **3**, 231–238.

KENSHALO, D. AND NAFE, J. (1963b) Cutaneous vascular system as a model temperature receptor. *Percept. Motor Skills*, **17**, 257–258.

MARUHASHI, J., MIZUGUCHI, K. AND TASAKI, I. (1952) Action current in single afferent nerve fibres elicited by stimulation of the skin of the toad and cat. *J. Physiol. (Lond.)*, **117**, 129–151.

MINUT-SOROKHTINA, O. P. (1972) *Physiology of Thermoreception*. Meditsina, Moscow. 268 pp. (In Russian).

PERL, E. R. (1968) Myelinated afferent fibres innervating the primate skin and their response to noxious stimuli. *J. Physiol. (Lond.)*, **197**, 593–615.

SEMENOV, S. P. (1965) *Morphology of Autonomic Nerve System and Interoreceptors*. State University Publishers, Leningrad, 160 pp. (In Russian.)

SOKOLOV, V. E. (1973) *Cutaneous Covering of Mammals*. Nauka, Moscow, 487 pp. (In Russian.)

ZAZYBIN, N. I. (1951) Innervation of extracellular substances. *Usp. sovr. biol.*, **31**, 427–432 (in Russian.)

ZEVEKE, A. V. AND KHAYUTIN, V. M. (1966) Measuring frequency spectrum of afferent impulses in a whole nerve trunk. *J. Physiol. (U.S.S.R.)*, **52**, 258–264.

ZEVEKE, A. V. AND GLADYSHEVA, O. S. (1969) Variation of frequency spectrum in myelinized afferent fibres of the Aδ group in the case of stimulation of skin receptors. *Dokl. Acad. Nauk USSR*, **189**, 1150–1153

ZEVEKE, A. V., MYADEROV, V. I., UTKIN, V. A. AND SHAPOSHNIKOV, V. L. (1973a) Medullated fibres of cat skin nerve with a slow conduction velocity. *Bull. exp. Biol. Med.*, **76**, 6–9 (in Russian).

ZEVEKE, A. V., MYADEROV, V. I., UTKIN, V. A. AND SHAPOSHNIKOV, V. L. (1973b) Conduction velocity in the nonmedullated nerve fibers of the skin nerve. *Bull. exp. Biol. Med.*, **76**, 6–9 (in Russian).

ZOTTERMAN, Y. (1939) Touch, pain and tickling: An electrophysiological investigation on sensory nerves. *J. Physiol. (Lond.)*, **95**, 1–28.

## DISCUSSION

TSIRULNIKOV: How do you correlate your results with the conceptions of specificity of receptors?

ZEVEKE: One cannot determine specificity of separate receptor units using the colliding impulses methods. We determined afferent flows from the whole cutaneous receptor field where impulses from both specific and polymodal receptors seemed to be recorded.

PERL: Why did you use the method that did not permit you to separate two fibres? Using the Douglas and Ritchie method you repeated their errors.

ZEVEKE: If you mean the determination of warm and cold fibres that must compensate the amplitude of evoked potential under variable temperature of skin then, considering the results of numerous authors, the hairy skin of cat's hindleg seems to have no warm receptors. We know of the limitation of the colliding impulses method and the criticism of this method in 1959. Indeed, this method does not allow the functional differentiation of two afferent fibres to be found. And it is not what we tried to do. Our report presents the dynamics of afferent flow in the whole nerve under various stimulations of skin receptors.

KHAYUTIN: The determination of nature of impulse flows in the whole nerve under stimulation of skin by four different stimuli appears to be very interesting indeed.

# The Structure and Function of the Infrared Receptors of Snakes

R. C. GORIS AND S. TERASHIMA

*Department of Physiology, Tokyo Medical and Dental University, Tokyo (Japan)*

## INTRODUCTION

In the animal kingdom, infrared receptors are known to be possessed only by certain snakes, *viz.*, the Boidae and the subfamily Crotalinae of the highly venomous family Viperidae. In the Boidae the receptors exist in a rather generalized form. In some, for example *Boa constrictor*, infrared reception is present in certain labial or snout areas without any externally visible organ. In others, there may be a series of pits along the upper lips, or along the lower lips, or across the snout, or various combinations of these series. All are innervated by various branches of the trigeminal nerve.

In the Crotalinae the receptors have acquired a much more highly specialized form (Fig. 1). In these snakes there is a prominent pit on each side of the face in the area between the nostril and the eye. The pit opening is generally smaller than the eye, but considerably larger than the nostril. The openings of the nostrils are generally directed sideways or backwards, but the pit openings are directed forward. Internally the pit expands to a diameter somewhat larger than the diameter of the external opening, and an extremely fine membrane divides the cavity into two chambers. This

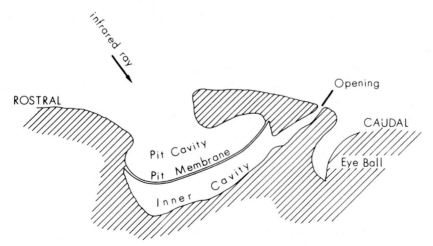

Fig. 1. Schematic sagittal section through the infrared receptor ("pit organ" or "pit") of a pit viper.

membrane is the sensory element of the pit. When illuminated by an external light source, it has the appearance of a tympanum without attached ossicles.


MATERIALS AND METHODS

In our laboratory we studied infrared reception in the following snakes: *Trimeresurus flavoviridis* and *T. okinavensis* from the Ryukyu Is., *Agkistrodon blomhoffi blomhoffi* from mainland Japan, and *A. blomhoffi brevicaudus* and *A. caliginosus* from the Korean peninsula.

The snakes were immobilized with tubocurarine chloride. For *T. flavoviridis* a dose of 0.13 mg/kg was used. For *T. okinavensis* as much as 200 mg/kg of body weight had to be used. The snakes of the genus *Agkistrodon* were even more difficult to immobilize. An initial large dose causes eventual death. Therefore, snakes of this genus were first anesthetized with Fluothane. The snake was put into a bottle of 5 liter capacity, and a cotton ball soaked in Fluothane was dropped into the bottle, which was then covered tightly. Usually the snake was immobilized within 5–6 min. Next a hole was opened in the pulmonary air sac by cutting through the intracostal muscles at an appropriate position. A stream of air was directed into the lungs through a cannula inserted into the glottis. The air was obtained from a very small aquarium pump, and was first bubbled through water for moisturization. Air flow was regulated with a valve. Once respiration was initiated, 0.075 mg of curare was injected intramuscularly, which is approximately 0.75–2.5 mg/kg of body weight, depending on the size of the snake. Some individuals required several such doses for complete immobilization.

As an infrared stimulus we used various incandescent lamps. However, the handiest and most easily used stimulus was the human hand. When recording was being done from the brain, the surest way to distinguish between infrared fibers and optical fibers was to put out the lights of the room and wave the hand in the receptive field of the pits. Only infrared fibers responded to such methods. For stimulation with pure infrared rays, a bandpass filter was inserted in front of the incandescent lamp.

In order to obtain slow potentials and action potentials from the sensory membrane of the pit, both metal and glass capillary electrodes were used. In order to obtain responses from the trigeminal nerve, single fibers were dissected out from the trunk bundle and lifted on a silver wire hook, taking care to keep the fiber moist. For obtaining responses from the tectum opticum, EEGs could be obtained with any metal wire; but for discrete, single-unit action potentials, it was necessary to use microcapillary glass electrodes filled with an electrolyte such as 3 $M$ KCl.


RECEPTOR STRUCTURE

*Macrostructure*

The sensory membrane is suspended inside the pit cavity. It is more or less concave in shape, and in *Trimeresurus flavoviridis* it is thinnest (15 μm) at the center, becoming thicker toward the edges, where it is attached to the walls of the cavity. The diameter of the membrane varies according to the species, but in *T. flavoviridis* it is about 7 mm. The membrane is innervated by the ophthalmic and supramaxillary divisions of the trigeminal nerve. The supramaxillary is divided into a deep and a superficial branch. The ophthalmic division enters the membrane dorsally, the superficial branch lateroventrally, and the deep branch medioventrally. Each branch breaks up into several nerve bundles as it enters the membrane. As these bundles progress towards the center of the membrane, they divide and subdivide to the point where they cease to be visible. A network of capillaries is also visible, but the orientation of the capillaries apparently is unrelated to the orientation of the nerve fibers.

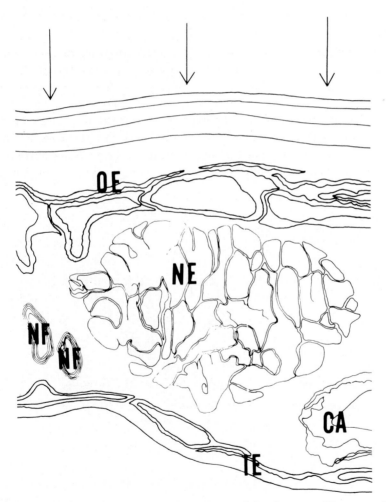

Fig. 2. Schematic cross-section of the sensory membrane of the pit organ. OE, outer epithelium; NE, nerve ending; CA, capillary; NF, nerve fiber; IE, inner epithelium. Arrows indicate arriving infrared radiation.

*Microstructure*

Seen in cross-section (Fig. 2), the membrane presents the aspects of a nerve layer sandwiched between two layers of epithelium. The outer, or external, epithelium is thicker than the epithelium on the inner side of the nerve layer, and the cornified layer of this outer epithelium is sloughed off together with the old epidermis of the whole body each time the snake sheds. The cornified layer of the inner epithelium is also shed at this time, passing through a pore in front of the eye. Immediately beneath the outer epithelium there is a single layer of non-overlapping free nerve endings. Below these lie the nerve bundles and the capillary bed. Among the free endings are numbers of cell nuclei, which seem at first sight to be the nuclei of receptor cells; in actuality, they are the nuclei of Schwann cells.

*Ultramicrostructure (Fig. 3)*

The myelinated nerve fibers which run along the bottom of the nerve layer of the membrane lose the myelin sheath abruptly at a certain point; beyond this point the axon begins to increase in volume and branch upwards. Then it divides into numerous fine branchlets. These branchlets entwine themselves among the fine processes given off by an aggregation of several Schwann cells, with the result that a terminal nerve mass is formed with the Schwann cells in the interior of the mass and the nerve branchlets on the exterior facing the outer chamber of the pit. Some of the branchlets are completely bare, while others are covered with a thin layer of Schwann cell

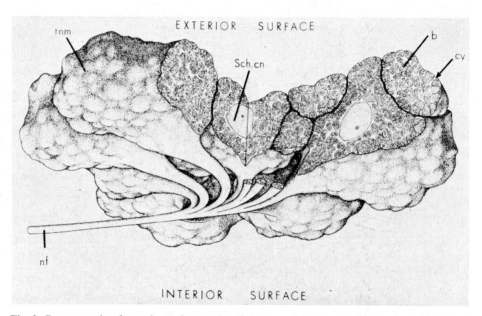

Fig. 3. Reconstruction from photomicrographs of a group of the terminal nerve masses which act as infrared receptors in the pit organ membrane. b, branchlet; cy, Schwann cell cytoplasm; nf, nerve fiber; Sch.cn, Schwann cell nucleus; tnm, terminal nerve mass.

cytoplasm. It seems that the Schwann cells have no direct part in the generation of response potentials. Mitochondriogenesis begins to occur at the point where the nerve fiber loses its sheath, and from this point on to the terminal nerve mass abundant mitochondria appear. The mass of these mitochondria replace the axoplasmic neuro-filaments to the extent that the neurofilaments become almost impossible to see. When strong infrared radiation is applied to the pit receptors, the mitochondria in the nerve endings have a configuration which is different from that of mitochondria before stimulation. The conglomeration of branchlets and Schwann cells ("terminal nerve mass") has a diameter of about 40 $\mu$m. The terminal nerve masses are arranged in a single layer without overlapping one another. Inside the pit membrane there are no synapses or tight junctions, and there are no terminal structures other than the abundant terminal nerve masses.

### COMPOSITION OF THE NERVES SUPPLYING THE RECEPTOR MEMBRANE

The three branches of the trigeminal nerve which supply the receptor membrane differ somewhat in number of fibers and fiber thickness from one species to another and from one individual to another. Bullock and Fox counted the number of nerve fibers in a rattlesnake, *Crotalus horridus*, of a total length of 965 mm. At a point several millimeters before entering the pit, the ophthalmic branch had 815 fibers, the superficial branch of the supramaxillary division 2921, and the deep branch 3538. This makes a total of 7274 nerve fibers entering the pit. Other individual specimens had totals of 8254, 6626, and 7410. These fibers varied from 3 to 16 $\mu$m in thickness, with the majority showing a thickness of about 7 $\mu$m. Nearly all of these fibers are warm fibers.

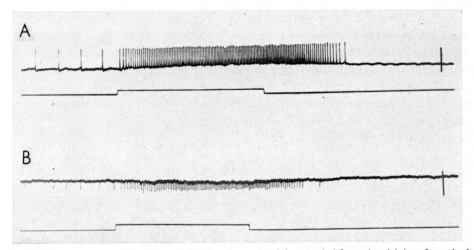

Fig. 4. Generator potentials with associated action potentials recorded from the vicinity of terminal nerve masses in the pit organ sensory membrane. A: positive-going potentials. B: negative-going potentials. Vertical line at right indicates 3 mV. Relation of the slow potential change to the super-imposed spikes and to the stimulus is clearly seen.

*References p. 170*

## ELECTROPHYSIOLOGY OF THE PIT MEMBRANE

It was not possible to record electric potentials from the intact membrane, but the outer cornified layer of the epidermis could be stripped off, and in this state a glass microelectrode could be pushed into the nerve layer, where both spike potentials and slow potentials could be recorded. The spike potentials often appeared imposed on the slow potentials (Fig. 4). Both were of the same polarity, which was negative-going in most cases. Depending on the position and depth of penetration of the electrode, at times only spike potentials, or only slow potentials could be recorded.

There was no latency in the slow potentials, and their amplitude changed in proportion to the stimulus intensity. When the membrane was irradiated evenly over its entire surface, slow potentials could be recorded from any location on the membrane. If a portion of the membrane was shaded, potentials could be recorded from the irradiated portion, but not from the shaded portion. These slow potentials were judged to be the generator potential of the infrared receptor, principally for the following reasons: (1) they were graded in proportion to the stimulus; (2) they were non-propagated, and recordable only from the membrane and (3) they were directly connected with the production of action potentials, as will be explained in the next paragraph.

Spike potentials were recorded either alone or in connection with the generator potential. When they were imposed on the generator potential, they appeared after a latency of 10–50 msec, depending on the intensity of the stimulus. Their frequency increased in proportion to the depth of the generator potential, and they disappeared together with it. When the electrode was inserted into the membrane in the vicinity of bundles of nerves, spike potentials alone were often recorded. In the absence of any particular stimulation, there was a background discharge averaging 4–5 spikes/sec, although units showing a frequency of as much as 10/sec were occasionally recorded. When an infrared stimulus was applied, this frequency increased in proportion to the intensity of the stimulus, up to a certain point, as will be described below for recordings from the peripheral nerve fibers. For example, when radiation of 9.74 mW/sq.cm was applied, the discharge increased to a frequency of 120/sec. If the stimulus was cut off at this point, the impulses decreased gradually for a short period of time and then ceased abruptly. Cessation was followed by several seconds of silence, after which background discharge resumed.

## ELECTROPHYSIOLOGY OF THE TRIGEMINAL NERVE

When a single fiber of the trigeminal nerve leading to the pit is dissected out and lifted on a metal electrode, three types of response patterns can be recorded. First, in the absence of any particular stimulus, a background discharge of 4–5 spikes/sec is recorded. Second, when a stimulus such as the human hand is brought into the field of the pit, a sharp increase in firing is recorded, which after a few seconds begins to show a certain amount of adaptation. If the stimulus is increased, say by increasing the voltage to an incandescent lamp in the receptive field, the firing increases still more, up to a rate of about 100/sec. When the stimulus is increased beyond this point, the third type of response is noted, namely, a sharp burst of firing at the onset of the stimulus, followed by a period of silence, followed by another burst of firing when the stimulus ceases.

When ice is brought into the response field of the pit, the ever-present background discharge disappears. When the ice is removed, a burst of responses occurs. This indicates that the environmental background also functions as a radiant heat stimulus, to which the pit gradually adapts. The pit responds to changes in the background radiation. Thus, even when ice is held for a long time in the field of the pit, adaptation gradually occurs; and when the ice is removed, the pit responds to the suddenly renewed warm radiation from the background.

It is interesting to compare the response of the pit warm fibers with that of the warm fibers of other animals. The warm fibers of animals such as the rat and the cat show a constant response to any particular temperature, and thus can function as detectors of the temperature of the internal environment. In contrast to this, because adaptation occurs, the snake cannot distinguish particular temperatures, for example, perceiving the difference between 20 °C and 30 °C. In other words, the information conveyed by the pit receptor is entirely about the external environment, and concerns external heat fluctuations.

## ELECTROPHYSIOLOGY OF THE TECTUM OPTICUM

### Evoked potentials

When the tectum opticum is exposed and an electrode is placed in contact with the surface of the tectum, an evoked potential of about 250 $\mu$V is recorded in response to an incandescent lamp placed in front of the snake and exposed at regular intervals with a camera shutter. If the snake's eyes are then covered with black paint, this large evoked potential disappears, indicating that it was an optical response. However, a smaller potential with fewer oscillations remains, which cannot be made to disappear unless both pits are filled with paint or a similar substance. Thus, this smaller potential is shown to be directly connected with the function of the pits.

### Localization

When a microelectrode is inserted perpendicularly into the tectum a layer of cells is encountered at a depth of about 200 $\mu$m which respond to infrared stimulation of the pits. Single units responding to infrared stimulation can be encountered both above and below this layer, but this layer is the place where mass (multiple-unit) response can most easily be recorded with a microcapillary electrode. This indicates a heavy concentration of cells or fibers responding to infrared stimulation. In the tectum opticum units responding to light, movement of the body joints, and vibration, and

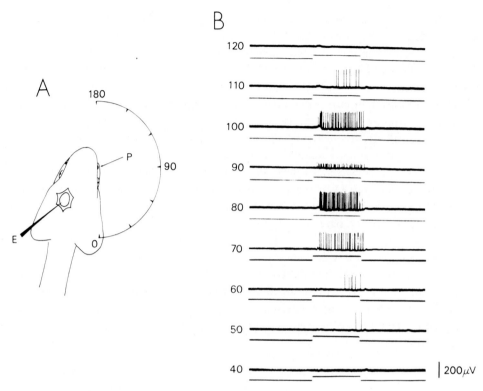

Fig. 5. Action potentials recorded from a single neuron in the tectum opticum when the stimulus source was moved in a horizontal arc as shown in A. E symbolizes the electrode; arrow P indicates the location of the pit organ. Numbers indicate the position of the stimulus in degrees. Lower trace of each position indicates the stimulus; duration is 1 sec. Lowered height of spikes at 90 degrees is due to slight movement of the electrode.

units whose normal stimulus is unknown can also be recorded. However, the existence of units which show interaction with infrared units has not yet been ascertained. We identify infrared units by the fact that they show a response to the movement of a hand in the response field of the pit, even in pitch darkness, but do not show any response to light movement or intensity fluctuations.

### Mode of response

The background discharge of infrared units in the tectum are lower in frequency and more irregular than peripheral discharge, and adaptation is faster. As a general rule discharge frequency increases when infrared stimulation is applied, but units responding only to ON, units responding to both ON and OFF, units showing slow adaptation, units showing habituation, etc. are also encountered. It seems that some of these response modes depend on the position and direction of the stimulus (Fig. 5), while some units may be unimodal.

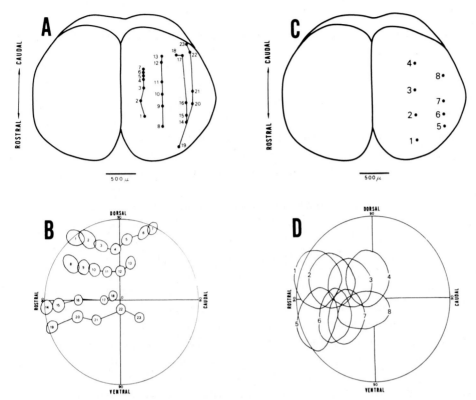

Fig. 6. Tectal organization of visual and infrared neurons in pit vipers. A and B: organization of visual neurons. A shows the two lobes of the tectum opticum, and the numbered dots indicate successive penetrations of the electrode. The numbered circles in B indicate the receptive fields of the neurons recorded by the corresponding penetrations of A. C and D show in the same way the topical organization of infrared neurons. The infrared receptive fields are much larger and more overlapping than visual fields.

## Laterality

Most units respond only to stimulation of the contralateral pit; however, bilaterally responding units, that is units which respond to stimulation of either the ipsilateral or the contralateral pit, are also encountered. It is not known whether there are also units which respond only to ipsilateral stimulation. The normal bilateral unit shows increasing discharge to increasing infrared stimulation, both on the ipsi- and contralateral sides. However, the mode of response is not the same for both sides. Generally, stimulation of one side will produce a response consisting of a relatively long pulse train, while stimulation of the opposite side will produce an ON burst followed by relatively few spikes. Both pulse trains and ON bursts may appear on either side, depending on the particular unit. In some types of bilateral units, heat stimulation of the ipsilateral side produces a *decrease* in background discharge, while ice produces an *increase* in background discharge. The ipsi- and contralateral response fields of this type of bilateral unit do not necessarily overlap in front of the snake. In fact, in one example measured, the two fields were separated by a space of 60 degrees in front of the snout.

## Receptive fields

In *Trimeresurus flavoviridis* the receptive field of individual units varied between 30 degrees and 80 degrees both in a vertical and horizontal sense, with an average of 58 degrees for the vertical and 55 degrees for the horizontal. In *Agkistrodon blomhoffi brevicaudus* the receptive fields showed an average of 35 degrees in both a horizontal and vertical sense. There is the possibility of an interspecific difference here, but it is not necessarily so, for the methods used to measure the two species were slightly different.

## Topical organization

As in other animals, so too in the pit vipers, visual responses in the tectum opticum show a retinotopic organization; that is, a light stimulus reaching a definite portion of the retina from a definite portion of the visual receptive field is recordable only in a clearly defined area of the tectum (Fig. 6A and B). The receptive field of the pits is reflected in the same way at the surface of the tectum (Fig. 6C and D). That is, the upper part of the receptive field is projected medially on the tectum, and the lower part laterally. The rostral part of the receptive field is projected rostrally on the tectum, and as the stimulus moves caudad, its projection on the tectum also moves caudad. While the visual fields recordable at each point on the tectum averaged about 10 degrees in diameter, infrared fields averaged about 60 degrees.

### SIGNIFICANCE OF THE PITS: ECOLOGICAL CONSIDERATIONS

Among the fishes and the reptiles, the tectum opticum is proportionately larger in those animals which rely primarily on vision for their daily activities. For example, it is known that the tectum opticum is larger in fish that normally live in clear water than in those that spend their lives in muddy water. It is also known that the tectum is larger in snakes that are active by day than in those that are primarily nocturnal. However, there are exceptions to this rule. *Trimeresurus flavoviridis* is a primarily nocturnal snake, yet it has a large, well-developed tectum. This can be explained by the fact that the brain cells which integrate the information from the pits are concentrated here. In *Agkistrodon blomhoffi brevicaudus* the receptive fields of the right and left pits overlap at a point slightly more than 1 cm in front of the snout. The angle of overlap is about 25 degrees. Therefore, within the area of overlap, it is possible for the snake to have stereoscopic perception of an object and to estimate its distance from the snake. However, it must not be thought that the sole function of the tectum opticum is depth perception in the area of overlap. There are single units in the tectum which respond over a field exceeding 180 degrees in extent. Among these units there are some bilateral units which have separate left and right receptive fields which do not overlap in front. The snake probably uses the pit receptors for the detection of meaningful moving objects in its field of infrared vision.

Just as it is possible for the human ear to detect and distinguish a musical melody from a background of noise, so it seems possible for the snake to detect and follow the movements of a discrete infrared source against a background of random noise radiation. Just as sound serves to attract the attention of animals (and men) who possess normal hearing, it seems possible that the units receiving information from the extreme periphery of the snake's infrared receptive field serve the purpose of attracting the attention of the snake to the movement of infrared objects in these areas.

Snakes feed on both cold-blooded and warm-blooded prey. In the case of birds and mammals, the body temperature, and consequently the heat radiation, is normally higher than the environmental background. In the case of reptiles, the body temperature is usually either higher or lower than the environment, depending on the preferred body temperature of the species. In the case of most amphibians, the body temperature is usually lower than the environment because of the evaporation of moisture from the skin. Thus, most of the prey animals of the snake will normally show a radiation difference with regard to the background. Thus the pit receptors provide the snake with an efficient means of detecting and capturing prey by means of an infrared image in situations where the other important senses such as the eyes are hampered, as in the darkness of the night.

## SUMMARY

The pit vipers (Serpentes, Crotalinae) possess in the loreal region of the face a pair of pits which function as infrared receptors. Inside each pit is a sensory membrane heavily innervated by branches of the trigeminal nerve. The receptors contained in the membrane are masses of nude nerve branchlets surrounding several Schwann cells at the tip of numerous non-myelinated nerve fibers. These "terminal nerve masses" lie just under the outer epithelium of the sensory membrane and face in the direction of incoming infrared radiation. In response to infrared stimulation, generator and action potentials have been recorded from the sensory membrane, action potentials from the peripheral nerves, and both action and evoked potentials from the tectum opticum of the brain. The peripheral nerves show spontaneous firing, which increases in response to infrared stimulation and decreases or disappears in response to a cold stimulus. Central neurons show similar firing patterns, but with faster adaptation and great sensitivity to movement. The receptive field of central neurons is about 50–60 degrees in diameter. On the surface of the tectum there is a topic organization of the receptive fields similar to the retinotopic organization of the visual system. It is concluded that the pits function as receptors supplementary to the visual system in situations where vision is hampered, as in the dark.

*References p. 170*

## REFERENCES

BARRETT, R. (1969) *Central Neural Response to Radiant Heat in Certain Snakes.* Doctoral Dissertation, University of California, Los Angeles.

BLEICHMAR, H. AND DE ROBERTIS, E. (1962) Submicroscopic morphology of the infrared receptor of pit vipers. *Z. Zellforsch.*, **56**, 748–761.

BULLOCK, T. H. AND BARRETT, R. (1969) Radiant heat reception in snakes. *Commun. Behav. Biol.* Part A. **1**, 19–29.

BULLOCK, T. H. AND DIECKE, P. J. (1956) Properties of an infrared receptor. *J. Physiol. (Lond.)*, **134**, 47–87.

BULLOCK, T. H. AND FOX, W. (1957) The anatomy of the infrared sense organ in the facial pit of pit vipers. *Quart. J. microsc. Sci.*, **98**, 219–234.

DE ROBERTIS, E. AND BLEICHMAR, H. (1962) Mitochondriogenesis in nerve fibers of the infrared receptor membrane of pit vipers. *Z. Zellforsch.*, **57**, 572–582.

GAMOW, R. I. AND HARRIS, J. F. (1973) The infrared receptors of snakes. *Sci. Amer.*, **228**, 94–100.

GORIS, R. C. AND NOMOTO, M. (1967) Infrared reception in oriental Crotaline snakes. *Comp. Biochem. Physiol.*, **23**, 879–892.

GORIS, R. C. AND TERASHIMA, S. (1973) Central response to infrared stimulation of the pit receptors in a Crotaline snake, *Trimeresurus flavoviridis. J. exp. Biol.*, **58**, 59–76.

HARRIS, J. F. AND GAMOW, R. I. (1971) Snake infrared receptors: thermal or photochemical mechanism? *Science*, **172**, 1252–1253.

LYNN, W. G. (1931) Structure and function of the facial pit of the pit vipers. *Amer. J. Anat.*, **49**, 97–139.

MASAI, H. (1975) Structural patterns of the optic tectum in Japanese snakes of the family Colubridae, in relation to habit. *J. Hirnforsch.*, **14**, 367–374.

MASAI, H. AND SATO, Y. (1965) The brain patterns in relation to behavior in fish hybrids. *Naturwissenschaften*, **52**, 43–44.

NOBLE, G. K. AND SCHMIT, A. (1937) Structure and function of the facial and labial pits of snakes. *Proc. Amer. phil. Soc.*, **77**, 263–288.

TERASHIMA, S., GORIS, R. C. AND KATSUKI, Y. (1968) Generator potential of Crotaline snake infrared receptor. *J. Neurophysiol.*, **31**, 682–688.

TERASHIMA, S., GORIS, R. C. AND KATSUKI, Y. (1970) Structure of warm fiber terminals in the pit membrane of vipers. *J. ultrastr. Res.*, **31**, 494–506.

WARREN, J. W. AND PROSKE, U. (1968) Infrared receptors in the facial pits of the Australian python *Morelia spilotes. Science*, **159**, 439–441.

## DISCUSSION

HENSEL: Did you account for the air temperature or the steady temperature of the membrane and did you make any experiments with changed background temperature of the membrane and perhaps observing different thalamic sensitivities as have been shown by Dubois?

GORIS: Yes, we did. The reaction was always relative, for example, if the air temperature was 23 °C, background temperature is supposedly 23 °C, anything less than 23 °C in the receptive field of the pit would cause a decrease in firing and an object of more than 23 °C would cause an increase in firing. And we tried this. We took a piece of heavy aluminum plate, heated the plate to 60 °C, then put it into the field of the pit and allowed the response to adapt to a normal level of spontaneous firing. The plate was 60 °C, at that temperature my hand, of course, is cooler than the plate. My hand was inserted between the plate and the pit. There was a decrease in firing just the same as if we have taken ice and put it in front of the pit at normal room temperatures.

BURGESS: Do you have any behavioral evidence that the snake can orient accurately to a thermal stimulus?

GORIS: Yes, plenty of them. Since the snake has scales over the eyes, it is very easy to blind the snake without causing any trauma. We have put heavy black paint on the eyes, then any warm stimulus or a stimulus that the snake could normally bite or strike at will cause a strike in spite of the fact that the snake is blind. The sensitivity is such that the snake is able to change the direction of its strike in mid-strike if you move the stimulus after he has initiated his strike.

SESSION IV

# MECHANORECEPTOR MECHANISMS

# Morphofunctional Properties of Pacinian Corpuscles

O. B. ILYINSKY, N. K. VOLKOVA, V. L. CHEREPNOV AND B. V. KRYLOV

*Laboratory of General Physiology of Reception, I. P. Pavlov Institute of Physiology, Academy of Sciences of the U.S.S.R., Leningrad (U.S.S.R.)*

The correlation between the functional aspects of tissue receptors and their structure is of great importance for an understanding of both the receptor activity and the functioning of the afferent systems of the inner organs and skin (Chernigovsky, 1960). The Pacinian corpuscles were taken for investigation as typical tissue receptors.

## METHODS

Experiments were carried out on single Pacinian corpuscles isolated from the mesentery and pancreas of cats. Receptor and action potentials were recorded by methods previously described (Ilyinsky, 1963 and 1966a). Mechanical stimulus with a special device (Ilyinsky and Kudrin, 1967) was applied to the receptors and displacements were recorded with the aid of an inductive system. In some cases following the electrophysiological part of the experiment the site of mechanical stimulation was labelled with ammoniacal silver prepared on $20\%$ AgNO$_3$. The structure of the Pacinian corpuscle was studied with an optical microscope (the Campos method) and an electron microscope (with fixation in $1\%$ OsO$_4$ in alkaline phosphate buffer, pH 7.1–7.4, and embedded in Araldite or Epon). Sections were contrasted with uranyl acetate and lead.

## RESULTS

### On- and off-responses

Pacinian corpuscles reacted with on- and off-responses to a long-lasting mechanical stimulus (Gray and Sato, 1953; Ilyinsky, 1962 and 1963), with thresholds and latencies varying not only in different, but in one and the same receptor. Analysis revealed (Ilyinsky, 1966a) that the off-responses were due to mechanical properties of the receptors capsule (whenever the receptor was decapsulated, the off-responses were absent).

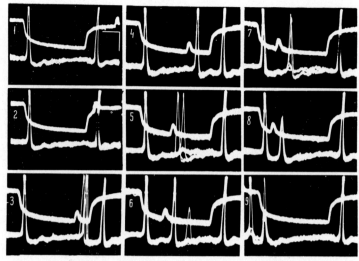

Fig. 1. Changes in the excitability of Pacinian corpuscles in the course of long-lasting deformation (Ilyinsky, 1966b). 1–9: successive changing responses to a short test stimulus of threshold intensity. Calibration: 4 msec and 200 $\mu$V.

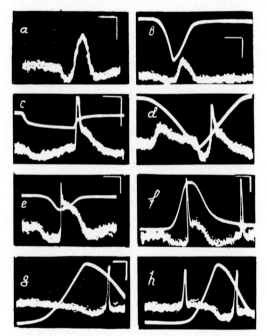

Fig. 2. Hyperpolarizing receptor potentials from 7 different corpuscles. From Ilyinsky, 1963 for a; 1965 for b, d and f; 1966c for e; 1966b for g and h.

The capsule of Pacinian corpuscles is a multilayer lamellar structure with a good elasticity. From this it follows that when a mechanical stimulus is applied to the receptor the nerve ending is compressed first in one direction, and later, when the stimulus is removed, the nerve ending, due to the elastic properties of the capsule, is deformed in a new direction perpendicular to the former one. This gives rise respectively to on- and off-responses. With a receptor of high excitability several spikes can be recorded in response to a stimulus of a great strength. In such a case the multiplied responses of the Pacinian corpuscle are due to repeated oscillations of capsular layers (Ilyinsky, 1965 and 1966a). With a long-lasting stimulation of moderate intensity the mechanical oscillation in the capsule leads only to undulating changes in receptor excitability (Fig. 1). Hyperpolarizing receptor potentials can also contribute to the appearance of the rhythmical discharges (post-hyperpolarizing responses; Ilyinsky, 1966b and c).

*Hyperpolarizing receptor potentials. Directional sensitivity*

Positive responses can appear along with depolarizing receptor potentials (Fig. 2) (Ilyinsky, 1963; Ozeki and Sato, 1965). More details concerning this type of response are given elsewhere (Ilyinsky, 1965).

It is known (see, for example, Pease and Quilliam, 1957) that the unmyelinated nerve ending in a Pacinian corpuscle has the shape of an elliptical cylinder. Again, on adequate stimulation, inner core displacements occur only in the radial direction (Hubbard, 1958). From these facts Hubbard concluded that the ratio of the two inner core axes should change at the moment of stimulation, thus leading (with constant volume of a cylinder) to a change in the surface of the nerve ending membrane. Therefore, it may be concluded that excitation of Pacinian corpuscles is based

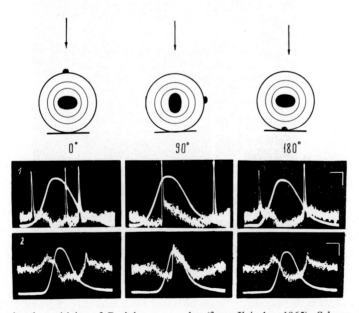

Fig. 3. Directional sensitivity of Pacinian corpuscles (from Ilyinsky, 1965). Scheme at the top: the relation between direction of the stimulus and position of the nerve ending. Bottom records: two different corpuscles. Action potentials in set 2 are blocked by procaine. Calibration: 4 msec; 1–10 $\mu$V (upper); 2–5 $\mu$V (lower record).

on the increase in the surface membrane area of the nerve ending. It should be noted, however, that it is only when the nerve ending is deformed along its minor transverse axis that the surface membrane area can increase, whereas the deformation of the nerve ending along its major axis leads to a decrease in area of the surface membrane. Proceeding from this idea it was proposed that depolarization might be the result of an increase in the surface area while the hyperpolarization might result from a corresponding decrease, *i.e.* there may exist in the Pacinian corpuscle a directional sensitivity (Ilyinsky, 1965).

According to this hypothesis a mechanical stimulus applied along the minor transverse axis results in the appearance of depolarizing receptor potential and action potential, whereas the hyperpolarizing response is due to stimulation applied along the major transverse axis of the nerve ending. When the Pacinian corpuscle is rotated along the longitudinal axis, the depolarizing responses change to hyperpolarizing and *vice versa* (see detail in Fig. 3). Conclusions based on the electrophysiological evidence were confirmed by the results of histological investigations (Ilyinsky and Volkova, 1966; Ilyinsky *et al.*, 1968). When the receptors were labelled as described above (see Methods), depolarizing responses in all cases were found to appear when the receptor

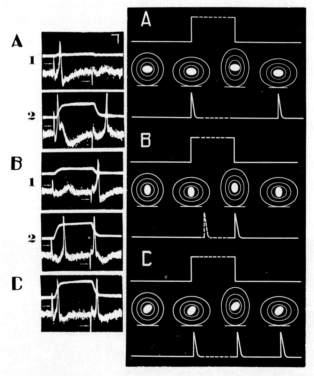

Fig. 4. Effect of the stimulus direction on the on- and off-responses (from Ilyinsky, 1966b). To the right: a scheme to explain the responses of Pacinian corpuscles to onset and offset of stimulation according to the position of a nerve ending. To the left: responses of receptors. In record 2 the stimulation amplitude was increased. A, B and C on the left correspond to the same notation on the right. Arrows: artefacts of stimulation. Calibration: 2 msec and 20 $\mu$V.

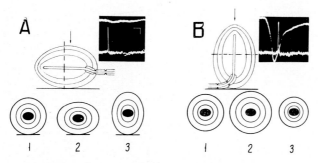

Fig. 5. Changes in thresholds with stimulus direction (from Ilyinsky et al., 1968). Top: records of responses to stimulus of threshold. Centre: position of receptors. Bottom: schemes to represent the cross-section. 1: without stimulation. 2: onset of stimulation. 3: end of stimulation. Calibration: 2 msec and 50 μV.

was stimulated along the minor transverse axis of its nerve ending, and primary hyperpolarization was observed only with a mechanical stimulus applied along the major transverse axis of the nerve ending. It should be remembered that the nerve ending is deformed twice due to the elastic properties of the capsule: the depolarization is followed by hyperpolarization and *vice versa*. This phenomenon explains, in particular, the observed variations in the latencies of the on- and off-responses (Fig. 4).

Experiments with stimulation along the longitudinal axis provide further support for the hypothesis that excitation of Pacinian corpuscles is based on the stretching of the surface membrane of the nerve ending (Fig. 5). Under the usual stimulation conditions the direction of mechanical strength is always perpendicular to the longitudinal axis of the nerve ending, and the threshold is low (Fig. 5A). If, however, the corpuscle is placed so that the direction of stimulation coincides with the longitudinal axis of the receptor (Fig. 5B), *i.e.* the receptor membrane is hard to stretch, the increase in threshold can be as much as 10 times or even more. Thus there is every reason to suppose that excitation of the Pacinian corpuscles is actually based on the stretching of the nerve ending surface membrane. As for the elliptical form of the nerve ending, the receptor's sensitivity to direction of stimulation applied is entirely due to this property. These results were confirmed by other authors (Nishi and Sato, 1968).

*Shape of the nerve ending and sensitivity of Pacinian corpuscles to mechanical stimulation*

We postulated on the basis of our results that the shape of the nerve ending in the Pacinian corpuscle has a direct bearing on the mechanism of activity of this mechanoreceptor. It was then reasonable to suppose that the nerve ending has an optimal shape, *i.e.* that one which offers the highest sensitivity of the system to mechanical stimulus. This problem was further approached by mathematical and morphological methods.

It may be assumed that at the moment of stimulation the volume and length of the nerve ending do not change. The degree of stretching of the membrane can then be

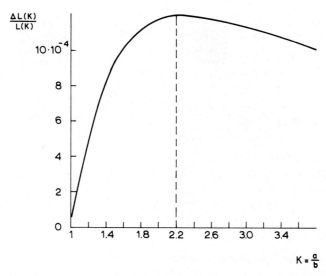

Fig. 6. The fractional change of perimeter with change of axes ratio for an ellipse of constant area.
Abscissa: k = a/b; ordinate:

$$\frac{\Delta L(K)}{L(K)} = \frac{1}{L(K)} \cdot \frac{dL(K)}{dK} \cdot \frac{\Delta K}{1!} + \frac{1}{L(K)} \cdot \frac{d^2L(K)}{dK^2} \cdot \frac{\Delta K^2}{2!}$$

where
$L(K) \approx \sqrt{\pi S} \cdot (\sqrt{K} + 1/\sqrt{K}) [1 + (K - 1)^2/4 \cdot (K + 1)^2 +$
$(K - 1)^4/64 \cdot (K + 1)^4 + (K - 1)^6/256 \cdot (K + 1)^6 + 25 \cdot (K - 1)^8/16384 \cdot (K + 1)^8]$
L(k), elliptical perimeter; $\Delta$L(k), its increment; a, semi-major axis; b, semi-minor axis; S, a given
area of an ellipse, here assumed to be a constant.

determined, in the final analysis, from changes in the perimeter of the transverse
section of the nerve ending, which is of an elliptical shape. Having denoted the perimeter of an ellipse as L, its change on stimulation due to changes in the major and
minor axes as $\Delta$L then the relationship between the relative perimeter change and
the axis ratio k = a/b (a and b being a semi-major and semi-minor transverse axis,
respectively) can be expressed as shown in Fig. 6. The digital computer analysis of
the relationship presented in Fig. 6 carried out in the second order of small quantities,
gave a maximum with k equal to about 2.2 (Ilyinsky *et al.*, 1968; Ilyinsky *et al.*,
1974). The variation of the axis ratio in a range $0.01 \leqslant \Delta K \leqslant 0.1$, which corresponded
to threshold values for receptor excitation (Loewenstein, 1965; Ilyinsky, 1966b),
gave the absolute increase in surface area as being from 7 (for $\Delta K = 0.1$) to 70 (for
$\Delta K = 0.001$) times more for the elliptical cylinder than for the circular cylinder of the
same volume.

To determine the actual shape of the nerve ending in the Pacinian corpuscle, the
transverse sections through receptors were studied with optical and electron microscopes (Ilyinsky *et al.*, 1968; Volkova and Cherepnov, 1971). The major and minor
transverse axes of the nerve ending were measured and the ratio a/b was calculated.
Optical microscopy showed that in the mid-region of the inner core in the corpuscle
of a regular form, $2a = 5.48 \pm 1.95\ \mu m$, $2b = 2.56 \pm 1.00\ \mu m$ and $a/b = 2.26 \pm 0.44$.
The corresponding results obtained with the electron microscope were: $2a = 5.73 \pm$

1.56 $\mu$m, 2b = 2.48 $\pm$ 0.77 $\mu$m and a/b = 2.35 $\pm$ 0.31, *i.e.* the results obtained by the different methods proved to be in agreement. As for the myelinated nerve fibre, its diameter varied from 4.0 $\pm$ 11.0 $\mu$m, the shape of its transverse section being close to a circle (K = 1.0 $\pm$ 0.1; measurements were made by an optical microscope).

Therefore, the unmyelinated nerve ending of the Pacinian corpuscle appears to have an optimum shape of an elliptical cylinder for which a minimum deforming force would produce a maximum change in surface area.

*The shape of the nerve ending as a result of bilaterally organized inner core (Ilyinsky and Volkova, 1966; Ilyinsky et al., 1968)*

The characteristic shape of the nerve ending described above is usually observed in the main, *i.e.* the middle, part of the unmyelinated nerve fibre. Investigation of a great number of transverse sections in series made it possible to find that it is not immediately after entering the inner core that the nerve ending assumes an elliptical shape. In the very beginning of the inner core where the latter is not yet bilaterally organized, the nerve ending, though without a myelinated sheath, is still of a circular shape. And it is not until the inner core is divided by a cleft into two halves that the transverse section of the nerve ending assumes elliptical shape. It is of interest to note that as soon as the nerve fibre loses its myelinated sheath it, though still circular in shape, becomes substantially narrower along the length of about 10–20 $\mu$m. It is possible that as the receptor potential is generated, the ionic current density across the membrane of this narrowed section of the fibre is larger compared with the neighbouring parts of the nerve, thereby promoting the impulse activity in receptor.

Studies of the ontogenetic development of Pacinian corpuscles (Volkova, 1972) also indicated a direct relationship between the shape of the unmyelinated nerve ending and the bilateral organization of the inner core. Thus, for instance, the inner core of the cat foetus Pacinian corpuscle is lacking a well developed cleft dividing the core into two halves, consequently the nerve fibre is circular in shape along the entire length of the receptor. The nerve ending assumes the elliptical form only in 9-week-old foetuses and in new-born kittens, with the development of the inner core. It is worth noting that in the other encapsulated mechanoreceptors bilateral organization of the inner part of the capsule is invariably accompanied by an elliptical shape of the nerve ending (Quilliam, 1966).

*Pacinian corpuscles ultrastructure (Cherepnov, 1968a, 1969; Ilyinsky et al., 1968)*

From the evidence above and the facts which have been gathered up to now (Gray and Sato, 1953; Loewenstein, 1965; Ilyinsky, 1965 and 1966c; Nishi and Sato, 1968), it can be concluded that Pacinian corpuscles are primary sensory mechanoreceptors. According to the classification of Davis (1961) the main specificity of primary sensory structures is their capability of generating receptor potentials and impulse activity in the same sensory neurone (see reviews by Ilyinsky, 1967 and 1972; Grundfest, 1971). However, in the opinion of some investigators (Lawrentiew, 1943; Portugalov,

1955; Munger, 1966), the inner core cells of the encapsulated receptors may also perform some sensory functions. This idea is based on morphological and histochemical studies which show that the so-called accessory cells surrounding the nerve ending are in a close contact with the sensitive ending of a nerve fibre. These cells

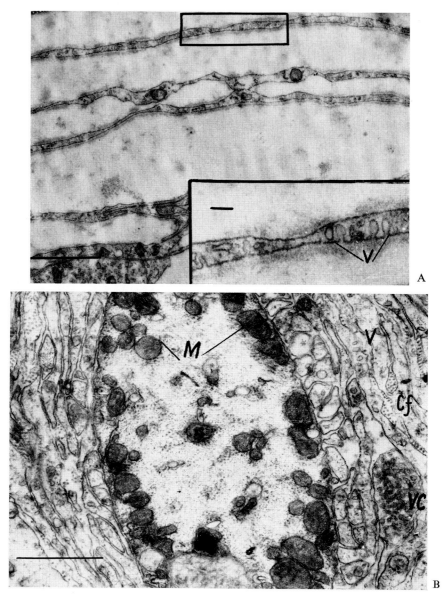

Fig. 7. Lamellar cells of outer capsule and inner core in Pacinian corpuscles (from Cherepnov, 1969). A: vesicles in cell processes of the outer capsule. A connection between vesicles membranes and lamellar cells protoplasmic membranes is observed under great magnification. B: central part of unmyelinated nerve endings with surrounding cell elements of the inner core (from Cherepnov, 1968a). V, vesicles; m, mitochondria; Cf, collagen fibres; ne, nerve ending; VC, vesicular clusters. Bar: 1 μm.

contain a great number of biologically active compounds. In various receptors, such as Grandry, Meissner and Krause corpuscles, these cells include synaptic-like vesicles (Pease and Pallie, 1959; Cauna and Ross, 1960; Quilliam, 1966). It was therefore of interest to look into the relationship between the inner core cells and unmyelinated nerve fibre. Other structures of Pacinian corpuscles were also studied with the electron microscope.

### Outer capsule

Each layer of the outer capsule is formed by several lamellar cells (containing mito-chondria), well developed granular endoplasmatic reticulum, Golgi apparatus and a great number of vesicles 40 nm in diameter. These vesicles are uniformly distributed in the cell (Fig. 7A). Capillaries, never observed in the inner core, can be easily traced between the layers of the outer capsule. The space between the layers is filled with intercellular liquid that contains a great number of collagen fibres, 20 nm in diameter.

### Inner core

The inner core in Pacinian corpuscles is known to be bilaterally organized and divided by a cleft 0.5–1.0 $\mu$m wide into 2 halves. The semi-circular layers of the inner core are formed by lamellae cells.

Processes of central cells are closely adjoining the nerve ending, the distance between the nerve ending membrane and adjacent processes being approximately 15 nm (Fig. 7B). The cytoplasm of lamellar cells processes is less abundant in cell organelles, though it contains a great number of vesicles 25–60 nm in diameter, with the same electron density of the inner content as cytoplasm (Fig. 7B). The number of vesicles in the cell processes does not depend on the distance from the nerve ending. No aggregations of vesicles are observed near either the nerve ending membrane or cytoplasmic membranes of the processes. Therefore, at present there are no reasons to believe that these vesicles may play a role as synaptic vesicles. This opinion is also supported by electron microscope investigations of Pacinian corpuscles subjected to vibration for a long period of time (Cherepnov, 1968b). Among the structural elements of the inner core separate rounded formations are to be met which are literally stuffed with vesicles 40–60 nm across and with electron-dense contents (Fig. 7B). These vesicles are either of a round or elongated shape. Vesicle-filled formations can closely approach the afferent nerve ending, but no structural changes in the nerve ending membrane and inner core cells were seen in this case. On the basis of the evidence obtained in electron microscope studies of the core in Pacinian corpuscles, a suggestion was made (Volkova and Cherepnov, 1967; Cherepnov, 1968a) that the above structures may well be efferent (additional) C-fibres of the receptors which were time and again reported on both in morphological and physio-logical works (Loewenstein et al., 1962). This problem remains to be studied more closely, though.

*Unmyelinated nerve ending*

The nerve ending loses its myelinated sheath before entering the inner core. In the inner core the now unmyelinated nerve ending is surrounded by a membrane, 7 nm thick, with increased electron density. The axoplasm close to a cleft contains electron-transparent vacuoles, 30 nm in diameter. There is a great number of mitochondria in the axoplasm of the nerve ending, especially at its distal part.

Mitochondrial distribution over the cross-section of the nerve ending varies in different receptors. In some cases they are uniformly distributed near the inner surface of the receptor membrane and in others, near the membrane region adjacent to the cleft. Abundance of mitochondria may be an indication of intensive metabolic processes in receptors.

The role of vesicular structures in the inner core and nerve ending of the Pacinian corpuscles is not yet clear. Most likely they appear as a result of high metabolic activity of receptor structures and represent pinocytosis (endo- and exocytosis) vesicles. Products of the metabolic activity of the nerve fibre must influence the surrounding cell structures and *vice versa*. For instance, it is well known that after the nerve fibre of the Pacinian corpuscle is cut and degenerated, the inner core cells undergo fast degeneration (Lee, 1936). However, there is no reason to suppose that the cell's metabolites perform any mediator function.

Our morphological findings do not agree with the notion that encapsulated mechanoreceptors are secondary sensory structures. The results of physiological and pharmacological experiments are in full agreement with this conclusion. Thus the latency time of depolarizing receptor potential measured at the body temperature of the animal at the point where the fibre leaves the corpuscle was 0.15 msec, and that calculated for the place of stimulation of a decapsulated fibre was about 0.05 msec (Ilyinsky, 1966b), being less than a minimum time for synaptic transmission.

The Pacinian corpuscle is the tissue mechanoreceptor which by the present time has received the most study. The question, however, suggests itself as to what extent the conclusions reached for this particular type of sensory structures are valid for the other receptor structures. Of course, such an extrapolation can, in principle, lead to erroneous inferences, but if working hypotheses are to suggest novel experiments then they can be thought of as well justified.

The Pacinian corpuscle can be considered as a primary receptor. An analogous conclusion also seems to be applicable to another tissue mechanoreceptor, one of the most complex — the muscle spindle (Katz, 1950; Ottoson and Shepherd, 1971). In spite of the fact that the other tissue mechanoreceptors have received less study, the information presented in the literature allows one to argue at least that most of the mechanoreceptors are also to be considered as primary sensory structures (Ilyinsky, 1967 and 1972).

Comparative analysis of different mechanoreceptor structures in Vertebrata indicates that starting from the structural and functional characteristics they can be divided into two groups: (1) the receptors of sense organs where the receiving element is a sensory hair-cell (which, according to Davis (1961), makes these receptors to be viewed upon as secondary sensory structures), and (2) receptors in body tissues (skin, muscles, inner organs, vessels etc.), where the receiving element is usually an afferent nerve fibre ending *per se* (Ilyinsky and Krasnikova, 1972). The basic functional distinction between the two groups is felt to lie in their sensitivity to adequate stimulation. Thus the range of threshold displacements for the secondary mechanoreceptors falls in the range from decimae of Angström units (the receptors from organs of heating in Mammalia (de Vries, 1956) to tens of Angström units (the receptors of the lateral-line (Kuiper, 1967). On the other hand, for primary tissue mechanoreceptors this range is from hundredths of a micron (in the case of Pacinian corpuscles (Loewenstein, 1965; Ilyinsky, 1966b; Gavrilov *et al.*, 1975) to tens and even hundreds of microns (the receptors of a free nerve ending type (Lindblom, 1963; Burgess *et al.*, 1968; Bessou *et al.*, 1971)).

Starting from this hypothesis one can explain some other facts to be found in the literature, *e.g.* those relative to the problem of efferent regulation of receptor activity. It should be apparent *a priori* that the receptor or structures with sensitivity equal to or approaching the theoretical value can be efficiently regulated, but with inhibitory influences. Indeed, it is the efferent influences of these types that are to be found in hair-cell mechanoreceptors of sense organs (see, for example, Fex, 1973; Flock and Russel, 1973). In contrast, receptors with a much lower sensitivity can be efficiently regulated not only by inhibitory but also by facilitatory influences. This is the case with tissue receptors some of which (the muscle spindle) can be even excited under the effect of efferent influences.

The concept presented above offers an explanation of the basic facts available at the present time concerning mechanoreceptor activity. Any other hypothesis should also account for these facts.

## SUMMARY

The off-responses and multiplied discharges of Pacinian corpuscle are due to oscillatory processes in the receptor capsule arising from mechanical stimulation. The hyperpolarizing receptor potentials and directional sensitivity of receptors are described. Directional sensitivity is associated with the elliptical shape of the nerve ending. The depolarizing receptor potential is shown to arise when the nerve ending is deformed along its minor transverse axis, an increase in the surface membrane area (*i.e.* stretching) occurring; the hyperpolarizing response appears when deformation is applied along the major transverse axis, the surface membrane area decreasing. The elliptical shape of the nerve ending (the ratio of the major and minor transverse axes being 2.2) effects a maximum sensitivity of corpuscle to mechanical stimulus. Such a form arises in the course of ontogenetic development and is associated with bilateral organization of the inner core.

No contacts of a synaptic type have been found between the inner core cells and the nerve ending membrane. A hypothesis is suggested in which all the tissue mechanoreceptors, or most of them, are considered to be the primary sensory units, their basic distinction from the secondary mechanoreceptors of sense organs lying in their lower sensitivity to mechanical stimulus.

*References p. 184–185*

REFERENCES

BESSOU, P., BURGESS, P. R., PERL, E. R. AND TAYLOR, C. B. (1971) Dynamic properties of mechano-receptors with unmyelinated (C) fibres. *J. Neurophysiol.*, **34**, 116–131.

BURGESS, P. R., PETIT, D. AND WARREN, R. M. (1968) Receptor types in cat hairy skin supplied by myelinated fibres. *J. Neurophysiol.*, **31**, 833–848.

CAUNA, N. AND ROSS, L. L. (1960) The fine structure of Meissner's touch corpuscles of human fingers. *J. biophys. biochem. Cytol.*, **3**, 467–482.

CHEREPNOV, V. L. (1968a) The ultrastructure of the inner core of Pacinian corpuscles. *J. evol. Biochem. Physiol.*, **4**, 91–96 (in Russian).

CHEREPNOV, V. L. (1968b) The effect produced by mechanical stimulation on ultrastructure of the inner core of Pacinian corpuscles. *Proc. Acad. Sci. U.S.S.R.*, **178**, 947–948 (in Russian).

CHEREPNOV, V. L. (1969) *Morpho-Physiological Investigation of Single Mechanoreceptors (Pacinian Corpuscles)*. Dissertation, Pavlov Physiology Institute, Leningrad. (In Russian.)

CHERNIGOVSKY, V. V. (1960) *Interoceptors*, Medgiz, Moscow (in Russian). English translation in *Russian Monographs on Brain and Behavior, Vol. 4*. Amer. Physiol. Association, Washington, D.C., 1967.

DAVIS, H. (1961) Some principles of sensory receptor action. *Physiol. Rev.*, **41**, 391–416.

FEX, J. (1973) Neuropharmacology and potentials of the inner ear. In A. MOLLER (Ed.), *Basic Mechanisms in Hearing*. Academic Press. New York, pp. 377–422.

FLOCK, A. AND RUSSEL, J. (1973) Efferent nerve fibres: postsynaptic action on hair cells. *Nature (Lond.)*, **243**, 89–91.

GAVRILOV, L. R., GERSHUNI, G. V., ILYINSKY, O. B., SIROTUK, M. G., TSIRULNIKOV, E. M. AND TSHEKANOV, E. E. (1975) Action focused ultrasound on skin and deep nerve structures of human arm. In A. IGGO AND O. B. ILYINSKY (Eds.), *Somatosensory and Visceral Receptor Mechanisms, Progress in Brain Research, Vol. 43*. Elsevier, Amsterdam, pp. 279–292.

GRAY, J. A. B. AND SATO, M. (1953) The properties of receptor potential in Pacinian corpuscles. *J. Physiol. (Lond.)*, **122**, 610–636.

GRUNDFEST, H. (1971) The general electrophysiology of input membrane electrogenic excitable cells. In W. LOEWENSTEIN (Ed.), *Handbook of Sensory Physiology, Vol. 1*. Springer, Berlin, pp. 135–165.

HUBBARD, S. J. (1958) A study of rapid mechanical events in mechanoreceptors. *J. Physiol. (Lond.)*, **141**, 198–218.

ILYINSKY, O. B. (1962) Local and action potentials of single mechanoreceptors (Vater–Pacinian corpuscle). *Proc. Acad. Sci. U.S.S.R.*, **142**, 488–490 (in Russian).

ILYINSKY, O. B. (1963) Properties of single mechanoreceptors (Vater–Pacinian corpuscles). *Sechenov physiol. J. U.S.S.R.*, **49**, 201–207 (in Russian).

ILYINSKY, O. B. (1965) Processes of excitation and inhibition in single mechanoreceptors (Pacinian corpuscles). *Nature (Lond.)*, **208**, 351–353.

ILYINSKY, O. B. (1966a) On and off responses of single mechanoreceptors. *Sechenov physiol. J. U.S.S.R.*, **52**, 99–107. English translation: *Fed. Proc.*, Translation Suppl. **26**, T948–T952 (1966–1967).

ILYINSKY, O. B. (1966b) *Physiology of Single Mechanoreceptors*. Dissertation, Pavlov Physiology Institute. Leningrad. (In Russian.)

ILYINSKY, O. B. (1966c) The electrophysiology of mechanoreceptors. In *Primary Processes in Receptor Elements of Sensory Organs*. Science, Leningrad. 154–171. (In Russian.)

ILYINSKY, O. B. (1967) *Mechanoreceptors*. Nauka, Leningrad. (in Russian).

ILYINSKY, O. B. (1972) The general physiology of the receptors. In *Handbook of Physiology of Sensory Systems, Vol. 2*. Science, Leningrad. pp. 30–56. (In Russian.)

ILYINSKY, O. B. AND KRASNIKOVA, T. L. (1972) Study of ionic composition of Pacinian corpuscle fluid in connection with their activity. *Sechenov physiol. J. U.S.S.R.*, **58**, 434–442.

ILYINSKY, O. B., KRYLOV, B. V. AND CHEREPNOV, V. L. (1975) The mathematical analysis of the structural properties of Pacinian corpuscles. In press.

ILYINSKY, O. B. AND KUDRIN, V. P. (1967) The methods of adequate, measured stimulation of the Mechanoreceptors. *Bull. exp. Biol. Med.*, **64**, 100–103 (in Russian).

ILYINSKY, O. B. AND VOLKOVA, N. K. (1966) Certain morphophysiologic traits of individual mechano-receptors (Pacinian corpuscles). *Proc. Acad. Sci. U.S.S.R.*, **171**, 494–497 (in Russian).

ILYINSKY, O. B., VOLKOVA, N. K. AND CHEREPNOV, V. L. (1968) Structure and function of Pacinian corpuscle. *Sechenov physiol. J. U.S.S.R.*, **54**, 295–302 (in Russian). English translation: *Neuroscience Translations*, **6**, 637–643 (1968–1969).

KATZ, B. (1950) Depolarization of sensory terminals and the initiation of impulses in the muscle spindle. *J. Physiol. (Lond.)*, **111**, 261–282.

KUIPER, J. W. (1967) Frequency characteristics and functional significance of the lateral line organ. In P. H. CANN (Ed.), *Lateral Line Detecters.* Ind. Univ. Press, Bloomington, Ind. pp. 105–121.

LAWRENTIEW, B. I. (1943) The sensitive innervation of the visceral organs. *J. gen. Biol.*, **4**, 232–252 (in Russian).

LEE, F. C. (1936) A study of the Pacinian corpuscle. *J. comp. Neurol.*, **64**, 497–522.

LINDBLOM, U. (1963) Phasic and static excitability of touch receptors in toad skin. *Acta physiol. scand.*, **59**, 410–423.

LOEWENSTEIN, W. R. (1965) Facets of a transducer process. *Cold Spr. Harb. Symp. quant. Biol.*, **30**, 29–43.

LOEWENSTEIN, W. R., GOTO, K. AND NOBAK, C. (1962) C-Fibre innervation of a mechanoreceptor. *Experientia (Basel)*, **18**, 460.

MUNGER, B. L. (1966) Chemical or physical nature of transduction. General discussion of Section 11. In A. V. S. DE REUCK AND J. KNIGHT (Eds.), *Touch, Heat and Pain, Ciba Foundation Symp.* Churchill, London. p. 197.

NISHI, K. AND SATO, M. (1968) Depolarizing and hyperpolarizing receptor potentials in the non-myelinated nerve terminal in Pacinian corpuscles. *J. Physiol. (Lond.)*, **199**, 383–396.

OTTOSON, D. AND SHEPHERD, J. M. (1971) Transducer properties and integrative mechanisms in the frog's muscle spindle. In W. LOEWENSTEIN (Ed.), *Handbook of Sensory Physiology, Vol. 1.* Springer, Berlin. pp. 442–499.

OZEKI, M. AND SATO, M. (1965) Changes in the membrane potential and the membrane conductance associated with a sustained depolarization of the non-myelinated nerve terminal in Pacinian corpuscles. *J. Physiol. (Lond.)*, **180**, 186–208.

PEASE, D. C. AND PALLIE, W. (1959) Electron microscopy of digital tactile corpuscles and small cutaneous nerves. *J. Ultrastruct. Res.*, **2**, 352–365.

PEASE, D. C. AND QUILLIAM, T. A. (1957) Electron microscopy of the Pacinian corpuscles. *J. biophys. Biochem. Cytol.*, **3**, 331–342.

PORTUGALOV, V. V. (1955) *Histology and Physiology of Nerve Endings.* Medzig, Moscow. (In Russian.)

QUILLIAM, T. A. (1966) Unit design and array pattern in receptor organs. In A. V. S. DE REUCK AND J. KNIGHT (Eds.), *Touch, Heat and Pain. Ciba Foundation Symp.* Churchill, London. pp. 86–116.

VOLKOVA, N. K. (1972) Formation of some structures of Pacinian corpuscle in ontogenesis. *Proc. Acad. Sci. U.S.S.R.*, **204**, 717–719 (in Russian).

VOLKOVA, N. K. AND CHEREPNOV, V. L. (1967) Structure of the inner core of Pacinian corpuscles. The third conf. anatomists and histologists, Bulgaria. pp. 25–26.

VOLKOVA, N. K. AND CHEREPNOV, V. L. (1971) Structure of Pacinian corpuscle. *Arch. Anat. Histol. Embryol.*, **60**, 101–105 (in Russian).

VRIES, DE H. (1956) Physical aspects of the sense organs. *Progr. biophys. Chem.*, **6**, 207–264.

## DISCUSSION

IGGO: Your analysis assumes that the whole circumference of the Pacinian terminal may be involved in mechanotransducer processes, whereas there is electron microscopic evidence that there seem to be small finger-like processes scattered around the edge. Does it make any difference to your analysis whether these small processes might be involved and not the whole circumference of the axon or of the terminal?

ILYINSKY: The nerve ending in the Pacinian corpuscle can really have the finger-like processes. They seem to be more abundant in the distal part of the nerve ending, *i.e.* in the region associated with its growth. In the middle and proximal parts of the receptor the processes are less common or, to be more precise, in many preparations they are not to be seen. Now, thresholds for impulse activity in response to mechanical stimulation are the lowest in the proximal and central parts of the receptor but not in its distal part. This fact can be accounted for if we assume that the area most favourable for firing the action potential is located in the proximal part of the receptors (see also W. R. Loewenstein, In *Handbook of Sensory Physiology, Vol. 1*, Springer, Berlin, 1971, pp. 269–290), so that excited areas of the terminal membrane which are unequally spaced from this region will make dissimilar contributions into the process of generation of the action potential. Thus the share of distal parts of the nerve ending in generation of impulse activity by the receptor is the lowest. Besides, we used in our experiments corpuscles of regular shape. Taken together these factors make it possible, while performing calculations, to neglect the finger-like processes. As discussed above there is a good agreement between the results of theoretical calculations and experimental morphological evidence. We cannot discard the possibility, though, that in some receptors the finger-like processes in question are able to essentially contribute to the pattern of excitation process. Thus, occasionally, the directional sensitivity in Pacinian corpuscles was lacking or poorly expressed and probably these cases should be explained by the abundance in the axonal processes.

BURGESS: Dr. Ilyinsky, you have shown very elegantly, I think, that in the Pacinian corpuscle the design of the receptor is appropriate for excitation by distention of the terminal. Do you feel that this is a general mechanism of excitation for the primary type of mechanoreceptor, for example, in the muscle spindle? Do you believe or do you have any evidence to suggest that it is also distention of the terminals in the muscle spindle which is the excitatory event?

ILYINSKY: Yes, I do. The facts now available in the literature, relating to a great variety of mechano-receptors, including the muscle spindle stretch receptors, vessel baroreceptors, tactile receptors etc., all speak in favour of the conception under discussion. Moreover, the capability of the nerve fibre of being excited by mechanical stimulation (F. J. Julian and D. E. Goldman, *J. gen. Physiol.*, **46**, (1962) 297) also supports this hypothesis.

CHUCHKOV: In the corpuscles of Herbst which share common features and properties with Pacinian corpuscles the nerve ending occasionally has a circular shape. What is your idea concerning the excitation mechanism in this case?

ILYINSKY: From analysis presented it follows that the shape of the nerve ending underlies the receptor sensitivity to a mechanical stimulus. This circumstance should be taken into account when considering the properties of tissue mechanoreceptor structures which are known to be of diversified shape and sensitivity. But it is felt that the mechanism underlying the excitation (the stretching of the receptor membranes in all the cases, including the corpuscle of Herbst), is essentially the same.

SANTINI: Elliptical shape of the nerve ending is not imperative in Pacinian corpuscles either. Thus I met the nerve ending of a triangular form.

CAUNA: It is known that there are Pacinian corpuscles with more than one axon (multiaxonal corpuscle).

MALINOVSKY: I would likewise note that at early stages of ontogenesis the nerve ending in Pacinian corpuscles can occasionally have a circular shape; in this case the initial stages of the inner core formation are to be observed. It is true, though, that in adult animals the nerve endings are always of an oval shape. Besides, I would like to make a comment. In our preparations we did not see vesicular packets in Pacinian corpuscles. Don't you think that their occurrence in your preparations may be accounted for by the oblique sectioning, resulting in the longitudinal cutting of cell elements of the inner core?

ILYINSKY: I have had an opportunity to note that a diversified shape of the nerve ending, their branching and other factors are not against the conception considered here that the excitation process in Pacinian corpuscles (and, I believe, in the other tissue mechanoreceptors as well) is due to the stretching of the membrane of their nerve endings. But the analysis of the processes of excitation in these cases would be much more complicated. As to the connection between the shape of the nerve ending and bilateral organization of the inner core, I would like to add that in Pacinian corpuscles of regular shape (and we saw to it that we worked with such preparations) with the inner core normally developed the nerve endings always have an elliptical shape. With an underdeveloped inner core, especially in the corpuscles at the formation stage, while the intracapsular pressure is still small, nerve endings of a form other than the elliptical one, usually circular, are really to be met. Elliptical shape of the nerve ending in bilaterally organized encapsulated receptors is well known in the literature (see Quilliam, 1966 in References). As to vesicular packets, I don't think that their occurrence is due to the oblique sectioning. Should they be considered as resulting from cutting, say, of an additional nerve fibre or axoplasmic processes of the main terminal, this question calls for further study.

# Effect of Acetylcholine and Catecholamines on Excitability of Pacinian Corpuscles

G. N. AKOEV, Yu. A. CHELYSHEV AND S. I. ELMAN

*I. P. Pavlov Institute of Physiology, Academy of Sciences of the U.S.S.R., Leningrad (U.S.S.R.)*

## INTRODUCTION

Physiological data indicate that the transducer mechanism in a Pacinian corpuscle is located on the surface membrane of the unmyelinated nerve terminal. There is ample evidence that deformation of receptor membrane results in an increase of permeability to sodium and potassium ions, leading to the generation of receptor potential (Gray and Diamond, 1957; Gray, 1959; Loewenstein, 1956, 1965, 1971; Ilyinsky, 1965 and 1967; Ilyinsky *et al.*, 1968). However, there exists a theory of chemical mediation in sensory receptor mechanisms (Vinnikov, 1946; Portugalov, 1955; Koelle, 1962), assuming that a certain transmitter, presumably acetylcholine, may be released from the inner core cells during mechanical stimulation of a corpuscle. The transmitter depolarizes the membrane thus leading to the appearance of a receptor potential. This view is based on the findings that the sensory mechanisms of mechanoreceptors is affected by acetylcholine and related drugs (Douglas and Gray, 1953; Chernigovsky, 1960; Ottoson, 1961; Paintal, 1964). The mechanism underlying the effects of acetylcholine is not as yet clear however.

Adrenaline and noradrenaline are transmitters in the sympathetic nervous system and apparently take part in efferent regulation of some tissue receptors. It is known that injection of catecholamines or sympathetic stimulation lead to an enhanced excitability in various mechanoreceptors (Loewenstein, 1956; Loewenstein and Altamirano-Orrego, 1956; Calma and Kidd, 1962; Chernetsky, 1964; Leitner and Perl, 1964; Nilsson, 1972; Akoev *et al.*, 1974). However, the mechanism of catecholamine influence on the receptors is obscure.

The Pacinian corpuscle provides a favourable preparation for comparative analysis of the drug effects upon two distinctly different membranes: the receptor membrane of the nerve ending and the membrane of the nodes of Ranvier. The aim of the present study was to look into the effects of acetylcholine and catecholamines upon the Pacinian corpuscles.

## METHODS

Experiments were performed on Pacinian corpuscles isolated from the cat's mesentery.

When the influence of drugs on receptor potential was studied, the receptors were decapsulated up to a central core. If the nodes of Ranvier were studied, the receptors were decapsulated by 10–15% and so the drugs influenced only the node of Ranvier, while the non-myelinated endings were protected by the connective tissue layers of the inner and outer capsules. Nerve endings of the decapsulated receptors were placed in a small chamber holding 0.2 ml, continuously perfused with Ringer–Locke solution. The myelinated axon was in another chamber separated from the first one by an air-gap of 200–300 $\mu$m. Potentials were recorded via non-polarizable electrodes across the air-gap with a condenser resistance coupled amplifier (Akoev and Elman, 1974). Stimuli were mechanical pulses of 2–5 msec duration with a frequency of 1–10/sec. In some cases (Figs. 1 and 3) the stimuli were applied to the platform on which the perfusion chamber was placed. The following drugs and ions were tested: acetylcholine chloride ($1 \times 10^{-6}$–$1 \times 10^{-3}$ g/ml); hexamethonium bromide ($1 \times 10^{-4}$ g/ml); D-tubocurarine chloride ($1 \times 10^{-6}$ g/ml); atropine sulphate ($1 \times 10^{-5}$ g/ml); adrenaline and noradrenaline hydrochloride ($1 \times 10^{-7}$–$2 \times 10^{-5}$ g/ml). All solutions were prepared *ex temporae*. To obtain a receptor potential uncomplicated by spike activity of the node, the preparation was treated with procaine at concentration of 0.1%. Data were obtained from 110 Pacinian corpuscles.

## RESULTS

*Effects of acetylcholine upon impulse activity of the receptor*

Acetylcholine in concentrations below $1 \times 10^{-5}$ g/ml was generally without effect on the corpuscle. In concentrations of $1 \times 10^{-4}$–$1 \times 10^{-3}$ g/ml the drug caused an increase in excitability of the receptor and the number of impulses per burst in response to mechanical stimuli (Fig. 1). Without adequate stimulation the appearance of impulse activity was not observed. It is well known that an action potential arises in the node of Ranvier whenever the generator potential reaches a critical amplitude (a firing threshold). Our results showed that in the solution with acetylcholine the firing threshold decreased (Fig. 2A).

*Effects of acetylcholine upon the receptor potential*

Acetylcholine in concentration below $1 \times 10^{-4}$ g/ml did not affect the receptor

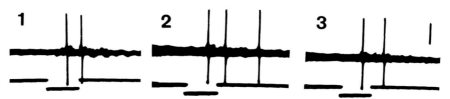

Fig. 1. Responses of Pacinian corpuscle in normal solution (1) and after 6 and 10 min (2 and 3 respectively) in acetylcholine solution ($1 \times 10^{-3}$ g/ml). Stimulus duration: 50 msec (lower trace), vertical bar: 50 $\mu$V.

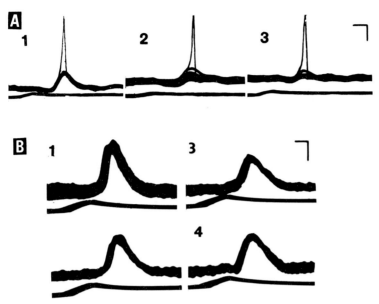

Fig. 2. A: effect of acetylcholine ($1 \times 10^{-3}$ g/ml) on firing level of the node of Ranvier. 1: response in normal solution; 2 and 3: responses after 15 and 30 min in acetylcholine solution, respectively. Vertical bar: 100 $\mu$V, horizontal bar: 2 msec. B: effect of acetylcholine ($1 \times 10^{-3}$ g/ml) on the receptor potential. 1: response in normal solution; 2 and 3: responses after 4 and 9 min in acetylcholine solution, respectively; 4: response after 16 min back in normal solution. Vertical bar: 50 $\mu$V, horizontal bar: 2 msec.

potential. In a concentration of $1 \times 10^{-3}$ g/ml the drug caused a decrease in receptor potential amplitude (Fig. 2B).

*Effects of MgCl$_2$*

Activity was not blocked if the receptors were continuously (30 min) perfused by a solution containing 20 m$M$ MgCl$_2$. The amplitude of receptor potential increased in such solutions.

*Effects of cholinolytic agents*

Responses of the receptors to mechanical stimulation were not blocked in a solution containing atropine ($1 \times 10^{-5}$ g/ml), hexamethonium ($1 \times 10^{-4}$ g/ml) and D-tubocurarine ($1 \times 10^{-6}$ g/ml). Sensitivity of the receptors remained unchanged in the presence of atropine and hexamethonium. D-Tubocurarine caused an increase in impulse activity and a decrease in receptor potential amplitude and firing threshold.

*Effects of catecholamines upon the spike activity*

Adrenaline and noradrenaline produced a temporary increase in the excitability of the receptors during the first 5–10 min and then the excitability decreased below the initial level (Fig. 3). The largest fall in threshold was 10–15% with adrenaline and 25% with noradrenaline. It was shown that adrenaline and noradrenaline caused an increase in firing threshold of the node of Ranvier.

*References p. 192–193*

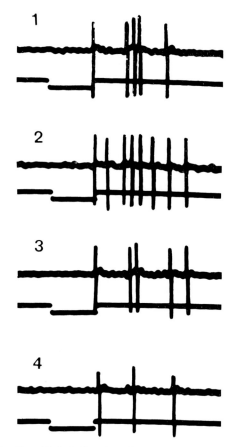

Fig. 3. Effect of adrenaline ($1 \times 10^{-6}$ g/ml) on impulse response of corpuscle. 1: in normal solution; 2–4: in adrenaline solution after 7, 14 and 17 min, respectively. Stimulus duration: (lower trace) 50 msec.

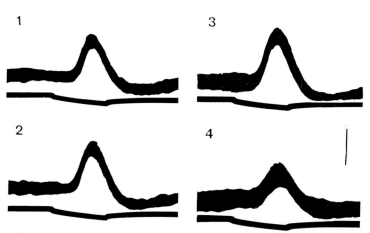

Fig. 4. Effect of adrenaline ($1 \times 10^{-5}$ g/ml) on the receptor potential. 1: response in normal solution; 2–4: responses in adrenaline solution after 2, 6 and 9 min respectively. Stimulus duration: (lower trace) 50 msec. Vertical bar: 100 $\mu$V.

*Effects of catecholamines upon the receptor potential*

Both the rate of rise and the amplitude of generator potentials increased after treatment with catecholamines at concentrations of $1 \times 10^{-7} - 2 \times 10^{-5}$ g/ml (Fig. 4). With adrenaline the receptor potentials were larger by 13.2% and with noradrenaline by 25.3%.

Under the given mechanical stimulus the receptor potential amplitude in solution with noradrenaline was larger than in the normal solution.


DISCUSSION


The present study confirmed the earlier observation that acetylcholine is able to excite terminals of the sensory nerves. The drug may act on the regenerative or receptor region of a corpuscle. The overall action of acetylcholine depends upon which of the two effects prevails. Our data showed that the receptor potential amplitude and the firing threshold are lower in the solution with acetylcholine. It seems reasonable to suppose that the second effect predominates and results in an increased excitability of the receptor. It may be assumed that the decrease in firing threshold of the node of Ranvier in acetylcholine solution can account for enhanced excitability of various mechanoreceptors to adequate stimuli.

It is known that the addition of cholinolytic agents to a normal solution leads to the blocking of transmission in cholinergic synapses. Our experiments indicate that these drugs fail to block the receptor response to mechanical stimuli.

Del Castillo and Engbaek (1954) showed that the addition of $Mg^{++}$ in small concentrations to the normal solution results in blocking of acetylcholine secretion from pre-synaptic endings. However, our data show that $Mg^{++}$ in concentrations up to 20 m$M$ does not block receptors responses to adequate stimuli; on the contrary, the receptor potential amplitude in such a solution increases. Therefore our results provide strong evidence against a physiological role of acetylcholine as a possible transmitter in the Pacinian corpuscle.

The evidence presented above shows that catecholamines produce a two-phase change in receptors excitability. These two phases are also observed in receptors with stimulation of the sympathetic nerves (Loewenstein, 1956; Calma and Kidd, 1962; Nilsson, 1972). The change in excitability of receptors in the catecholamine solution may be due to the altered excitability either of the receptor's membrane or the node of Ranvier. Our analysis shows that in catecholamine solution the excitability of the nodes of Ranvier falls and the receptor potential amplitude rises. It is thus possible that the increase in receptor potential amplitude compensates for the decreased excitability of the node of Ranvier, the excitability of the receptor as a whole being enchanced.

It has been recently shown that catecholamines hyperpolarize the nerve cells through activation of adenyl cyclase (Kebabian and Greengard, 1971; Siggins et al., 1973). Therefore, it may be assumed that catecholamines may cause an increase in membrane potential of a nerve ending in a similar way, thereby increasing receptor potential amplitude and receptor sensitivity.

The presence of post-ganglionic sympathetic fibres in the inner core region of the Pacinian corpuscle has recently been shown by electron microscopic methods and the Falck–Hillarp fluorescence histochemical technique (Cherepnov, 1968; Santini, 1969; Santini *et al.*, 1971). Electrical stimulation of these fibres results in an enhanced sensitivity of receptors (Goto and Loewenstein, 1961). The efferent regulation of the receptor sensitivity *in vivo* can probably be performed through the same mechanism as with the catecholamines *in vitro*, *i.e.* by increasing the amplitude of receptor potential. To summarize, our results indicate that some drugs (acetylcholine) have a primary effect on the excitability of the regenerative region of the receptor while some others (catecholamines) act upon the generator mechanism.

## SUMMARY

The effect of acetylcholine, cholinolytics and catecholamines on the electrical activity of the Pacinian corpuscle was studied on isolated decapsulated preparations.

Acetylcholine ($1 \times 10^{-3}$–$1 \times 10^{-4}$ g/ml) was found to enhance the excitability of the receptors due to an increased excitability of the node of Ranvier. In acetylcholine solutions the amplitude of the generator potential decreased. Cholinolytic drugs (atropine, hexamethonium and D-tubocurarine) did not block the response of the receptor to mechanical stimuli. The results obtained provide strong evidence against a physiological role of acetylcholine as a transmitter in Pacinian corpuscle. Adrenaline and noradrenaline enhanced the excitability of receptors by 10–15% due to an increase in the amplitude of generator potential.

## REFERENCES

AKOEV, G. N. AND ELMAN, S. I. (1974) Potassium ions and electrical activity of single mechanoreceptors (Pacinian corpuscles). *Sechenov physiol. J. U.S.S.R.*, **60**, 55–61 (in Russian).

AKOEV, G. N., CHELYSHEV, YU. A. AND ELMAN, S. I. (1974) Effect of catecholamines on the excitability of single mechanoreceptors (Pacinian corpuscles). *J. Neurophysiol.*, **6**, 312–317 (in Russian).

CALMA, I. AND KIDD, G. L. (1962) The effect of adrenaline on muscle spindle in cat. *Arch. ital. Biol.*, **100**, 381–393.

CHEREPNOV, V. L. (1968) The ultrastructure of the inner core of the Pacinian corpuscles. *J. comp. Biochem. Physiol.*, **4**, 91–96 (in Russian).

CHERNETSKY, K. E. (1964) Sympathetic enhancement of peripheral sensory input in the frog. *J. Neurophysiol.*, **27**, 493–515.

CHERNIGOVSKY, V. N. (1960) *Interoceptors*. Medgiz, Moscow. (In Russian.)

DOUGLAS, W. W. AND GRAY, J. A. B. (1953) The excitant action of acetylcholine and other substances on cutaneous sensory pathway and its prevention by hexamethonium and D-tubocurarine. *J. Physiol. (Lond.)*, **119**, 118–128.

DEL CASTILLO, J. AND ENGBAEK, L. (1954) The nature of the neuromuscular block produced by magnesium. *J. Physiol. (Lond.)*, **124**, 370–384.

GOTO, K. AND LOEWENSTEIN, W. R. (1961) An accessory small nerve fiber in a mechanoreceptor. *Biol. Bull.* **121**, 391.

GRAY, J. A. B. (1959) Initiation of impulses at receptors. In J. FIELD (Ed.), *Handbook of Physiology. Section I, Neurophysiology, Vol. 1.* Amer. Physiol. Soc., Washington, D.C. pp. 123–145.

GRAY, J. A. B. AND DIAMOND, J. (1957) Pharmacological properties of sensory receptors and their relation to the autonomic nervous system. *Brit. med. Bull.*, **13**, 185–188.

ILYINSKY, O. B. (1965) Processes of excitation and inhibition in single mechanoreceptors (Pacinian corpuscles). *Nature (Lond.)*, **208**, 351–353.

ILYINSKY, O. B. (1967). *Mechanoreceptors.* Nauka, Leningrad. (In Russian.)

ILYINSKY, O. B., VOLKOVA, N. K. AND CHEREPNOV, V. L. (1968-9) Structure and function of Pacinian corpuscle. English translation in *Neuroscience Translations.* 6, 637–643.

KEBABIAN, J. W. AND GREENGARD, P. (1971) Dopamine-sensitive adenyl cyclase role in synaptic transmission. *Science*, **174**, 1345–1349.

KOELLE, C. B. (1962) A new general concept of neurohumoral functions of acetylcholine and acetylcholinesterase. *J. Pharm. Pharmacol.*, **14**, 65–90.

LEITNER, J.-M. AND PERL, E. R. (1964) Receptors supplies which respond to cardiovascular changes and adrenaline. *J. Physiol. (Lond.)*, **175**, 2, 54–274.

LOEWENSTEIN, W. R. (1956) Modulation of cutaneous mechanoreceptors by sympathetic stimulation. *J. Physiol. (Lond.)*, **132**, 40–60.

LOEWENSTEIN, W. R. (1965) Facets of transducer process. *Cold Spr. Harb. Symp. quant. Biol.*, **30**, 29–43.

LOEWENSTEIN, W. R. (1971) Mechano-electric transduction in the Pacinian corpuscle. Initiation of sensory impulses in mechanoreceptors. In W. R. LOEWENSTEIN (Ed.), *Handbook of Sensory Physiology. Vol. 1.* Springer, Berlin. pp. 269–290.

LOEWENSTEIN, W. R. AND ALTAMIRANO-ORREGO, R. (1956) Enhancement of activity in a Pacinian corpuscle by sympathomimetic agents. *Nature (Lond.)*, **178**, 1292–1293.

NILSSON, B. Y. (1972) Efiect of sympathetic stimulation on mechanoreceptors of cat vibrissae. *Acta physiol. scand.*, **85**, 390–397.

OTTOSON, D. (1961) The effect of acetylcholine and related substances on the isolated muscle spindle. *Acta physiol. scand.*, **53**, 276–287.

PAINTAL, A. S. (1964) Effects of drugs on vertebrate mechanoreceptors. *Pharmacol. Rev.*, **16**, 341–380.

PORTUGALOV, V. V. (1955) *Histology and Physiology of Nerve Ending.* Medzig, Moscow. (In Russian.)

SANTINI, M. (1969) New fibres of sympathetic nature in the inner core region of Pacinian corpuscle. *Brain Res.*, **16**, 535–538.

SANTINI, M., IBATA, Y. AND PAPPAS, G. D. (1971) The fine structure of the sympathetic axons within the Pacinian corpuscle. *Brain Res.*, **33**, 279–287.

SIGGINS, C. R., BATTENBERG, E. F., HOFFER, B. J., BLOOM, F. E. AND STEINER, A. L. (1973) Noradrenergic stimulation of cyclic AMP in rat Purkinje neurons: an immunocytochemical study. *Science*, **179**, 585–588.

VINNIKOV, J. A. (1946) Contribution to the study of the ontophylogenetic classification of receptors (organ of sense) of the vertebrates. *J. gen. Biol.*, **7**, 347–368 (in Russian).

## DISCUSSION

CHERNIGOVSKY: I have three questions to ask Dr. Akoev. (1) Why did you use such high concentrations of acetylcholine? (2) If acetylcholine is not a transmitter how then do you explain the excitation in a Pacinian corpuscle? (3) If acetylcholine is not involved in a primary process how do you explain the fact that application of acetylcholine to tissue receptor does excite the nerve ending?

AKOEV: (1) In our experiments the acetylcholine concentration was $10^{-3}$–$10^{-4}$ g/ml. It is the concentration that most of the authors used dealing with the impulse activity in mechanoreceptors. The results obtained in our study also comply with those obtained by the authors who used acetylcholine in the above concentrations. It should be noted that the very fact that acetylcholine should be used in so high a concentration is a further indication that there is no specific sensitivity to this substance in Pacinian corpuscle. (2) The results obtained in our experiments indicate that acetylcholine is not involved in excitation process. As for the mechanism responsible for transformation of the energy of a mechanical stimulus into that of the electrical response, this question is far from being settled now. (3) Our evidence indicates that the excitatory action of acetylcholine is due to its effect upon the node of Ranvier.

# Functional Organization of Mechanoreceptors

O. B. ILYINSKY, T. L. KRASNIKOVA, G. N. AKOEV AND S. I. ELMAN

*I. P. Pavlov Institute of Physiology, Academy of Sciences of the U.S.S.R., Leningrad (U.S.S.R.)*

Great attention is now being paid to investigation of the composition of the medium surrounding sensory structures. In 1954 Smith and co-workers showed that endolymph of the inner ear of guinea pig has a high potassium concentration. This observation has been confirmed by other investigators in different species (Murray and Potts, 1961; Simon *et al.*, 1973). The lateral-line hair cells of fish have been also shown to be surrounded by a specific medium with a relatively high potassium concentration (Ilyinsky and Krasnikova, 1971; Fänge *et al.*, 1972). Further it has been demonstrated that hyperpotassium medium in labyrinth receptors (Konishi *et al.*, 1966) and lateral-line receptors (Katsuki and Hashimoto, 1969) appears to enhance the receptor sensibility to mechanical stimulation.

However, data concerning the ionic composition of the medium surrounding tissue mechanoreceptors and the role of this composition in receptor functioning have not been available up to now. It is reasonable to believe that the fluid in Pacinian corpuscles, which are typical mechanoreceptors, may also have an unusual content. This conclusion can be drawn from the evidence concerning the character of the post-hyperpolarizing responses to mechanical stimulation of the corpuscle (Ilyinsky, 1965, 1966b and 1970).

The present study deals with the post-hyperpolarizing responses of Pacinian corpuscles, the ionic content of their inner medium and its possible physiological role.

## METHODS

### Electrophysiological methods

Experiments were carried out on Pacinian corpuscles isolated from the cat's mesentery or pancreas and intact receptors with normal blood circulation (Ilyinsky, 1966a and 1970). In order to study the effect of ionic composition of the medium around the corpuscle, the latter was decapsulated up to the inner core and then continuously perfused with test solution (Akoev and Elman, 1974).

### Analytical methods

Potassium and sodium concentrations within the Pacinian corpuscle fluid were studied.

The receptors were removed from surrounding tissues either in Krebs–Henseleit's solution or in blood plasma (T = 35°C). Pacinian corpuscle fluid was taken under vaseline oil after the receptors had been decapsulated or merely perforated by a sharp needle. Intracapsular fluid and blood plasma samples for potassium and sodium analyses were 0.2–0.4 $\mu$l. Analysis of the ionic content of the samples was performed by the method of total emission flame photometry using the single-channel integrating ultramicro flame photometer. The lowest amount to be reliable assessed was $1 \times 10^{-14}$ moles for potassium and $1 \times 10^{-13}$ moles for sodium, the accuracy of the method being 8–10%. The potassium concentration in mesentery fluid was analyzed by the electrometric method using potassium-selective membrane electrodes.

## RESULTS

### *Post-hyperpolarizing responses*

Mechanical stimulation of Pacinian corpuscles results in both depolarizing and hyperpolarizing responses (Ilyinsky, 1965 and 1966b; Ilyinsky *et al.*, 1968; Nishi and Sato, 1968). Typical responses are to be seen in Fig. 1. In this volume, Ilyinsky and co-workers (1975) discuss the mechanism of these responses, which is due to the structure of Pacinian corpuscles. In the present study we deal with some specific hyperpolarizing reactions only. After the hyperpolarizing receptor potential (RP) the impulse activity usually appeared. Action potential (AP) was preceded by the depolarizing receptor potential. However, with hyperpolarizing responses appearing before the depolarizing RP the firing threshold was lower (Fig. $1_{1-3}$). In some receptors with low sensitivity the action potentials did not appear at all at the moment of stimulation and were observed only after the hyperpolarizing RP (Fig. $1_{4,6,7}$). Occasionally the decrease in the amplitude of hyperpolarizing RP was followed by rhythmical discharge (Fig. $1_{5-7}$). In such a discharge each AP was due to a negative deflection of the local response, *i.e.* here hyperpolarization resulted in oscillation of the depolarizing RP. It should be emphasized that this phenomenon could also be observed with gradually increasing stimulus of moderate amplitude, *i.e.* when there was practically no mechanical oscillation in the receptor capsule. If the receptor was damaged, the hyperpolarizing RP was followed by an action potential with greater amplitude, *i.e.* the functional condition of the receptor improved (Fig. $1_8$). The above phenomena were observed with both isolated and intact preparations with normal blood circulation.

It may be assumed that the effect of hyperpolarizing RP was identical to the influence of the anodal current upon various excitable structures, *e.g.* nerve fibres (Frankenhaeuser and Widen, 1956; Tasaki, 1959; Ooyama and Wright, 1961), crayfish stretch receptors (Jansen *et al.*, 1971), etc. It is well known that the background depolarization is one of the main conditions for the appearance of anode-break (post-hyperpolarizing) responses. This type of response can be due either to the cathodic current (Ooyama and Wright, 1961; Jansen *et al.*, 1971) or an increase

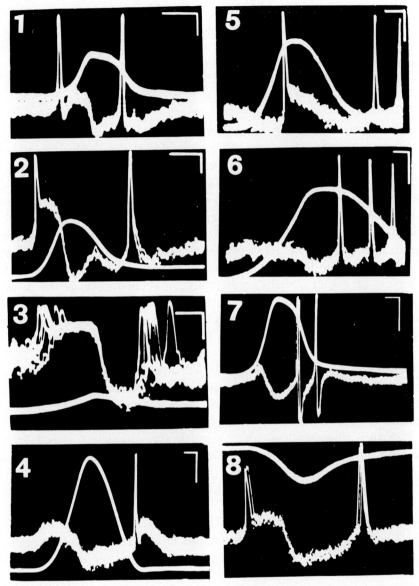

Fig. 1. Post-hyperpolarizing responses of Pacinian corpuscles. Eight different receptors. Vertical bar ($\mu$V) for 1, 2, 4–8 shows 50 $\mu$V and for 3, 30 $\mu$V. Horizontal bar (msec) for 1–7 shows 4 msec and for 8, 2 msec.

in the extracellular potassium concentration (Frankenhaeuser and Widen, 1956; Tasaki, 1959; Ooyama and Wright, 1961), or merely to the natural conditions (Kuffler and Eyzaguirre, 1955; Jansen *et al.*, 1971), etc.

Pacinian corpuscle post-hyperpolarizing responses to adequate stimulation resembled the anode-break responses. Therefore, the possibility of background depolarization should be taken into account. The lowered value of membrane potential can probably result from metabolic processes or the specific ionic content of the medium around the nerve ending. Metabolic processes in Pacinian corpuscles are impossible to study with the techniques available at present, but it is possible to obtain information about the ionic content of the medium.

### *Potassium and sodium content in Pacinian corpuscle fluid*

The intracapsular fluid in a Pacinian corpuscle is a viscous transparent substance. The flame photometric microanalysis showed that the potassium concentration varied from 3.40 to 13.90 mEq/litre in the intracapsular fluid and from 1.20 to 4.40 mEq/litre in the blood plasma, being always lower ($3.41 \pm 0.61$; $P < 0.001$) in the plasma of the same animal (Table I) (Ilyinsky and Krasnikova, 1972). The sodium concentration in both cases was approximately the same.

The question can be raised, however, whether the elevated potassium concentration in the capsular fluid may not result from release of potassium ions from the lamellar cells due to damage of the receptor. Decapsulation of the receptor to different levels or puncture of it with a sharp needle failed, however, to change the potassium concentration in the capsular fluid. The lamellar cells of the outer capsule of the Pacinian corpuscle are extremely elongated flat structures with small amounts of cytoplasm, the viscosity of cytoplasm in the lamellar cells being much higher than that in the Pacinian corpuscle fluid. In order to have the intracapsular fluid un-contaminated by cytoplasm of the lamellar cells whilst decapsulating the corpuscle, the lamellae were immediately removed from the intralamellar fluid.

According to the electrometric analysis, the potassium ion concentration in the mesenteric tissue fluid and in the blood plasma was practically the same. The result then is that the potassium concentration in Pacinian corpuscle fluid is 2–2.5 times higher than that in the blood plasma or mesentery tissue fluid in the same animal.

### *Effect of increase in potassium concentration (Akoev and Elman, 1974)*

#### *Impulse activity*

The enhancement of potassium concentration to 11.2–22.4 m$M$/litre decreased the threshold by 50–60% and increased the number of impulses per burst in response to

TABLE I

POTASSIUM AND SODIUM CONTENT OF THE PACINIAN CORPUSCLE FLUID AND THE BLOOD PLASMA

Values are means $\pm$ standard deviation.

| Element | Number of animals | Pacinian corpuscle fluid | Blood plasma | Difference | P |
|---------|-------------------|--------------------------|--------------|------------|---|
| Potassium | 14 | $6.19 \pm 0.72$ | $2.78 \pm 0.38$ | $3.41 \pm 0.61$ | $<0.001$ |
| Sodium | 7 | $114 \pm 10.4$ | $125.6 \pm 10.0$ | $11.1 \pm 6.7$ | $>0.05$ |

equal mechanical stimuli (Fig. 2). In the potassium-rich solution the firing threshold slightly decreased. The immersion of receptors in the potassium-rich solution for a long time resulted in the appearance of spontaneous activity and decrease in the action potential amplitude. Back in the normal solution, the receptor sensitivity and AP amplitude were restored.

*Depolarizing receptor potential*

Increasing potassium ion content from 5–6 m$M$/litre to 11.2 m$M$/litre gradually decreased the receptor potential amplitude (Fig. $3_{1,2}$). Fig. 3 (right) shows the receptor potential–stimulus strength relationship in the normal and potassium-rich solution. It will be seen that a 2-fold increase in potassium concentration resulted

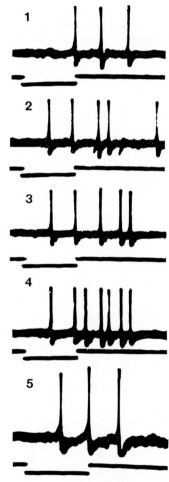

Fig. 2. Effect of increase in potassium concentration (11.2 m$M$/litre) on impulse response of cor-puscle. 1, in normal solution; 2–4 in potassium-rich solution at 4, 8 and 22 min respectively; 5, recovery back in normal solution (41 min). Stimulus duration: 50 msec. Receptor was stimulated with mechanical shocks applied to the platform on which the chamber with receptor was placed. In this case the stimulus oscillated and the receptor responded with several action potentials.

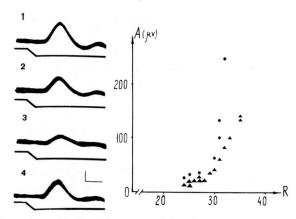

Fig. 3. Left: the changing amplitude of receptor potential in potassium-rich solution (11.2 m*M*/litre). 1, response in normal solution; 2 and 3, response in potassium-rich solution at 7 and 11 min respectively; 4, recovery back in normal solution (11 min). Vertical bar: 50 $\mu$V. Horizontal bar: 2 msec. Right: plot of amplitude of receptor potential (ordinate) *versus* intensity of mechanical stimulus (abscissa) in relative units in normal solution (filled circles) and in potassium-rich solution (11.2 m*M*/litre, 39 min) (filled triangles).

in a decrease in maximal amplitude of receptor potential, no shift of the curve along the abscissa occurring.

*Effects of a potassium-free solution*

Two phases of excitability changes were observed in a potassium free solution: at first it lowered because of an increase of the firing threshold and then it rose when the receptor potential amplitude increased. However, the extent of enhancement in sensitivity was higher in the potassium-rich solution than in the medium of low potassium ion content.

*Effect of removal of sodium ions*

Removal of sodium ions from the external solution abolished the nerve impulse and reduced receptor potential to 10% of its original value. This result agrees with the evidence obtained by other authors (Diamond *et al.*, 1958).

DISCUSSION

The evidence presented above indicates that potassium concentration in the Pacinian corpuscle fluid is higher than in the blood plasma or in the mesentery tissue fluid. Therefore the corpuscle fluid cannot be regarded as an ultrafiltrate of the blood plasma. Electrophysiological experiments showed that increasing potassium concentration in the perfusing solution, within the limits of the concentrations found in the Pacinian corpuscle, results in the enhancement of receptor mechanosensitivity. Analogous results were obtained by Nishi (1968) for Pacinian corpuscles and by Kidd *et al.* (1971) for muscle spindles. Enhancement in excitability was observed only with moderate increases in potassium concentration. High potassium concentrations (28 m$M$/litre) were found to block the impulse activity. The Pacinian corpuscle fluid thus appears to have the right potassium content to enhance the receptor excitability according to physiological requirements.

The enhanced sensitivity of the receptor may be accounted for by the effect of potassium ions on either regenerative or generative parts of receptor. The overall effect of potassium ions depends on which of the two effects prevails. In potassium-rich solution the higher extent of excitability is due to the regenerative part of the receptor.

According to morphological studies, one or two nodes of Ranvier lie within the outer capsule and are immersed in the intracapsular fluid (Quilliam and Sato, 1955; Ilyinsky, 1966b). Therefore, all the regenerative structures of the receptor are immersed into the fluid with elevated potassium concentration and this fact appears to account for post-hyperpolarizing responses.

Our data show that the tissue mechanoreceptors, as well as secondary mechanoreceptors of the sense organs, have a specific medium with elevated potassium content. It is likely that the main difference between these two types of receptors lies in their sensitivity (Ilyinsky and Krasnikova, 1972). Threshold displacements for tissue mechanoreceptors are known to be 2–4 orders higher than those for secondary mechanoreceptors of the sense organs. But within each receptor type there are sensory structures with high and low sensitivity. For the tissue mechanoreceptors examples are Pacinian corpuscles and free nerve endings, respectively, and for the secondary mechanoreceptors examples are the labyrinth receptors and lateral line receptors. Such a difference in sensitivity of the two types of receptors is apparently due to the functional and structural organization of these receptors. However, it may well be that the tissue mechanoreceptors and secondary mechanoreceptors of the sense organs developed in principally similar ways: by complicating and perfecting accessory structures and by establishing their own inner medium.

## SUMMARY

Post-hyperpolarizing responses in Pacinian corpuscles recorded by conventional electrophysiological techniques are described. With post-hyperpolarizing responses, thresholds for impulse activity have been found to be lower than otherwise.

The elevated concentration of potassium ions in the intracapsular fluid of Pacinian corpuscles may be one of the factors favouring the appearance of post-hyperpolarizing responses. According to microflame photometry, the potassium concentration in the capsular fluid is 6.19 $\pm$ 0.72 mEq/litre, *i.e.* 2–2.5 times greater than the potassium concentration either in the blood plasma or in the intertissue fluid surrounding the Pacinian corpuscles in the mesentery.

Electrophysiological analysis has demonstrated that application of hyperpotassium solutions, where potassium concentration was 2–3 times higher than that in the blood plasma, results in an enhanced excitability of the corpuscle (by 50–60%) due to a decrease in the firing threshold.

The suggestion is made that there may exist a general factor — the hyperpotassium medium — favouring the enhancement of sensitivity both in the primary tissue mechanoreceptors and in the secondary mechanoreceptors of the sense organs.

## REFERENCES

AKOEV, G. N. AND ELMAN, S. I. (1974) Potassium ions and electrical activity of single mechano-receptors Pacinian corpuscles. *Sechenov physiol. J. U.S.S.R.*, **60**, 55–61 (in Russian).

DIAMOND, J., GRAY, J. A. B. AND INMAN, D. R. (1958) The relation between receptor potentials and the concentration of sodium ions. *J. Physiol. (Lond.)*, **142**, 382–394.

FÄNGE, R., LARSSON, A. AND LIDMAN, U. (1972) Fluids and jellies of the acusticolateralis system in relation to body fluids in *Coryphaenoides rupestric* and other fishes. *Marine Biol.*, **17**, 180–185.

FRANKENHAEUSER, B. AND WIDEN, L. (1956) Anode break excitation in desheathed frog nerve. *J. Physiol. (Lond.)*, **131**, 243–247.

ILYINSKY, O. B. (1965) Processes of excitation and inhibition in single mechanoreceptors (Pacinian corpuscles). *Nature (Lond.)*, **208**, 351–353.

ILYINSKY, O. B. (1966a) On and off responses of single mechanoreceptors. *Sechenov physiol. J. U.S.S.R.*, **52**, 99–107. English translation in *Fed. Proc.* Transl. Suppl., **26**, t948–t952 (1966–1967).

ILYINSKY, O. B. (1966b) Certain aspects of the receptive formation. *Sechenov physiol. J. U.S.S.R.*, **52**, 360–369 (in Russian).

ILYINSKY, O. B. (1970) Posthyperpolarizing responses of Pacinian corpuscles. *Proc. Acad. Sci. U.S.S.R.*, **190**, 472–475 (in Russian).

ILYINSKY, O. B. AND KRASNIKOVA, T. L. (1971) On the composition of the fluids surrounding some mechano- and electroreceptor structures in Elasmobranchia. *J. evol. Biochem. Physiol.*, **7**, 570–575 (in Russian).

ILYINSKY, O. B. AND KRASNIKOVA, T. L. (1972) Study of ionic composition of Pacinian corpuscle fluid in connection with their activity. *Sechenov physiol. J. U.S.S.R.*, **58**, 434–442 (in Russian).

ILYINSKY, O. B., VOLKOVA, N. K. AND CHEREPNOV, V. L. (1968) Structure and function of Pacinian corpuscle. *Sechenov physiol. J. U.S.S.R.*, **54**, 295–302. English translation in *Neuroscience Translations*, **6**, 637–643. (1968–1969).

ILYINSKY, O. B., VOLKOVA, N. K., CHEREPNOV, V. L. AND KRYLOV, B. V. (1975) Morphofunctional properties of Pacinian corpuscles. In A. IGGO AND O. B. ILYINSKY (Eds.), *Somatosensory and Visceral Receptor Mechanisms, Progress in Brain Research, Vol. 43.* Elsevier, Amsterdam, pp. 173–186.

JANSEN, J. K. S., NIA, A., ORMSTAD, K. AND WALLE, L. (1971) On the innervation of the slowly adapting stretch receptor of the crayfish abdomen. An electrophysiological approach. *Acta physiol. scand.*, **81**, 273–285.

KATSUKI, J. AND HASHIMOTO, T. (1969) Shark pit organs: enhancement of mechanosensitivity by potassium ions. *Science*, **166**, 1287–1289.

KIDD, G. L., KUCERA, J. AND VAILLANT, C. H. (1971) The influence of the interstitial concentration of $K^+$ on the activity of muscle receptors. *Physiol. bohemoslov.*, **20**, 95–108.

KONISHI, T., KELSEY, E. AND SINGLETON, G. T. (1966) Effect of chemical alteration in the endolymph on the cochlear potential. *Acta oto-laryng. (Stockh.)*, **62**, 393–404.

KUFFLER, S. W. AND EYZAGUIRRE, C. (1955) Synaptic inhibition in an isolated nerve cell. *J. gen. Physiol.*, **39**, 155–184.

MURRAY, R. W. AND POTTS, W. T. W. (1961) The composition of the endolymph, perilymph and other body fluids of elasmobranchs. *Comp. Biochem. Physiol.*, **2**, 65–75.

NISHI, K. (1968) Modification of the mechanical threshold of the Pacinian corpuscle after the perfusion with solutions of varying cation content. *Jap. J. Physiol.*, **18**, 216–231.

NISHI, K. AND SATO, M. (1968) Depolarizing and hyperpolarizing receptor potentials in nonmyelinated nerve terminal in Pacinian corpuscles. *J. Physiol. (Lond.)*, **199**, 383–396.

OOYAMA, H. AND WRIGHT, E. B. (1961) Anode break excitation on single Ranvier node of frog nerve. *Amer. J. Physiol.*, **200**, 209–218.

QUILLIAM, T. A. AND SATO, M. (1955) The distribution of myelin on nerve fibres from Pacinian corpuscles. *J. Physiol. (Lond.)*, **129**, 167–176.

SIMON, E. J., HILDING, D. A. AND KASHGARIAN, M. (1973) Micropuncture study of the mechanism of endolymph production in the frog. *Amer. J. Physiol.*, **225**, 114–118.

SMITH, C. A., LOWRY, O. H. AND WU, M. L. (1954) The electrolytes of the labyrinthine fluids. *Laryngoscope (St Louis)*, **64**, 141–153.

TASAKI, I. (1959) Demonstration of two stable states of the nerve membrane in potassium rich media. *J. Physiol. (Lond.)*, **148**, 306–331.

## DISCUSSION

KHAYUTIN: Do you not think that it would be more correct to class with the category "the tissue mechanoreceptors" only those which have a direct contact with the tissue fluid?

KRASNIKOVA: On the basis of the information available at present on morphology and physiology of receptors, the term "the tissue receptors" should seemingly embrace all the receptors located in tissues as opposed to the receptors of the sense organs. As for mechanoreceptors they appear to be divided into two groups: the tissue receptors and the mechanoreceptors of the sense organs.

ANDRES: A muscle spindle inner fluid has a direct communication with a peripheral nerve. I wonder if there are concentration differences between the outside of the perineural sheaths and the inside of the muscle spindle?

KRASNIKOVA: We have no evidence concerning the ionic content of the intracapsular fluid in the muscle spindle. From the results reported by Brzezinski (Acta histochem., 12 (1961) 277–278) it follows, however, that this fluid differs from the lymph by a higher content of the acid mucopolysaccharides and thus also has a specific composition.

BURGESS: Outer lamellae of the Pacinian corpuscles are continuations of the perineural sheaths of peripheral nerves, I believe. Do you have any evidence concerning whether the content of fluid inside the peripheral nerve is different than in blood, perhaps, showing higher potassium?

KRASNIKOVA: No, we have not, since we did not study the ionic content of the fluid of perineural sheath of the peripheral nerve supplying the Pacinian corpuscle. The data on the elevated potassium concentration in the intracapsular fluid of Pacinian corpuscles presented above, and those mentioned while discussing a possibility of specificity of the fluid composition in the capsule of muscle spindle, give good reasons to believe, though, that at the boundary between the peripheral nerve and receptor there are certain systems responsible for the specific content of the medium around the receptor nerve ending.

IGGO: Is it possible that the statistical difference between the concentration of the potassium ions in the capsular fluid and in blood plasma arises because you are working with the low potassium concentration in the fluid so that only a small leakage of cell cytoplasm content would cause a relatively large change in potassium content of your fluid in contrast to sodium content?

KRASNIKOVA: When taking the samples of Pacinian corpuscle fluid we perforated only the outer, *i.e.* the densest, receptor capsule lamellae, that resulted in a release of a big amount of capsular fluid, or else we decapsulated the receptor removing as many as about 30 lamellae of the outer capsule which were perforated with a sharp needle by one puncture through all the lamellae. A mean amount of fluid taken from a capsule of moderate size ($200 \, \mu m \times 500 \, \mu m$) is about $0.20 \times 10^{-3}$ ml. Calculations based on morphological evidence show that the cytoplasmic volume from 30 lamellae of the outer capsule is about $0.13 \times 10^{-6}$ ml. Even with all cytoplasm of lamellar cells leaked into the sample to be analyzed, the cytoplasmic volume does not exceed $6.5 \times 10^{-4}$ of the volume of intracapsular fluid. Potassium concentration in cytoplasm is about 120–150 mEq/litre and that in blood plasma about 3–5 mEq/litre. If the fluid of the Pacinian corpuscle is considered as an analogue of plasma, potassium concentration in receptor fluid after mixing with cytoplasm will increase by only 0.1 mEq/litre. Our results, though, show that potassium concentration in Pacinian corpuscle fluid is 2–2.5 times higher than that in blood plasma. Again, it should be mentioned that never in the course of preparation were the lamellar cell structures all damaged, mixing of cytoplasm with receptor fluid actually being much less than that assessed above.

# General Properties of Mechanoreceptors that Signal the Position of the Integument, Teeth, Tactile Hairs and Joints

P. R. BURGESS

*Department of Physiology, University of Utah College of Medicine, Salt Lake City, Utah 84132 (U.S.A.)*

Two factors may be considered when discussing the properties of receptors that signal the position of some part of an animal's body. The first concerns the features of individual receptors that ensure accurate specification of a position. The second has to do with the way in which different receptors collaborate to indicate a particular position among the various positions that the body part can occupy. The following discussion is concerned primarily with the second point, but will begin with a brief consideration of the properties that individual receptors should have if they are to provide an accurate position signal.

## PROPERTIES OF INDIVIDUAL RECEPTORS SIGNALLING POSITION

In order for a receptor to give an accurate indication of the position of a structure, its discharge should be a function of the position of the structure only, and should not vary with the time that a particular position has been held, the rate or direction of the movement used to reach that position, or how frequently the structure has been placed in the position. Otherwise, the position signal is degraded.

## POSITION CODING BY POPULATIONS OF RECEPTORS

### General considerations

Three ways will be presented whereby the position of a structure could be specified by a population of receptors. The first uses "spatially tuned" receptors, the second uses populations of "opponent" receptors, and the third uses a "full range" receptor population.

Spatially tuned receptors are illustrated in Fig. 1. Four individual receptors are shown, each responding over a particular portion of the range. Some respond in the central portions of the range, and others at the edges. In this and all subsequent illustrations the discharge shown is that which is present after all movement has ceased and the structure is stationary. If a number of receptors were added to those

SPATIAL TUNING

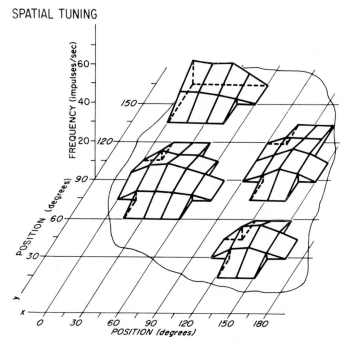

Fig. 1. In this and subsequent figures, the x and y axes define an arbitrary space the extent of which is indicated by the curved solid line. It is assumed that some structure (such as a joint) can occupy any position within this space. The coordinates are given in degrees but any convenient coordinates could be used. The four receptors illustrated in this figure are "spatially tuned". The discharge of an individual receptor increases as the structure is displaced, reaches a peak, and then decreases as the structure is moved further in the same direction, except in the case of the receptor in the upper left hand corner which is situated at the edge of the range. The discharge illustrated is that occurring after movement ceases and the structure is stationary.

shown in Fig. 1, covering the whole of the space that the structure can occupy, any position could be specified by the particular group of receptors activated. This is akin to the way in which a cutaneous stimulus is localized and one would expect, therefore, that spatially tuned afferent fibers would be "somatotopically" distributed within the central nervous system.

Opponent receptor populations are illustrated in Fig. 2. In this case, positions which progressively deviate from some intermediate location produce an increasing discharge in one receptor population and decreasing activity in the opponent population. Positions on the opposite side of the intermediate location evoke the converse pattern of activity. Only two receptors are shown in Fig. 2, signalling positions on the y axis. It is probable, particularly in mammals, that in place of each receptor there actually would be a population of receptors with varying thresholds and input–output slopes. Two additional populations of opponent receptors would be needed to signal positions along the x axis.

Full range receptors bear some resemblance to the opponent system except that only one of the two opponent populations is present and the thresholds of the re-

A. OPPONENT POPULATIONS

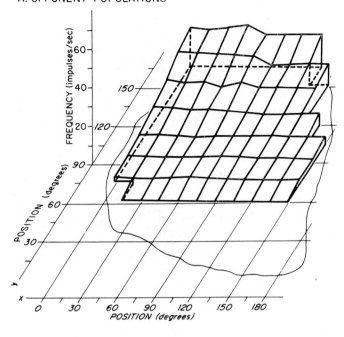

B.

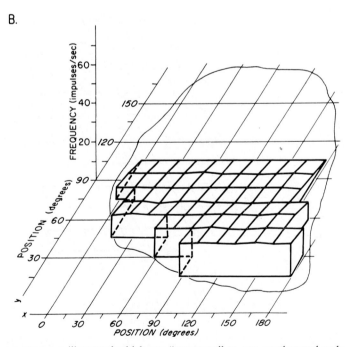

Fig. 2. Two receptors are illustrated which are "opponent" to one another and code positions on the y axis. Positions that increase the discharge of one receptor decrease the discharge of the other. The format of the figure is the same as Fig. 1.

## A. FULL RANGE RECEPTORS

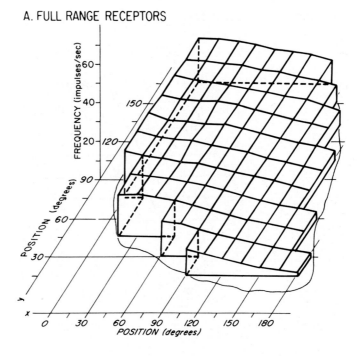

### B.

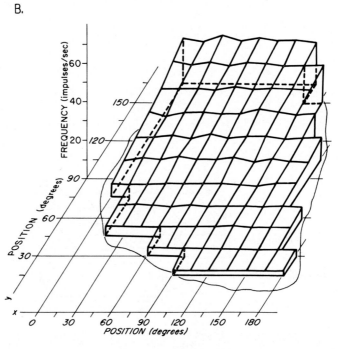

Fig. 3. Two "full range" receptors are shown. In A, coding positions are on the x axis, and in B, on the y axis. These receptors change their discharge as the structure is displaced from a position at one extreme of the range to a position at the opposite extreme in the appropriate direction. The format of the figure is described in Fig. 1.

ceptors are such that they discharge at a progressively increasing frequency as the structure is positioned from one extreme of the range to the other. Full range receptors coding positions along the x and the y axes are shown in Fig. 3A and 3B respectively.

Having presented some of the major ways in which position information might be signalled, the discussion will now turn to the codes actually used in nature. How the position of mammalian joints is indicated will be considered first since recent evidence suggests a reconsideration of traditional views concerning this problem.

### Signal for joint position in mammals

In recent years, it has generally been thought that the receptors signalling joint position are located in the articular tissues proper, *i.e.* the capsules and ligaments of the joint, and that the receptors are spatially tuned (Skoglund, 1973). However, studies of the cat knee joint have now led to a questioning of these views for two reasons. First, receptors in articular tissues provide little information about the position of the joint over most of its working range. Instead, their activity is largely confined to positions at the edge of the range (Burgess and Clark, 1969; Clark and Burgess, unpublished observations). Second, none of the few receptors whose activity extends appreciably into the range have been found to discharge at peak frequency in the central portions of the range, as would be required for a code using spatially tuned receptors (Clark and Burgess, unpublished observations). The first consideration led us to hypothesize that the receptors which signal joint angle lie not in articular tissues but in muscles, a suggestion which is consistent with recent psychophysical observations (Goodwin *et al.*, 1972; Eklund, 1972). If this hypothesis is correct (and it may only apply to proximal joints like the knee and hip) the position code used to signal joint angle employs opponent populations of receptors since each movement at a joint is controlled by both agonist and antagonist muscles and the evidence indicates that receptors in both must be used to cover the full range of positions, at least under passive conditions (Simon, Randić and Burgess, unpublished observations).

### Position codes for other structures

Position signalling with opponent populations is widely used by animals. Among the mammals, tactile hairs (Fitzgerald, 1940), teeth (Pfaffman, 1939) and the skin (Chambers *et al.*, 1972) are known to employ this principle. Among the arthropods, joint position is usually signalled by opponent receptor populations, although in a few cases full range populations may be used (Table I). In the case of a half to full range receptor population, there is always the possibility that an opponent population exists which has yet to be discovered. For example, the well known muscle receptor organs that lie beneath the dorsal exoskeleton of the crayfish and related crustaceans and which are activated by abdominal flexion (Wiersma *et al.*, 1953) are now known to form an opponent system with receptors in the sheath of the ventral nerve cord

## TABLE I

The position code has been referred to as half to full range in those cases where the studies have not been sufficiently quantitative to specify precisely how much of the range is covered. It was clear in every instance, however, that the response was not of the end position type, where activity occurs only at or near the extremes of the range. Receptors are considered to signal with a bipositional code if the same fiber is active at two positions and is inactive at positions in between. The sensitivity of receptors under efferent control will be a function of the relevant motor output. The position code has been given for passive conditions, i.e. when the limb is moved by an outside force and the efferent output is minimal. Golgi tendon organs and apodeme sensory neurons are so situated that they register the forces acting on the large muscle masses of the limbs and hence their response will be determined by the load against which the muscles contract rather than by the position of the limb. Muscle spindles, myochordotonal organs and muscle receptor organs, on the other hand, incorporate specialized muscles which are small and do not contribute appreciable force to the support or movement of the limbs. These specialized muscles lie in parallel with the large muscle masses and thus change their length with alterations of limb position. The designation of half to full range applies in the absence of appreciable motor output to the muscles in the receptors. In the presence of more motor outflow the range would expand.

| Receptor group | Phylum or subphylum | Location of sensory endings | Neural code for position | Reference |
|---|---|---|---|---|
| | Vertebrata | muscle spindles | opponent | Matthews, 1931 |
| | | tendons (Golgi tendon organs) | opponent: end position | Houk et al., 1971 |
| Receptors Closely Associated with Muscle and Under Efferent Control | Arthropoda | myochordotonal organs | half to full range | Cohen, 1963; Clarac, 1968 |
| | | muscle receptor organs | half to full range | Wiersma et al., 1953; Bush and Roberts, 1971 |
| | | apodemes (apodeme sensory neurons) | opponent | Bowerman, 1972 |
| | | | opponent: end position | Macmillan and Dando, 1972 |
| | Vertebrata | joint ligaments and capsules | opponent: end position, bipositional: end position | Burgess and Clark, 1969 and unpublished |
| Receptors in Connective Tissue Structures Spanning Joints | Arthropoda | chordotonal organs | opponent, half to full range | Wiersma and Boettiger, 1959; Bush, 1965 |
| | | elastic strands | half to full range | Finlayson and Loewenstein, 1958; Bush and Roberts, 1971 |
| | | nerve cord sheath | full range | Grobstein, 1973 |
| | | hair plates | opponent, half to full range | Pringle, 1938; Mittelstaedt, 1957 |
| Receptors Located in Surface Structures At or Near Joints | Arthropoda | beneath joint membranes | opponent | Pringle, 1956; Bowerman and Larimer, 1973 |
| | | | half to full range | Wyse, 1971 |
| | | | spatially tuned | Barber, 1960 |
| | | lyriform organs | opponent | Pringle, 1955 |

which are sensitive to abdominal extension (Grobstein, 1973). Some individual chordotonal organs have opponent receptor populations, others have half to full range receptors. The latter, however, are often paired at a single joint so that together they provide an opponent signal (Wiersma, 1959; Bush, 1965). Elastic strands which individually have half to full range receptors may be similarly paired (Finlayson and Loewenstein, 1958). Some of the proprioceptive organs in the more distal joints of arthropods have full range populations without any obvious opponent receptors (Wiersma, 1959; Wyse, 1971). It may be that in such cases distal joint positions are signalled with a full range code. Less precise tonic information is likely to be required about the positions of distal joints than of more proximal joints (see Sherrington, 1900).

In only one instance has a spatially tuned receptor population been proposed. Barber (1960) reported this type of code for the coxo-trochanteral joint of the *Limulus* walking leg. At the more distal femoro-tibial joint in the same animal Pringle (1956) described opponent populations, and at the still more distally located tibio-tarsal joint Wyse (1971) found a full range signal. It seems reasonable to conclude that spatially tuned populations, if present at all, are rare, even though joint receptor structures of quite different morphology are employed by different animals.

CONCLUSION

Opponent populations of receptors serve to code the positions of the parts of an animal's body in most cases, although the animals may be quite distantly related phylogenetically. Sometimes full range populations may be used, perhaps when less precision is required. There could be a number of reasons why these populations of receptors have evolved. It may not be easy to produce spatially tuned receptors given the patterns of distortion that occur in tissues when structures are positioned at different locations. The opponent and full range codes could be more "economical" than spatial tuning in terms of the numbers of central neurons required, since there is no necessity to somatotopically map a large number of afferent channels from one joint within the central nervous system, although different joints would presumably be distinguished by different central connections. Since most structures occupy an intermediate position at rest, an opponent system, depending on the exact thresholds and input–output functions of the receptors, can be minimally active at the rest position. This is not possible with a system of full range receptors and may serve a simple energy conservation function. Since receptors signalling position are rarely ideal in their behavior in the sense described in the first section of this paper, the presence of two populations functioning reciprocally could provide a more accurate position signal than a single full range population with similar properties. For example, if the receptors show directional sensitivity, discharging when the structure is moving in a direction which excites the endings but not in the reverse direction, full range receptors would give no signal as the structure is moved in the latter direction throughout the range. This could occur through only a part of the range with

an opponent system and would be eliminated completely if the two opponent populations overlapped over the entire range. Other as yet unknown advantages of opponent
receptors may be revealed as the central processing of position information becomes
known.

## SUMMARY

Receptors that signal the position of some part of an animal's body are usually
organized in an "opponent" fashion. The activity of one population of receptors
increases as the body part deviates progressively from some intermediate (rest)
position toward one extreme of the range and the activity of another (the opponent)
population of receptors decreases. The converse pattern of activity occurs when the
body part deviates from the rest position in the opposite direction. This is the method
whereby receptors signal the positions of joints, teeth, vibrissae and the skin in
mammals. Joint position in arthropods is also signalled in this fashion. In a few cases,
one of the opponent receptor populations may be absent. Rarely has it been reported
that individual receptors respond over only a limited portion of the range at intermediate positions. It is apparent, therefore, that position signalling with opponent
populations is widely used by animals that are distantly related phylogenetically.

## REFERENCES

BARBER S. B. (1960) Structure and properties of *Limulus* articular proprioceptors. *J. exp. Zool.*,
  **143**, 283–321.
BOWERMAN, R. F. (1972) A muscle receptor organ in the scorpion postabdomen. I. The sensory
  system. *J. comp. Physiol.*, **81**, 133–146.
BOWERMAN, R. F. AND LARIMER, J. (1973) Structure and physiology of the patella–tibia joint receptors
  in scorpion pedipalps. *Comp. Biochem. Physiol.*, **46A**, 139–151.
BURGESS, P. R. AND CLARK, F. J. (1969) Characteristics of knee joint receptors in the cat. *J. Physiol.
  (Lond.)*, **203**, 317–335.
BUSH, B. M. H. (1965) Proprioception by chordotonal organs in the merocarpopodite and carpo-
  propodite joints of *Carcinus maenas* legs. *Comp. Biochem. Physiol.*, **14**, 185–199.
BUSH, B. M. H. AND ROBERTS, A. (1971) Coxal muscle receptors in the crab: the receptor potentials
  of S and T fibres in response to ramp stretches. *J. exp. Biol.*, **55**, 813–832.
CHAMBERS, M. R., ANDRES, K. H., DUERING, M. VON AND IGGO, A. (1972) The structure and function
  of the slowly adapting type II receptor in hairy skin. *Quart. J. exp. Physiol.*, **57**, 417–445.
CLARAC, F. (1968) Proprioception by the ischio-meropodite region in legs of the crab *Carcinus
  mediterraneus* C. *Z. vergl. Physiol.*, **61**, 224–245.
COHEN, M. J. (1963) The crustacean myochordotonal organ as a proprioceptive system. *Comp.
  Biochem. Physiol.*, **8**, 223–243.
EKLUND, G. (1972) Position sense and state of contraction; the effects of vibration. *J. Neurol.
  Neurosurg. Psychiat.*, **35**, 606–611.
FINLAYSON, L. H. AND LOEWENSTEIN, O. (1958) The structure and function of abdominal stretch
  receptors in insects. *Proc. roy Soc. B*, **148**, 433–449.
FITZGERALD, O. (1940) Discharges from the sensory organs of the cat's vibrissae and the modification
  in their activity by ions. *J. Physiol. (Lond.)*, **98**, 163–178.
GOODWIN, G. M., McCLOSKEY, D. I. AND MATTHEWS, P. B. C. (1972) The contribution of muscle
  afferents to kinaesthesia shown by vibration induced illusions of movement and by the effects of
  paralysing joint afferents. *Brain*, **95**, 705–748.

GROBSTEIN, P. (1973) Extension-sensitivity in the crayfish abdomen. I. Neurons monitoring nerve cord length. *J. comp. Physiol.*, **86**, 331–348.

HOUK, J. C., SINGER, J. J. AND HENNEMAN, E. (1971) Adequate stimulus for tendon organs with observations on mechanics of ankle joint. *J. Neurophysiol.*, **34**, 1051–1065.

MACMILLAN, D. L. AND DANDO, M. R. (1972) Tension receptors on the apodemes of muscles in the walking legs of the crab, *Cancer magister*. *Mar. Behav. Physiol.*, **1**, 185–208.

MATTHEWS, B. H. C. (1931) The response of a single end organ. *J. Physiol. (Lond.)*, **71**, 64–110.

MITTELSTAEDT, H. (1957) Prey capture in mantids. In B. T. SCHEER (Ed.), *Recent Advances in Invertebrate Physiology*. Univ. of Oregon Publications, Eugene, Oreg., pp. 51–71.

PFAFFMANN, C. (1939) Afferent impulses from the teeth due to pressure and noxious stimulation. *J. Physiol. (Lond.)*, **97**, 207–219.

PRINGLE, J. W. S. (1938) Proprioception in insects. III. The function of the hair sensilla at the joints. *J. exp. Biol.*, **15**, 467–473.

PRINGLE, J. W. S. (1955) The function of the lyriform organs of arachnids. *J. exp. Biol.*, **32**, 270–278.

PRINGLE, J. W. S. (1956) Proprioception in *Limulus*. *J. exp. Biol.*, **33**, 658–667.

SHERRINGTON, C. S. (1900) The muscular sense. In E. A. SCHÄFER (Ed.), *Textbook of Physiology*. Macmillan, New York, pp. 1002–1025.

SKOGLUND, S. (1973) Joint receptors and kinaesthesis. In A. IGGO (Ed.), *Handbook of Sensory Physiology, Vol. II*. Springer, New York, pp. 111–136.

WIERSMA, C. A. G. (1959) Movement receptors in decapod Crustacea. *J. mar. biol. Ass. U.K.* **38**, 143–152.

WIERSMA, C. A. G. AND BOETTIGER, E. G. (1959) Unidirectional movement fibres from a proprioceptive organ of the crab, *Carcinus maenas*. *J. exp. Biol.*, **36**, 102–112.

WIERSMA, C. A. G., FURSHPAN, E. AND FLOREY, E. (1953) Physiological and pharmacological observations on muscle receptor organs of the crayfish, *Cambarus clarkii* Girard. *J. exp. Biol.*, **30**, 136–150.

WYSE, G. A. (1971) Receptor organization and function in *Limulus* chelae. *Z. vergl. Physiol.*, **73**, 249–273.

## DISCUSSION

ZEVEKE: Do the cutaneous receptors participate in the signalling of limb position?

BURGESS: We believe that they do not participate in signalling limb position because it is possible to anesthetize the skin around the joint without any impairment in limb position information. That was one reason. Second reason. The information about skin position is poor. If you displace the skin and hold it displaced, the sensation of displacement disappears after about a minute. So, this is different than the joint. In the case of the joint the awareness continues for many minutes in the absence of movement. Therefore, for these two reasons we believe that skin receptors do not participate in limb position sense.

CAUNA: I am not challenging your views, but I think we have to realize that we have to be very good gross anatomists to carry out our work successfully because many muscles act upon two and three or more joints and there is again the question of action: active movement or passive movement and action with or without gravity and lifting weight so that in your experiments you have to take all this into account.

BURGESS: Yes, I agree that the coding of limb position under a variety of different circumstances must be a complex phenomenon and that the system must be able to compensate for different patterns of movements, different loading conditions and different rates of movement across several joints. We originally preferred to think that the receptors which signal the position of the limb were in the joints and would be free from interference from load changes, from factors concerned with the rates and patterns of movements of different joints. That has the appeal of simplicity, I agree. Now, we can understand how the muscle spindles can give the signal. If the central nervous system knows the $\gamma$-efferent activity to the spindles then it can read the spindle discharge in terms of absolute muscle length and at every joint we do have muscles that control just that one joint. In fact, for every movement at every joint there is an agonist and antagonist group of muscle fibers available to provide a signal.

IGGO: There are two points I should like to take up with you. I think the first one is your assumption. For the sake of simplicity you have ignored the fact that any slowly adapting receptors which could provide information about the joint position on any of your schemes all have dynamic sensitivity which you omit from your theoretical interpretation. The second point is partly in response to Dr. Zeveke's question about the possible role of cutaneous receptors. It is known that in the skin there are receptors which can maintain a steady discharge, particularly in primates, for a very long time, for half an hour or longer. I think the fact that the central processing of the cutaneous sensation ignores this continuous background information is not a sufficient reason to exclude the possibility that central processing for joint information may use it.

BURGESS: Let me just say very quickly that I agree with Professor Iggo that the dynamic sensitivity of the joint receptors, muscle receptors, cutaneous receptors, whichever are involved here, certainly cause difficulty, and that is why I spent some time in the beginning describing the ideal properties of receptors that signal position, but, of course, these ideal properties are not present. How this is accomplished by the central nervous system remains to be determined. But we are doing some experiments on the skin, which we can talk about privately, which I think may give some insight into the way of how these dynamic responses of position receptors are handled by the central nervous system. The evidence that the skin is not involved in coding position really comes from the fact that you can anesthetize skin and there is no impairment of limb position sense.

LINDBLOM: I have just a short comment on the eventual contribution of cutaneous receptors. In a study by Valbo and Teckni on the human receptors with recording from the median nerve they recorded from slowly adapting type II units with the receptive field located around the nails, and it was possible to relate the discharge frequencies from these units directly to the angular position at a distant phalange and they suggested that in special situations, as for the distant joints, skin receptors might contribute. My second comment would be that, perhaps, one should also consider unknown efferent discharges in thin efferents and this is because you can find, in conditions with diseases in peripheral nerves, a situation where large fibers are injured and, for instance the vibratory sensation, impaired, but the joint sensation is retained.

TSIRULNIKOV: I would like to know your opinion in connection with this. Your hypothesis is very interesting. Do you relate position sensations only to stationary or to dynamic states? The fact is known that if the human hand is stationary for a long period of time, the sensation of the position of the fingers is lost.

BURGESS: We worked on the knee-joint (the sensation of the knee joint position is not lost). This should be distinguished from the situation in the hand, and I think that it is an important distinction to make.

ZELENA: Your idea that position of the joints is signalled by muscle receptors is very logical. I think it might be rewarding to develop it more on the quantitative basis. We know that the extensors and flexors, agonist and antagonist muscles differ in number and density of receptors and individual muscles have different contents of muscle receptors, but we do not know why. I wonder if one makes the sum, if it could give some sense? You have speculated about the knee, if you allow me to speculate about the ankle. Physiologically flexors have a very high number of muscle spindles, the anterior tibia muscles have about 30 spindles in the rat, the extensor digitorial muscle has about 35 spindles and the small ext. hallucis has 4 spindles. Physiologically extensors have a large mass of muscle fibers, but the density of receptors is smaller. So, it probably also contributes to the determining of the position.

BURGESS: Thank you for that information and for that perspective on the problem. I certainly would be in agreement that similar numbers of receptors should be available for both extension and flexion coding. It is interesting that the number of receptors available appears to be equal even if the mass of the muscles is different.

# The Mechanoreceptors of the Sinus Hair Organ on the Cat's Foreleg

BENGT Y. NILSSON

*Department of Physiology, Karolinska Institutet, Stockholm (Sweden)*

## INTRODUCTION

In addition to the comparatively short and thin hairs making up the general hair coat, most mammalian species have morphologically distinct tactile hairs which are recognized by their larger size and by the presence of a large blood sinus in the hair follicle. The vibrissae are a well-known type of these so-called sinus hairs. Almost a century ago British zoologists discovered a group of hairs resembling vibrissae on the forelegs of many mammals (Bland-Sutton, 1887; Beddard, 1902). These hairs, which are located on the volar side just above the paw, are found especially in those species using their forefeet not only for locomotion but also to catch prey, to hold the food or to climb. The carpal hair group is common among rodents and carnivora (rabbits and dogs being two exceptions), and it is absent in ungulates. However, the exact functional significance of these hairs is unknown. As they are equally well developed in animals of both sexes they are generally not considered as a secondary sexual character. A well-developed blood sinus enclosing the hair root proper makes the carpal hairs morphologically similar to the vibrissae (Frédéric, 1905; Fritz, 1909).

The carpal sinus hair organ in the cat was rediscovered in the course of studies of more deeply situated mechanoreceptors of the cat's foreleg (Skoglund, 1960). Subsequent morphological and physiological studies have shown that the cat's carpal hairs in certain respects are similar to vibrissae but that they have clearly different properties as well (Nilsson and Skoglund, 1965; Nilsson, 1968, 1969a and b).

## MORPHOLOGICAL STUDIES

The carpal sinus hair organ in the cat consists of a tuft of 4–6 coarse hairs 20–30 mm in length, which protrudes above the general fur hairs. On account of the large follicular blood sinuses the hair organ is easily palpated as a small elevation in the skin about 4 mm in diameter. This skin area is supplied by relatively large branches from the ulnar nerve and artery.

Histological sections (Fig. 1) show the group of hair follicles with their characteristic blood-filled cavities enclosed by strong connective tissue walls. The lower part

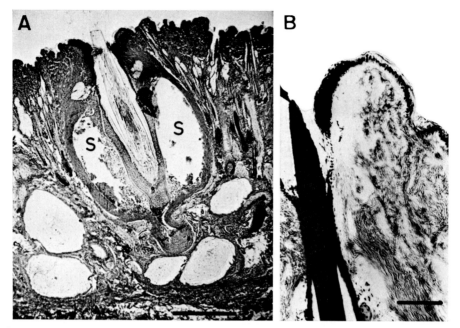

Fig. 1. Longitudinal sections of carpal sinus hairs. A: five Pacinian corpuscles situated close to the external wall of the blood sinus (S). Calibration bar = 0.5 mm. B: the hair disk at the follicle mouth is immediately adjacent to the sinus hair. Calibration bar = 0.1 mm.

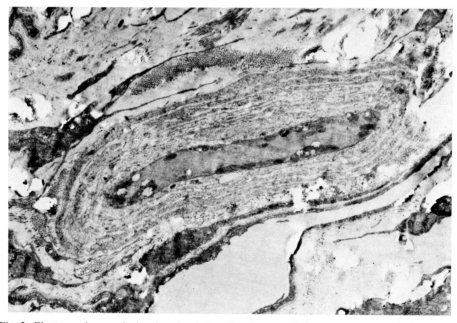

Fig. 2. Electron micrograph showing simple lamellated corpuscle in cavernous part of blood sinus. × 6600. (In collaboration with Å. Flock.)

of each sinus is filled with a cavernous tissue while the upper portion, the ring sinus, is filled with blood. From the internal mesenchymal sinus wall a "ring wulst" projects into the ring sinus. The hair follicle is densely innervated by means of several small bundles of nerve fibers which, after penetrating the lower part of the external sinus wall, pass through the cavernous tissue to reach the hair root proper. The nerve fibers then ascend in the inner sinus wall, symmetrically arranged around the hair root.

A section through the upper part of the follicle shows a network of winding varicose fine nerve fibers in the internal mesenchymal sinus wall while other fibers penetrate the glassy membrane to form Merkel cell-neurite complexes in the external root sheath. Electron microscopic studies (Flock and Nilsson, unpublished observations) revealed the presence of a simple type of lamellated corpuscles in the cavernous sinus (Fig. 2). Adrenergic nerve endings in the lower sinus and in the internal sinus wall were described by Fuxe and Nilsson (1965).

Thus, these studies have established fundamental similarities in the pattern of follicular innervation between the carpal sinus hairs and vibrissae (cf. Andres, 1966; Patrizi and Munger, 1966). There are, however, in the immediate surroundings of the hair follicles three pronounced differences.

(1) Several Pacinian corpuscles are found in the cat's carpal sinus hair organ surrounding the lower parts of the hair follicles (Fig. 1) (Fritz, 1909; Nilsson and Skoglund, 1965).

(2) Movements of vibrissae are elicited by contractions in fast striated facial muscles (Lindquist, 1973), whereas the carpal hairs are connected to a strong smooth pilomotor musculature (Nilsson, 1968). Slow contractions in these muscles induce a piloerection which further raises the tactile hairs above the general hair coat.

(3) A typical hair disk is found at the mouth of each carpal sinus hair follicle (Fig. 1B). This area shows a thickened epithelium, a richly vascularized subepidermal tissue and a row of Merkel cell–neurite complexes at the base of the epidermis (Nilsson, 1969b). In this respect the carpal sinus hairs resemble the tylotrich hairs (Straile, 1960). Hair disks have not been described in connection with cat vibrissae. Mann (1968), however, demonstrated the presence of this structure at the vibrissae of the American opossum.

PHYSIOLOGICAL STUDIES

*Methods*

A full account of the technique has been given in a previous paper (Nilsson, 1969a). The experiments were carried out on cats anesthetized with Nembutal. Guard and down hairs in the vicinity of the carpal sinus hairs were cut short. The afferent nerve was dissected free in the proximal part of the lower leg and impulse activity was recorded from thin filaments with chlorided silver wire electrodes. The mechano-receptors were stimulated by manual bending of the hairs. For a quantitative analysis the hairs were displaced at various amplitudes and velocities by a specially designed mechanical stimulator. Stimulation amplitudes up to 450 $\mu$m were used, the velocities normally ranging from 0.5 to 63 mm/sec. The movement of the stimulator probe was usually parallel to the skin surface and approximately at right angles to the hair shaft. The contact point was 2–3 mm above the follicle mouth.

## *Results*

An initial mechanical stimulation of the carpal sinus hair organ with a hand-held probe showed that responses from at least four main types of afferent units could be distinguished: (1) slowly adapting responses from sinus hair follicle receptors; (2) slowly adapting responses emanating from the hair disk receptors; (3) rapidly adapting discharges from extremely vibration-sensitive receptors, *i.e.* Pacinian corpuscles and (4) rapidly adapting responses from receptors within the sinus hair follicle. In addition the afferent nerve included fibers from the surrounding skin area carrying rapidly adapting discharges from ordinary hair follicle receptors and slowly adapting responses from cutaneous SA type I receptors (Iggo and Muir, 1969).

### *(1) Slowly adapting sinus hair receptors*

Many afferent units of this type had a regular spontaneous activity which varied in frequency up to 20 impulses/sec. Each nerve fiber supplied only one sinus hair while each hair was innervated by several afferent fibers. Often recordings from thin filaments showed two and sometimes three afferent units activated by movements of one and the same sinus hair.

The sinus hair receptors usually displayed a directional sensitivity giving high

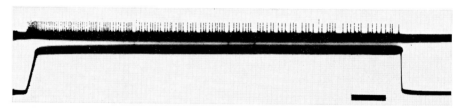

Fig. 3. Response obtained in slowly adapting sinus hair unit (upper trace) to movement of hair at a constant velocity of 14.4 mm/sec up to an amplitude plateau of 450 $\mu$m (lower trace) Time calibration bar 100 msec.

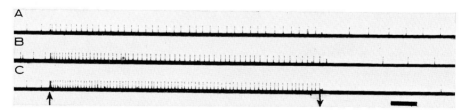

Fig. 4. Responses obtained in slowly adapting sinus hair unit to static displacement of a hair at three different amplitudes each about 1 sec in duration. Onset and end of stimuli at arrows. A: 150, B: 325 and C: 500 $\mu$m. Time calibration bar 100 msec. (Note increase in post-excitatory pause with increasing stimulus intensity.)

frequency bursts of impulses on displacements within a quadrant. Movements in the opposite direction gave no response or an inhibition of a spontaneous activity present. On controlled displacements with the aid of the mechanical stimulator a very high frequency dynamic discharge was recorded throughout the movement (Fig. 3). In the subsequent static plateau, when the hair was held in a bent position, there was an initial rapid decline in impulse frequency followed by a very slowly adapting discharge. Impulse intervals in this phase were either quite regular (Fig. 4) or more irregular (Fig. 3).

The recordings shown in Fig. 4 demonstrate that the frequency of the static response is dependent on the displacement amplitude. An analysis of responses from 15 afferent units showed that a plot of impulse frequency *versus* displacement amplitude gave the best fit to a straight line on log–log coordinates, indicating that the stimulus–response relation can be described by a power function.

The dynamic phase of the mechanical stimulation elicits a response with gradually diminishing impulse intervals. The frequency attained in the final part of the displacement is higher the faster the movement, and the receptors are thus velocity-dependent. A maximal impulse frequency of 900–1000 impulses/sec was evoked by fast longitudinal movements, that is by pushing the hair shaft into the skin. The dynamic threshold on this type of movement was less than 10 $\mu$m while the threshold on sideways displacements varied between 10 and 75 $\mu$m.

The size of the dynamic response was calculated as the difference in impulse frequency between the discharge at the end of the movement and the discharge during the subsequent plateau phase. Also the dynamic stimulus–response relation seemed to be approximated by a power function. Most of the afferent fibers had conduction velocities in the range 54–78 m/sec.

Gottschaldt *et al.* (1973) recorded afferent discharges from vibrissae receptors and were able to distinguish two main types of slowly adapting units. The characterization was based *i.a.* on differences in spontaneous discharge, in regularity of interspike intervals and in adaptation to a maintained stimulus. These two kinds of afferent units were considered to have the properties of slowly adapting type I and type II cutaneous receptors (Iggo and Muir, 1969). Gottschaldt *et al.* also found experimental evidence for a similar separation of responses from carpal sinus hairs into two groups. Thus, the difference in interspike interval regularity seen in Figs. 3 and 4 may be an expression of this bimodal organization.

## (2) Slowly adapting responses from hair disk receptors

The hair disk was always found on the lateral side of the sinus hair and its receptors were excited by hair deflections in this direction. As they did not respond to medial displacements or longitudinal pushes on the hair they were easily distinguished from sinus hair afferent units. Each nerve fiber never supplied more than one hair disk. No spontaneous activity was recorded. Quantitative mechanical stimulation established the velocity-dependent dynamic and amplitude-dependent static responses which are characteristic of type I units.

*(3) Pacinian corpuscles*

Responses from the Pacinian corpuscles were characterized by a low threshold 1:1 discharge on vibratory stimulation applied either to the skin adjacent to the hair organ or to the sinus hairs. A particular afferent unit could be excited from each of the tactile hairs without obvious threshold differences. The course of the threshold–frequency curve was typically U-shaped and a regular response was usually obtained for frequencies up to 300–400 c/sec. Square wave stimuli elicited on- and off-responses.

*(4) Rapidly adapting sinus hair receptors*

Besides responses from Pacinian corpuscles, another type of rapidly adapting discharge could be discerned. These units did not respond to transmitted vibrations but only to rapid movements of one particular sinus hair. On high velocity stimulations the impulse intervals were brief and regular, on slower movements the impulse frequency was lower and the interspike intervals were of increasing duration during the later part of the movement. No discharges were set up during the static displacements, but a short off-response could be obtained when the hair was released from the deflected position. These units did not show a directional sensitivity.

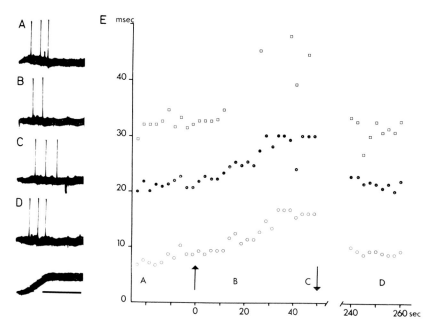

Fig. 5. A–D: sensory unit responses to rapid deflections of cat vibrissae before (A) and during stimulation of cervical sympathetic trunk at 10/sec (B and C) and about 3 min after end of stimulation the initial response has recovered (D). Below, recording of movement. Time calibration bar 50 msec. E: graphical representation of latencies from onset of each mechanical stimulus to first (○), second (●) and third (□) dynamic spikes. Mechanical stimuli (velocity 14.4 mm/sec, amplitude plateau 450 μm) delivered at 2.5 sec intervals. Arrows show onset and end of sympathetic stimulation. Times for recordings in A–D are indicated.

## *Effects of sympathetic stimulation on sinus hair receptors*

The demonstration of adrenergic nerve terminals within the follicles of the carpal sinus hairs as well as within those of vibrissae (Fuxe and Nilsson, 1965) raised the question whether sinus hair receptors are influenced by sympathetic activity in the same way as certain other types of mechanoreceptors (Loewenstein, 1956; Hunt, 1960; Chernetski, 1964). However, electrical stimulation of sympathetic fibers innervating the carpal skin area caused a strong contraction in the pilomotor muscles of the sinus hairs and the concomitant piloerection made studies of changes in receptor excitability impracticable. Therefore these studies were carried out on the vibrissae which lack smooth pilomotor muscles.

Electrical stimulation of the cervical sympathetic trunk at frequencies of 5–10 c/sec changed the responses from several slowly adapting vibrissae receptors (Nilsson, 1972). The dynamic responses to repeated identical deflections of a vibrissa were altered in a way indicating a slightly decreased excitability during a period of sympathetic stimulation; the impulse intervals increased in length and/or the number of impulses elicited during the movements was diminished (Fig. 5). These effects appeared after a delay of 10–25 sec and were fully reversible on cessation of the electrical stimulation.

Stimulation frequencies below 2–3 c/sec gave no change in the receptor response. Intravenous injection of phentolamine 5 mg/kg body weight abolished the sympathetic influence. Clamping of the ipsilateral carotid artery did not change the receptor response nor the effect of sympathetic stimulation.

The sympathetic modulation of the static response was small and varying; these effects were probably not significant.

## DISCUSSION

These morphological and physiological studies have shown that the carpal sinus hairs constitute the main component in a unique receptor complex comprising (1) sinus hair follicle receptors of a main type detecting both velocity and position and a second type showing purely velocity-dependent responses, (2) hair disk receptors sensitive to both velocity and position of hair deflections and (3) Pacinian corpuscles responding to very small, rapid mechanical transients. Each of these receptors may be excited by movements of a sinus hair. It is probable that the combined information from the different receptors may give a more distinct perception of hair movements. How this afferent impulse flow is treated in the central nervous system is largely unknown; however, slowly adapting responses from carpal sinus hair receptors have been recorded in cat thalamic nuclei (Curry, 1972; Gordon and Manson, 1973).

If, for example, the cat's foreleg is moved in such a way that the long and stiff sinus hairs make contact with an object, the beginning of the resulting hair deflection is signalled by on-responses from the Pacinian corpuscles (*cf.* Fig. 6), while information about deflection velocity, amplitude and direction is carried by impulse discharges

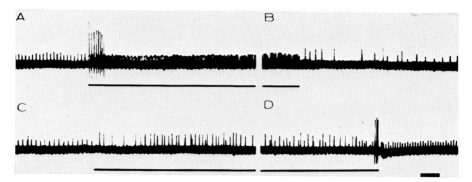

Fig. 6. Deflections of a carpal sinus hair inducing responses in three different fibers. A: abrupt lateral deflection (indicated by black line). B: slow return to resting position. C: slow medial deflection. D: rapid return of hair to normal position. Rapid movements (A and D) excite a Pacinian corpuscle (large spikes). Lateral deflection (A and B) accelerates activity in a spontaneously active hair follicle unit (small spikes) followed by a silent pause at the end of the stimulus. This unit is inhibited by a medial deflection (C and D), which instead activates another hair follicle unit (intermediate spikes). Time calibration bar 100 msec.

from slowly adapting sinus hair and hair disk receptors. Supplementary information on deflection velocity is given by rapidly adapting sinus hair receptors. The adequate "physiological" stimuli for the carpal sinus hair organ are unknown, but it is probable that they are more complex than the simple mechanical pulses used in this analysis of the receptor properties. These stimuli may be composed of vibrations and small movements superimposed on more or less static displacements of the hairs. In view of the combination of a number of receptors possessing different properties the carpal sinus hair organ provides a material well suited for analysis of such complex stimuli.

SUMMARY

The follicles of the cat's carpal sinus hairs are supplied by free nerve endings and Merkel cell–neurite complexes. Simple lamellated corpuscles lie within the cavernous blood sinus. Slowly adapting sinus hair follicle units showed a directional sensitivity and responded to mechanical stimulation with a high-frequency velocity-dependent dynamic impulse discharge and an amplitude-dependent static response. A few sinus hair follicle mechanoreceptors were of fast adapting type. Pacinian corpuscles located close to the external sinus walls responded to vibratory stimuli. Hair disks immediately lateral to each sinus hair gave slowly adapting discharges. The functional significance of the unique combination of four mechanoreceptor types with different response properties within the carpal sinus hair organ is emphasized. Adrenergic nerve fibers have been demonstrated within cat sinus hair follicles. Electrical stimulation of the cervical sympathetic trunk produced small but repeatable changes in the dynamic responses of slowly adapting mechanoreceptors of cat vibrissae follicles.

ACKNOWLEDGEMENT

The permission from the Editors of *Acta physiologica scandinavica* to publish some of the figures is gratefully acknowledged.

## REFERENCES

ANDRES, K. H. (1966) Über die Feinstruktur der Rezeptoren an Sinushaaren. *Z. Zellforsch.*, **75**, 339–365.

BEDDARD, F. E. (1902) Observations upon the carpal vibrissae in mammals. *Proc. zool. Soc. Lond.*, **3**, 127–136.

BLAND-SUTTON, J. (1887) On the arm glands of the Lemurs. *Proc. zool. Soc. Lond.*, **27**, 369–372.

CHERNETSKI, K. E. (1964) Sympathetic enhancement of peripheral sensory input in the frog. *J. Neurophysiol.*, **27**, 493–515.

CURRY, M. J. (1972) The exteroceptive properties of neurones in the somatic part of the posterior group (PO). *Brain Res.*, **44**, 439–472.

FRÉDÉRIC, J. (1905) Untersuchungen über die Sinushaare der Affen, nebst Bemerkungen über die Augenbrauen und den Schnurrbart des Menschen. *Z. Morphol. Anthropol.*, **8**, 239–275.

FRITZ, F. (1909) Über einen Sinnesapparat am Unterarm der Katze nebst Bemerkungen über den Bau des Sinusbalges. *Z. wiss. Zool.*, **92**, 291–305.

FUXE, K. AND NILSSON, B. Y. (1965) Mechanoreceptors and adrenergic nerve terminals. *Experientia (Basel)*, **21**, 641–642.

GORDON, G. AND MANSON, J. (1973) Quoted by WAITE, P. M. E., The responses of cells in the rat thalamus to mechanical movements of the whiskers. *J. Physiol. (Lond.)*, **228**, 541–561.

GOTTSCHALDT, K.-M., IGGO, A. AND YOUNG, D. W. (1973) Functional characteristics of mechanoreceptors in sinus hair follicles of the cat. *J. Physiol. (Lond.)*, **235**, 287–315.

HUNT, C. C. (1960) The effect of sympathetic stimulation on mammalian muscle spindles. *J. Physiol. (Lond.)*, **151**, 332–341.

IGGO, A. AND MUIR, A. R. (1969) The structure and function of a slowly adapting touch corpuscle in hairy skin. *J. Physiol. (Lond.)*, **200**, 763–796.

LINDQUIST, C. (1973) Contraction properties of cat facial muscles. *Acta physiol. scand.*, **89**, 482–490.

LOEWENSTEIN, W. R. (1956) Modulation of cutaneous mechanoreceptors by sympathetic stimulation. *J. Physiol. (Lond.)*, **132**, 40–60.

MANN, S. J. (1968) The tylotrich (hair) follicle of the American opossum. *Anat. Rec.*, **160**, 171–179.

NILSSON, B. Y. (1968) Activity of the pilomotor muscles of single tactile hairs in the cat. *Acta physiol. scand.*, **74**, 348–358.

NILSSON, B. Y. (1969a) Structure and function of the tactile hair receptors on the cat's foreleg. *Acta physiol. scand.*, **77**, 396–416.

NILSSON, B. Y. (1969b) Hair discs and Pacinian corpuscles functionally associated with the carpal tactile hairs in the cat. *Acta physiol. scand.*, **77**, 417–428.

NILSSON, B. Y. (1972) Effects of sympathetic stimulation on mechanoreceptors of cat vibrissae. *Acta physiol. scand.*, **85**, 390–397.

NILSSON, B. Y. AND SKOGLUND, C. R. (1965) The tactile hairs on the cat's foreleg. *Acta physiol. scand.*, **65**, 364–369.

PATRIZI, G. AND MUNGER, B. L. (1966) The ultrastructure and innervation of rat vibrissae. *J. comp. Neurol.*, **126**, 423–435.

SKOGLUND, C. R. (1960) Properties of Pacinian corpuscles of ulnar and tibial location in cat and fowl. *Acta physiol. scand.*, **50**, 385–386.

STRAILE, W. E. (1960) Sensory hair follicles in mammalian skin: the tylotrich follicle. *Amer. J. Anat.*, **106**, 133–147.

## DISCUSSION

SANTINI: I appreciate that you had found an inhibitory effect of sympathetic stimulation similar to my own findings. Did you use longer stimulation periods? I suggest that the effect is maximal at a later stage.

NILSSON: I have not stimulated the sympathetic nerves for longer periods than one minute. I also want to point out that the sympathetic modulation of the vibrissae receptors was less pronounced and of longer latency than the modulation of the Pacinian corpuscles in your experiments.

ZEVEKE: Did you measure the mechanical properties of the skin, and are these properties changed during the sympathetic stimulation?

NILSSON: I chose the vibrissae for these experiments as they, in contrast to the carpal sinus hairs, do not have smooth pilomotor muscles. No measurements of the proposed kind have been made, but visual inspection through a microscope revealed no changes in the skin and no movements of the vibrissae or other adjacent hairs.

AKOEV: Does the sympathetic stimulation induce any excitation?

NILSSON: No initial excitatory phase was seen during stimulation of the sympathetic nerves. However, my experimental set-up may not have detected very small and transient changes in the mechanical threshold.

IGGO: Are the small lamellated corpuscles within the carpal hair sinuses a frequent finding?

NILSSON: The electron microscopic material is too small to allow any definite conclusions, but these corpuscles have been an occasional finding, and I also believe that they are scanty as responses from rapidly adapting sinus hair units probably associated with these corpuscles have been recorded in a limited number.

SANTINI: I am very glad to see that Dr. Nilsson also has evidence for some kind of action of sympathetic innervation on a sensory system and I think it might be worthwhile to look with a longer time scale at this type of sympathetic innervation, as I did in the case of the Pacinian corpuscle. I wonder whether you have added to your report in Acta physiol. scandinavica last year some more experiments within the range of a few minutes.

NILSSON: No, I have not done these studies.

SANTINI: I think that this is quite an important point because these sympathetic effects are of a certain latency and are long lasting.

NILSSON: Yes, it would be interesting to do, but I think that your responses came a bit earlier than 15 sec. That is right?

SANTINI: Yes. In the case I saw in the Pacinian corpuscle, as I have shown yesterday in the presentation, the latency for the effects is quite short, within 2 or 3 sec. The peak of the effect takes a longer time, but the drop in the discharge frequency has been already observed in the first few seconds.

NILSSON: I noticed the same latency of the effect in the muscle spindles, which is shorter than the latencies that Hunt described.

SANTINI: I designed the experiments in order to affect the spinal ganglion cells supplying the two groups, the group II or the group I afferent fibers to the muscle spindle receptors. There is a combined stimulation of both the spindle and the spinal ganglion cells. When I injected noradrenaline to the spinal ganglion cells innervating muscle spindles, then there was some evidence for very clear-cut short latencies.

AKOEV: How can you explain that you did not observe an excitation effect on the receptors when sympathetic nerves were stimulated, though different authors showed on various mechanoreceptors that the excitation phase preceded the inhibition phase?

NILSSON: We have not seen initial excitation, and maybe our set-up did not detect the small changes in the threshold. We saw only inhibition and as I have reported, the inhibition was rather small, so I think we should be a bit cautious about evaluating these results.

ZEVEKE: Have you observed on sympathetic nerve stimulation any changes in physical state of the skin, in particular in the region where the receptors studies were situated? The skin becomes more dense due to pilomotor contractions. Have you measured the physical state of the skin or its oscillatory movements at hair bending?

NILSSON: Yes, that was one of the reasons why we chose vibrissae and not a carpal hair, because in the carpal hairs great changes are produced by pilomotor contractions and in the vibrissae we did not see any movement of the hairs or, by inspection, we did not see any changes in the skin; there are no pilomotor muscles in the face vibrissae which are only moved by very fast facial muscles. I do not think that the effect can be explained in this way.

IGGO: This is a question of fact concerning the presence of small lamellated corpuscles in the sinus follicles, and I understood that Dr. Andres had not seen them in the carpal sinus hairs and you have not described them. Are they very common in carpal hairs compared with the cat vibrissae in which I think they are more abundant?

NILSSON: I have no experience on the cat vibrissae and I do not think they are very common in the carpal hairs because we have only seen very few of them and also those types of receptors, rapidly adapting receptors, are also very few.

ANDRES: May I answer this question. These lamellated endings of Pacinian-like corpuscles are very few in my material too, but in each sinus hair I find some of them. There are about 100 myelinated fibers which go to a single sinus hair and only a few of them belong to these lamellated endings.

NILSSON: Do I understand that you did find those lamellated corpuscles in the carpal hair?

ANDRES: I did not look at the carpal hairs, only at sinus hairs.

NILSSON: And they are not very common in sinus hair?

ANDRES: In every sinus hair there are few lamellated endings. But if you compare these findings with 100 myelinated fibers, they are very few.

NILSSON: That is my impression, if you regard the type of units, that this type is very uncommon.

CAUNA: I have a brief question which I want to address to Dr. Nilsson and Dr. Andres in respect to the lamellar structures they observed. I wonder how much attention they have paid to the details. Are those structures actually borne upon the end of the axons or, perhaps, at some preterminal segment? In my experience I have found that such structures, such lamellation, are occasionally found over the preterminal segments. The axon goes through and may even attain a myelin sheath.

ANDRES: These lamellated structures were observed in cats and rats. In cats the lamellation is very narrow like in a core of Pacinian corpuscles, there is no free terminal ending in the connective tissue but in rats the lamellae are very few and the end of the terminal goes free into the connective tissue. I did not see the lamellations in the axons with myelin sheaths. In rats we think the endings are branched, but not in cats and in this way they are similar to the lamellated endings in the frog. In the frog and in the snakes the lamellated endings have free terminals which go out of the lamellation but only to a short distance.

# Adaptation in Mechanoreceptors of Amphibian Skin

W. T. CATTON

*Physiology Department, Medical School, The University, Newcastle upon Tyne (Great Britain)*

The mechanoreceptive terminals in the dermal and epidermal layers of frog and toad skin consist largely of free nerve endings, with widespread overlapping distribution (*e.g.* Whitear, 1955). They show a wide range of adaptation rates to prolonged steady stimuli (*e.g.* Catton, 1958; Lindblom, 1958). The capsule of the Pacinian corpuscle has been regarded as a high-pass mechanical filter, giving to this receptor organ the property of very rapid adaptation (*e.g.* Hubbard, 1958; Loewenstein and Skalak, 1966), such that only one or two spikes may be fired at the onset of the stimulus. But many receptors in frog skin ("tactile receptors") show similar rapid adaptation, along with others which are more slowly adapting. Recent anatomical studies have revealed the presence of highly organised encapsulated endings in the skin of *Rana esculenta*, resembling the structure of mammalian Pacinian corpuscles (Düring and Seiler, 1974). These corpuscles were found in all skin areas, but were densest near the tips of the digits.

The existence of these structures was not known when the work now to be described was performed, but this fact is not considered to invalidate the theoretical basis or the conclusions reached.

Thus it was proposed (Catton and PeToe, 1966) that mechanical "slip" of the terminal, with respect to the surrounding tissue, can largely account for the adapta-

$$S = \tau \dot{x}(1 - e^{-t/\tau}).$$

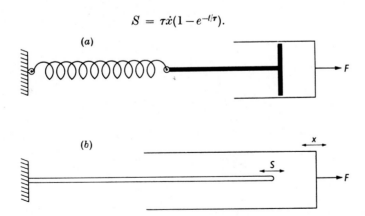

Fig. 1. a: series visco-elastic model. b: force F, moves skin cylinder through distance x, and sensory terminal moves through distance S.

tion shown by skin mechanoreceptors; a quantitative theory was developed. A little earlier, Catton (1966) had shown that a brief delay occurs in the mechanical mode of stimulation, and that this delay varied with stimulus parameters. This conclusion was reached by comparing the latencies of responses, recorded close to the receptor, to mechanical and electrical pulse stimulation of the same receptor.

The concept of "slip" led to the consideration of a simple series visco-elastic model (Fig. 1), in which the force extending the terminal was dependent on viscous drag, and the restoring force was the elastic property of the axon terminal. Analysis of such a model yields the following relation between velocity of skin movement (dx/dt) and resulting change in length of the terminal (S). Thus

$$S = \tau \, dx/dt \left( 1 - \exp\left( -\frac{t}{\tau} \right) \right) \tag{1}$$

where $\tau$ is a time constant and t is the time taken for S to reach its new and final value. $\tau$ depends on the coefficient of viscosity of the coupling fluid and on the geometry of the terminal itself.

The firing of the spike is assumed to occur when S reaches a threshold value S′, at time t′ (see Fig. 2). The steeper the rise of the stimulus (dx/dt) the sooner is S′ (and hence t′) attained, which corresponds with the experimental observation that the response latency shortens as the stimulus slope becomes steeper. An alternative statement of Equation 1 is thus:

$$dx/dt = \frac{S'}{\tau \left( 1 - \exp\left( -\frac{t'}{\tau} \right) \right)} \tag{2}$$

Stimulus slope was plotted against latency for a large number of skin receptors (experimental results). Computer solutions of Equation 2 were obtained for different chosen values of S′ and $\tau$; these constants could not be known beforehand. An approximation for S′ was given by the threshold amplitude for a very steep slope, where "slip" is least, and by the restriction that S′ is always less than X (skin dis-

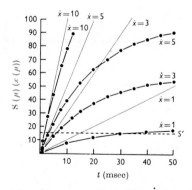

Fig. 2. S (and x) plotted against time, for a range of velocities (ẋ) from 1 to 10 $\mu$m/msec, as calculated from the basic equation. The $\tau$ value was 20 msec and S′, the arbitrary threshold, was set at 15 $\mu$m.

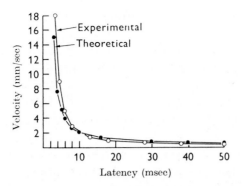

Fig. 3. Experimental slope–latency curve for a frog skin receptor, compared with theoretical curve derived from the basic equation, after compensation for afferent conduction time. ($S' = 5\ \mu$m; $\tau = 40$ msec.)

placement). The constant $\tau$ was estimated by taking an arbitrary value of $t'$, being that intercept on the time axis corresponding to twice the critical slope, and designated $t_c$. It was shown that $t_c = 0.693\ \tau$.

With these data it was possible to obtain very close fits with experimental slope–latency curves (Catton and PeToe, 1966) (Fig. 3). However, this is not an absolute proof that visco-elastic behaviour explains adaptation. A different process, such as accommodation of the receptor terminal, could obey a similar law with respect to stimulus slope and lead to a similar result. This was not investigated, but instead some experiments were performed to test the mechanical hypothesis. Thus whole skin–nerve preparations were treated with tissue-destroying enzymes, such as collagenase, hyaluronidase and trypsin. After an appropriate time for enzyme action the responses were tested again and there were found to be changes in slope–latency curves and in critical slopes in accordance with expectations from the visco-elastic model. Such treatments would not be expected to affect accommodative properties, but only mechanical linkage.

Both dynamic and static excitability changes were produced by long duration mechanical deflections (Catton, 1962). The static change was assumed to be due to an additional elastic coupling between terminal and tissue, so that in a prolonged deflection the terminal was held in some degree of steady extension. In this type of experiment, using long *subliminal* stimuli, it was found that enzyme treatments resulted in a marked decline in the static phase, indicating a loosening in the elastic bonding (Catton and PeToe, 1966). Where both viscous and elastic *coupling* is assumed the mathematical analysis is more complex and theoretical prediction is not possible in a quantitative manner.

In addition to the publications mentioned above there will appear a further account in a forthcoming book, "*Frog Neurobiology*", to be published by Springer Verlag, 1975. Mechanoreceptor adaptation in a wider context is discussed in a recent review (Catton, 1970).

*References p. 230*

## SUMMARY

The mechanoreceptors in amphibian skin are found to show a wide range in rates of adaptation to constant stimuli. Whereas most of the sensory terminals are free nerve endings, some lamellated corpuscles have recently been found, and these are probably the fast adapting "touch" receptors.

By comparing the latencies of responses to electrical and mechanical stimulation of the same receptor it was shown that there is a brief delay in mechanical excitation.

A theory of "slip" was proposed to explain this delay, and the behaviour of a series visco-elastic model was analysed. The model predicted that response latency would vary with slope of stimulus. This relationship was studied experimentally on skin receptors, and the slope–latency curves plotted were compared with curves derived from the analysis of the model. Good fits could be obtained when allowance was made for conduction time in the sensory axon, and when selection was made of two constants. One of these represented threshold extension of the terminal, the other was a time constant. The values selected were always within physiological range. Treatment with tissue-destroying enzymes, expected to increase the degree of "slip", produced changes in slope–latency curves in accord with the theory.

Experiments on the excitability changes under long subliminal conditioning pulses demonstrated both a dynamic and a static phase. The latter was ascribed to elastic (in addition to viscous) coupling between tissue and terminal. Again, enzyme treatment caused changes which would be expected from theory. A model which included an elastic coupling element yielded equations with too many unknown constants to enable quantitative theoretical predictions to be made.

## REFERENCES

CATTON, W. T. (1958) Some properties of frog skin mechanoreceptors. *J. Physiol. (Lond.)*, **141**, 305–322.

CATTON, W. T. (1962) The effects of subliminal stimulation on the excitability of frog skin tactile receptors. *J. Physiol. (Lond.)*, **164**, 90–102.

CATTON, W. T. (1966) A comparison of the responses of frog skin receptors to mechanical and electrical stimulation. *J. Physiol. (Lond.)*, **187**, 23–34.

CATTON, W. T. (1970) Mechanoreceptor function. *Physiol. Rev.*, **50**, 297–318.

CATTON, W. T. AND PETOE, N. (1966) A visco-elastic theory of mechanoreceptor adaptation. *J. Physiol. (Lond.)*, **187**, 35–50.

DÜRING, M. VON AND SEILER, W. (1974) The fine structure of lamellated receptors in the skin of *Rana esculenta*. *Z. Anat. Entwickl.-Gesch.*, **144**, 165–172.

HUBBARD, S. J. (1958) A study of rapid mechanical events in a mechanoreceptor. *J. Physiol. (Lond.)*, **141**, 198–218.

LINDBLOM, U. F. (1958) Excitability and functional organisation within a peripheral tactile unit. *Acta physiol. scand.*, **44**, Suppl. 153, 5–82.

LOEWENSTEIN, W. R. AND SKALAK, R. (1966) Mechanical transmission in a Pacinian corpuscle. An analysis and a theory. *J. Physiol. (Lond.)*, **182**, 347–378.

WHITEAR, M. (1955) Dermal nerve endings in *Rana* and *Bufo*. *Quart. J. micr. Sci.*, **96**, 343–349.

## DISCUSSION

ANDRES: I should ask you what diameter have the fibers, from which you made your recordings. In your morphological experiments we had two types of fibers from mechanoreceptors in the skin, the one with a very large diameter and another of one-half of this.

CATTON: I did not in fact measure the diameter of fibers in the skin nerves but most of the experiments were on large fibers.

ANDRES: Though we have had 4 different types of the endings in the skin, only one is published. Three other types were stretch receptors too.

# Touch Perception Threshold in Terms of Amplitude and Rate of Skin Deformation

U. LINDBLOM*

*Department of Neurological Rehabilitation, Karolinska Sjukhuset, 104 01 Stockholm (Sweden)*

The tactile threshold was measured on the finger tips of normal adults using half cycle sinusoidal mechanical pulses from a minishaker (Brüel and Kjaer 4810) monitored by a Wave Tek stimulator (Model 112). The pulse frequency was varied to produce various slow and rapid displacements in imitation of natural tactile stimuli which would be composed of different rates, as well as different amplitudes, of deformation. The stimuli were applied to the skin perpendicularly from below via a 2 mm diameter blunt-ended plastic probe, the movement of which was recorded by means of a cylindrical condenser and a capacitance meter and displayed on a storage oscilloscope. The movement amplitude was calibrated in $\mu$m and measured on the oscilloscope together with the steepness of the tangent of the rising phase of the pulses, which was taken as a measure of the rate of skin displacement. The subjective threshold was determined with the method of limits.

The threshold for the rapid pulses (from 400 down to 10 Hz) was of the order of 5 $\mu$m. At 5 Hz, corresponding to a displacement rate of about 0.2 mm/sec, the threshold was about 10 $\mu$m. With pulses around 1 Hz, a steep rise in threshold occurred and simultaneously the tactile character of the sensation disappeared. This is illustrated

FIG. 1

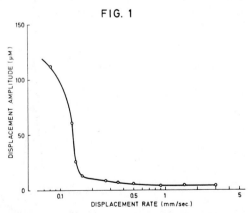

Fig. 1. Relation between threshold amplitude and estimated displacement rate on stimulation of finger pulp of normal adult with single half cycle sinusoidal mechanical pulses.

* Present address: Department of Neurology, Huddinge University Hospital, Huddinge, Sweden.

in Fig. 1, where the conspicuous threshold rise is seen in the 0.1–0.2 mm/sec rate region.

The threshold gap, *i.e.* the difference between the lowest amplitude which was felt on at least three consecutive stimulations and the highest amplitude which was never felt, varied considerably on successive determinations and increased with distraction or fatigue. On average, however, the gap was a fraction of between 22 and 34% of the absolute threshold value.

The low threshold on rapid pulse stimulation indicates that this sensation is mediated by the Pacinian corpuscles (PC receptors), which are the only known receptors which can be excited by such discrete stimulation of primate glabrous skin (Lindblom and Lund, 1966; Talbot *et al.*, 1968). In this type of skin, the threshold of the rapidly adapting receptors (RA receptors, probably Meissner's corpuscles, see Jänig, 1971) is above 50 $\mu$m (Knibestöl, 1973) and can thus only be relevant for tactile sensation on suprathreshold stimulation.

The threshold rise in the 0.15 mm/sec rate region indicates a transition from PC to other receptors. It is doubtful if the latter could be RA receptors because of their critical slope (Lindblom, 1965; Knibestöl, 1973) and it seems more probable that the higher perceptual threshold on stimulation with slow pulses is mediated by the slowly adapting intracutaneous glabrous skin receptors (SA receptors, see Iggo, 1963; Vallbo and Hagbarth, 1968; Knibestöl and Vallbo, 1970; Jänig, 1971; Kenton *et al.*, 1971; Pubols *et al.*, 1971; Knibestöl, 1975).

Preliminary tests were made on patients with various types of central or peripheral lesion in the nervous system. Significant threshold increases were commonly recorded. This is illustrated in Fig. 2 which is from a patient with a traumatic median nerve lesion which had been sutured three years earlier. Fig. 2A shows the threshold for rapid pulse stimulation on the index finger of the healthy side, and Fig. 2B the increased threshold and threshold gap of the corresponding finger on the affected side. In this case sensation was clearly impaired even on routine clinical examination, and the threshold measurements implied only a quantification. In other cases, however, such as incipient uremic neuropathy, a threshold elevation was observed before any

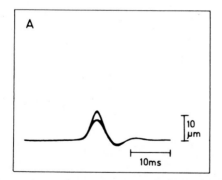
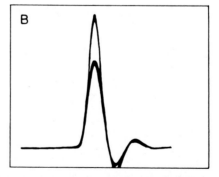

Fig. 2. Records from capacitance meter showing normal tactile threshold and threshold gap of pad of left index finger (A), and increased threshold (both the absolute value and the threshold gap) on right index finger (B); from a patient with right-sided sutured median nerve lesion.

signs could be detected by usual clinical means. It is likely that the threshold parameters, as well as the suprathreshold intensity functions that so far have not been studied, will appear to be differentially affected by different types of lesion to the nervous system. The method provides a sensitive means of assessing even subclinical lesions in the nervous system.

## SUMMARY

On the finger tips the touch perception threshold was about 5 $\mu$m on stimulation with rapidly rising mechanical pulses. The low value indicates that the threshold sensation for touch is mediated by Pacinian corpuscles. With slow pulse stimulation the threshold rose sharply when the displacement rate fell below 0.2 mm/sec. The threshold difference limen was a fraction of the absolute value of the threshold amplitude. The stimulation technique provided a quick and sensitive method for clinical testing of impaired sensibility.

## ACKNOWLEDGEMENT

The investigation was supported by the Swedish Medical Research Council (Project B74-14X-4256-01).

## REFERENCES

IGGO, A. (1963) An electrophysiological analysis of afferent fibres in primate skin. *Acta neuroveg. (Wien)*, **24**, 175–180.

JÄNIG, W. (1971) Morphology of rapidly and slowly adapting mechanoreceptors in the hairless skin of the cat's hind foot. *Brain Res.*, **28**, 217–231.

KENTON, B., KRUGER, L. AND WOO, M. (1971) Two classes of slowly adapting mechanoreceptor fibres in reptile cutaneous nerve. *J. Physiol. (Lond.)*, **212**, 21–44.

KNIBESTÖL, M. (1973) Stimulus–response functions of rapidly adapting mechanoreceptors in the human glabrous skin area. *J. Physiol. (Lond.)*, **232**, 427–452.

KNIBESTÖL, M. (1975) Stimulus–response functions of slowly adapting mechanoreceptors in the human glabrous skin area. *J. Physiol. (Lond.)*, **245**, 63–80.

KNIBESTÖL, M. AND VALLBO, Å. B. (1970) Single unit analysis of mechanoreceptor activity from the human glabrous skin. *Acta physiol. scand.*, **80**, 178–195.

LINDBLOM, U. (1965) Properties of touch receptors in distal glabrous skin of the monkey. *J. Neurophysiol.*, **29**, 966–985.

LINDBLOM, U. AND LUND, L. (1966) The discharge from vibration-sensitive receptors in the monkey foot. *Exp. Neurol.*, **15**, 401–417.

PUBOLS, L. M., PUBOLS, B. H., JR. AND MUNGER, B. L. (1971) Functional properties of mechanoreceptors in glabrous skin of the raccoon's forepaw. *Exp. Neurol.*, **31**, 165–182.

TALBOT, W. H., DARIAN-SMITH, I., KORNHUBER, H. H. AND MOUNTCASTLE, V. B. (1968) The sense of flutter-vibration: comparison of the human capacity with response patterns of mechanoreceptive afferents from the monkey hand. *J. Neurophysiol.*, **31**, 301–334.

VALLBO, Å. B. AND HAGBARTH, K.-E. (1968) Activity from skin mechanoreceptors recorded percutaneously in awake human subjects. *Exp. Neurol.*, **21**, 270–289.

## DISCUSSION

SCHEKANOV: How can you explain the higher threshold of tactile sensation in the palm in comparison with the finger tips?

LINDBLOM: There may be two explanations. One may be that it is another kind of receptor, perhaps, very low threshold rapidly adapting. I do not know that. The other explanation is that the Pacinian corpuscles, if they are responsible for the palmar threshold sensation, are located a little bit deeper or in a slightly softer tissue, so that the mechanical coupling to this stimulus probe will be looser, and therefore we will have the higher threshold.

SCHEKANOV: It is known that the receptive fields of the Pacinian corpuscles are very large, they may spread through the whole hand. How can you explain the ability of the patient to localize a stimulus if the Pacinian corpuscles are responsible for the threshold of tactile sensation?

LINDBLOM: This is a very relevant question, because it is very easy with a vibratory stimulus supplied to the glaborous skin to excite Pacinian corpuscles as you say at a long distance from the stimuli site. However, with these discrete stimuli the subjective response was localized not exactly to the point of the applied probe but to the palm. So, I think this localization of the stimulus effect as far as the particular responses are concerned, is dependent upon the small size of the stimulus and as soon as one increases the amplitude of vibration, this spread will increase.

CATTON: I have heard of a technique for exposing Meissner's corpuscles of the finger tips which I imagine you can stimulate directly by shaving off a little epidermis. I think Dr. Cauna knows this technique and would like to comment on this. We did try some experiments with this technique, but were not very successful.

CAUNA: Well, that procedure is very simple. You shear off the epidermis in a small area of the finger tip exposing the tips of the epidermal papillae. You do not have to touch the core, because of capillary bleeding, of course, you should wait a little. Then you put a drop of methylene blue of low concentration and you can design some holder for the finger or for the whole arm and the Meissner corpuscles are nicely visible, they are about 20–40 $\mu$m in diameter and easily accessible. Therefore the stimulation is possible.

# On the Effect of Electrical Stimulation of the Dorsal Column System on Sensory Thresholds in Patients with Chronic Pain

U. LINDBLOM* AND B. A. MEYERSON

*The Departments of Neurological Rehabilitation and Neurosurgery, Karolinska Sjukhuset, 104 01 Stockholm (Sweden)*

The development of a method for intermittent, electrical stimulation of the dorsal columns of the spinal cord in man (DCS) has provided a new approach for the treatment of chronic pain (Shealy *et al.*, 1970; Nashold and Friedman, 1972). The background for this method is the pain gate theory (Melzack and Wall, 1965) and it is assumed that the large fiber systems which are activated by the electrical stimulation, anti- or orthodromically, exert an inhibitory influence on the mechanisms for pain transmission. It is conceivable that stimulation applied to the dorsal aspect of the spinal cord would interfere not only with pain mechanisms but also with those modalities of sensation which are specifically mediated by the dorsal columns. The present report deals with quantitative effects of DCS on the thresholds for vibration, touch and cutaneous pain. Special attention is paid to the time course of these effects and the relation to the effect on spontaneous pain.

The material consisted of four patients who had had dorsal column electrodes implanted for 6–16 months. A short case history will be given of the patient illustrated in Table I and Figs. 1 and 2. This patient was a 40-year-old man who has suffered for the past three years from causalgia in the left lower thorax following a transthoracic vagotomy. There was a marked hyperesthesia in the area of maximal pain. In addition to the superficial causalgic pain there was a deep, stabbing ache. DCS resulted in an almost instantaneous reduction of the pain. There was a complete relief of the superficial pain within 3 min and the deep pain was abolished after about 5 min of stimulation. There was a post-stimulatory pain relief lasting about 4 hr. On examination 16 months after the electrode implantation the DCS was still found to be equally efficient for pain relief.

For the assessment of cutaneous pain threshold the skin was pinched with a flat forceps and the exerted pressure was recorded by means of a strain gauge and calibrated in g/sq.mm. Half cycle sinusoidal mechanical pulses were used for tactile stimulation (Lindblom, 1975) and a 100 Hz sine wave as vibratory stimulus (Goldberg and Lindblom, 1975). The threshold for both types of stimulation was measured with the method of limits and expressed in $\mu$m displacement amplitude. Control mea-

---

* Present address: Department of Neurology, Huddinge University Hospital, Huddinge, Sweden.

TABLE I

CUTANEOUS PAIN THRESHOLDS IN g/sq.mm BEFORE AND AFTER DORSAL COLUMN STIMULATION WITH
IMPLANTED ELECTRODES IN A PATIENT WITH CHRONIC POST-OPERATIVE PAIN.

PAIN TRESHOLD (g/mm$^2$)
Dorsal Column Stimulation

|  | Before | After |
|---|---|---|
| Painful trunk area | 8.0 | 35.5 |
| Normal trunk skin | 30.5 | 44.0 |
| Carpal skin | 55.0 | 65.1 |
| Tarsal skin | 60.2 | 75.1 |

surements before and after DCS revealed that none of the thresholds were influenced by the presence of spontaneous pain.

To obtain pain relief the patients deliberately set the DCS to a voltage which produced paresthesias spreading below the level of the implanted spinal electrode. A stimulus voltage subliminal for paresthesias could reduce, but not abolish spontaneous pain. The threshold for induced cutaneous pain was not significantly altered by DCS except when tested within the hyperesthetic area of the lower thorax in the patient described above. In this case the abnormally low threshold for pain was increased to normal values as a result of DCS (Table I). As seen in Table I a slight general pain threshold elevation cannot be excluded but this possibility needs further study. The normalization of the pain threshold in the hyperesthetic area persisted for several hours, *i.e.* as long as the pain relief, after cessation of DCS. This result may be compared with the observation made by Wall and Sweet (1967) that, with peripheral nerve stimulation, a prolonged pain relief may be obtained provided the stimulated nerve is the site of injury.

The thresholds for tactile and vibratory sensation were measured on the pulp of one finger of both hands and on the foot soles. The values obtained in the hands, *i.e.* above the level of the implanted spinal electrode, were never influenced by the DCS whereas a marked effect could be observed in the feet. Fig. 1 shows the effect of DCS at three different intensities, all supraliminal for paresthesias, on the tactile threshold measured in the left foot. Apparently there is a relationship between the intensity of DCS and the magnitude of the threshold elevation. There was also a residual threshold elevation lasting about 20 min as can be seen following the first period of stimulation.

The influence of DCS on vibratory thresholds in the tarsal regions is illustrated in Fig. 2. The vibrator was applied in the region where paresthesias could be provoked during DCS. It appears in the figure that when the voltage of the DCS was subliminal for paresthesias there was already an elevation which became more pronounced with supraliminal stimulation. The effects were more marked on the left side, which may

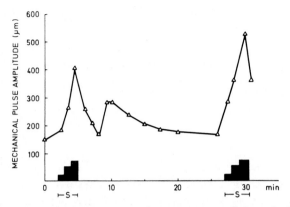

Fig. 1. Effects of DCS on the threshold for tactile stimulation applied on the left foot sole. DCS was performed on two occasions (S) and with three different intensities (black columns), all being supraliminal for paresthesias.

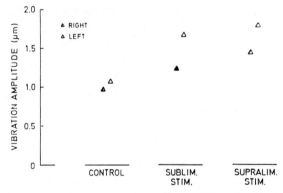

Fig. 2. Effect of DCS on the threshold for vibratory stimulation applied to the tarsal regions. Stimulus intensity of the DCS was adjusted to a level subliminal and supraliminal for paresthesias.

be due to the fact that in this case the spinal electrode was intentionally located slightly to the left which was the side of spontaneous pain.

The elevation of thresholds for vibratory and tactile stimuli during DCS may be due to a blocking effect of the artificial impulse discharge which will travel both orthodromically and antidromically. The antidromic discharge may collide with the afferent discharge set up by the natural stimulus, or block the receptors (Lindblom, 1958). However, the post-stimulatory effects of the DCS, which may last for up to 15 min, can hardly be accounted for by refractoriness or other events in the peripheral neuron. It is, therefore, reasonable to assume that the orthodromic discharge set up by the DCS interferes with the afferent impulses at the synaptic relays. The threshold increase observed on subliminal stimulation, *i.e.* when paresthesias were not elicited in the stimulated region, indicates a similar mechanism.

There was a discrepancy between the prolonged effect of DCS on spontaneous pain and hyperesthesia and the relatively short-lasting effect on tactile and vibratory thresholds. Therefore, it is reasonable to assume that different mechanisms are

*References p. 240*

responsible for the effects of DCS on spontaneous pain and on senses such as touch and vibration.

The relative inefficiency of the DCS to influence the threshold for cutaneous pain induced by mechanical stimulation warrants other testing methods in order to find a reliable correlate to the pain relieving effect of DCS.

## SUMMARY

Four patients who had dorsal column electrodes implanted for the relief of chronic pain were examined for the influence of dorsal column stimulation on the spontaneous pain and on the thresholds for touch, vibration and cutaneous pain induced by pinching. In these patients stimulation of the dorsal columns resulted in an almost instantaneous abolition of spontaneous pain. The relief of pain outlasted the period of stimulation by several hours. The normal threshold for induced cutaneous pain was not significantly changed either during or after dorsal column stimulation. The thresholds for tactile and vibratory sensations were increased during dorsal column stimulation, the increase being correlated to the intensity of the stimulation. There was a post-stimulatory effect lasting up to 20 min. The results indicate that different mechanisms may account for the effect of dorsal column stimulation on the spontaneous pain and on the sensory thresholds. A more extensive report will appear shortly (Lindblom and Meyerson, 1975).

## ACKNOWLEDGEMENTS

The study was supported by grants from the Swedish Foundation against Multiple Sclerosis and the Swedish Medical Research Council (B74-14X-4256-01 and B75-14X-4505-01).

## REFERENCES

GOLDBERG, M. AND LINDBLOM, U. (1975) The vibration threshold in terms of displacement amplitude. In preparation.

LINDBLOM, U. F. (1958) Excitability and functional organization within a peripheral tactile unit. *Acta physiol. scand.* **44**, Suppl. 153, 1–84.

LINDBLOM, U. (1975) Touch perception threshold in human glabrous skin in terms of displacement amplitude on stimulation with single mechanical pulses. *Brain Res.*, **82**, 205–210.

LINDBLOM, U. AND MEYERSON, B. A. (1975) Influence on touch, vibration and cutaneous pain of dorsal column stimulation in man. *Pain*, in press.

MELZACK, R. AND WALL, P. D. (1965) Pain mechanisms: a new theory. *Science*, **150**, 971–979.

NASHOLD, B. S., JR. AND FRIEDMAN, H. (1972) Dorsal column stimulation for control of pain. Preliminary report on 30 patients. *J. Neurosurg.*, **36**, 590–597.

SHEALY, C. N., MORTIMER, J. T. AND HAGFORS, N. R. (1970) Dorsal column electroanalgesia. *J. Neurosurg.*, **32**, 560–564.

WALL, P. D. AND SWEET, W. H. (1967) Temporary abolition of pain in man. *Science*, **155**, 108–109.

## DISCUSSION

CATTON: Do you classify your data as the result of peripheral effects of dorsal column stimulation or the central effect?

LINDBLOM: I think that they are both. One effect is peripheral and very simple, and that is the anti-dromic blocking of the afferent fibers which could occur at any level between the entry zone and the receptor by the antidromic impulses which are by necessity elicited by stimulation. But I also think that there is a central effect if you mean the tactile vibratory threshold. Here is the picture which shows the effect on the tactile threshold of dorsal column stimulation. During a very slight dorsal column stimulation there are actually two threshold values which are lower than any other values suggesting a facilitation, and during a slightly more intense stimulation there was a transient increase followed by the recovery to the prestimulation level. Similar changes could be observed at the higher stimulus level while a strong stimulus caused a sustained elevation,, but these changes I think also indicate a central effect of the stimulation.

CATTON: Why does the effect of a short stimulation period appear to last so long, why is there the long duration after-effect?

LINDBLOM: I have no explanations whatsoever. It is only an indication that the mechanism behind the pain is way off from the usual functions.

# Modes of Excitation of Respiratory Tract Receptors

J. G. WIDDICOMBE

*Department of Physiology, St. George's Hospital Medical School, Tooting, London SW17 0QT (Great Britain)*

## INTRODUCTION

Surface-acting chemical and mechanical irritants applied to different parts of the respiratory epithelium can elicit powerful reflexes of many different patterns — sneezing, coughing, apnoeas, etc. (Widdicombe, 1964 and 1974; Fillenz and Widdicombe, 1971; Tomori *et al.*, 1973). These reflexes are due to stimulation of epithelial "irritant receptors". Although these nervous end-organs have been studied histologically we know little about the structure of the receptors in different sites, their relationships to their environments (cellular and tissue elements), and the various local changes which stimulate or inhibit them. The receptors will be referred to as "irritant receptors" if they respond to intra-luminal irritants. Other endings which are localized in the epithelium but do not respond to those irritants which have been tested will be called "epithelial receptors".

The aim of the study of receptor physiology must be the correlation of receptor structure with behaviour. This is very incomplete for the irritant endings, and for several groups it is not even possible to identify the histological appearance of the surface receptors with the physiological patterns of activity in afferent nerve fibres. For these types of ending important progress must await the sure histological identification of the receptors which have been studied physiologically by action potential recording.

## PROPERTIES OF IRRITANT AND EPITHELIAL RECEPTORS

### *General properties*

The main method for studying the physiology of the receptors is by recording action potentials from single fibres from individual receptors, and by testing the conditions which set up or change this impulse traffic. There seems to be no study of receptor potentials or of the mode of initiation of action potentials in the endings themselves. Where fibre discharge patterns can be correlated confidently with the histological appearance of an epithelial ending (*i.e.* we are sure which type of receptor causes the afferent discharge), we can postulate the way in which a receptor is activated or inhibited by chemical or mechanical changes in the immediate environment of the end-organ, but even here the evidence is very indirect.

All the receptors studied, from nose to small bronchi, have many features in common: all are mechanosensitive; nearly all are sensitive to chemical "irritants"; nearly all are rapidly adapting to a maintained mechanical stimulus, (i.e. their firing frequency slows considerably or stops altogether within a few seconds); most of them have very irregular, probably random, discharge patterns; and many of the endings show an "off-response" when the stimulus is removed.

In spite of these similarities of behaviour, the receptors show clear differences in their relative sensitivities to various chemical excitants. When stimulated the different groups of ending cause widely different reflex responses, both quantitatively and qualitatively.

Some of these differences can be explained by the fact that there are two types of respiratory tract epithelium: the ciliated columnar cell layer of the nose, trachea and

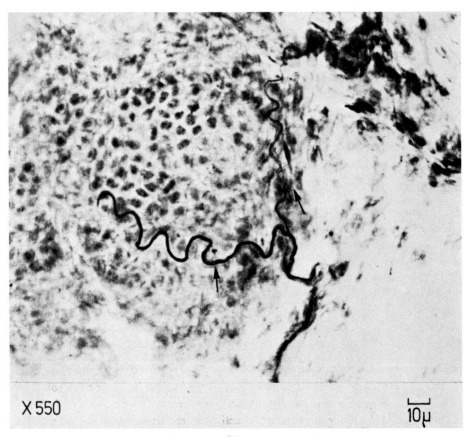

X 550                                                                          10μ

Fig. 1. Frozen section of cat epipharyngeal region showing nerve fibres ramifying among epithelial cells. Schofield's silver stain. Photograph by Mrs. A. M. White. (From Fillenz and Widdicombe, 1971.)

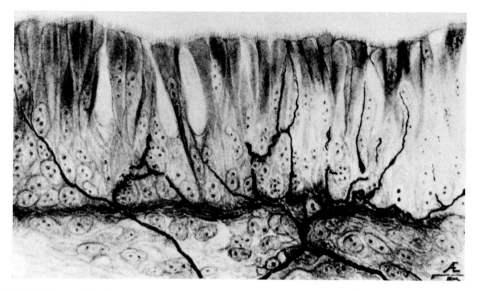

Fig. 2. Picture of an irritant receptor with nerve terminals ramifying between columnar epithelial cells of the trachea.

bronchi, and the squamous cell layer of the epipharynx, pharynx and vocal cords. Histologically, receptors in the two types of epithelium show obvious differences (Figs. 1 and 2).

### Nasal irritant and epithelial receptors

Nasal receptors are of clear physiological significance, but have been less studied than those lower in the respiratory tract. Their investigation is complicated firstly by the presence of olfactory endings, and the relationship between the latter and "irritant" receptors is not clear; and secondly by the relative difficulty of the surgical approach to the afferent nerve fibres. For these reasons no review of their properties is possible.

### Epipharyngeal epithelial receptors

Mechanical stimulation of the epipharyngeal mucosa (behind and above the soft palate, at the back of the nose) causes a highly specific reflex consisting of brief inspiratory efforts, bronchodilatation and hypertension, the "aspiration reflex" (Tomori and Widdicombe, 1969). Histologically there are nerve endings under the squamous cell epithelium which may mediate this reflex (Fig. 1). They appear less complex structurally than the tracheal and irritant receptors. Recording of action potentials in glossopharyngeal single nerve fibres from these receptors shows that they are sensitive to mechanical deformation by a catheter, a jet of air and distension of the pharynx, but not to chemical substances such as ammonia and histamine (Fig. 3). This chemical insensitivity could be due to their situation beneath the squamous cell

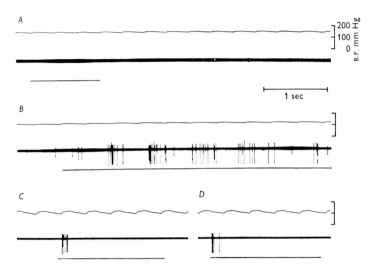

Fig. 3. Blood pressure and action potentials in a strand of the pharyngeal branch of the glosso-pharyngeal nerve during stimulation of the epipharynx. A: 3 ml ammonia vapour at signal; no response. B: mechanical stimulation with nylon fibre during signal; transient discharges with each movement of the thread. C and D: air flow at 6 litre/min through a catheter in the left nostril; rapidly adapting discharges at the start of air flow only. Long horizontal bars mark the duration of each stimulus. (From Nail *et al.*, 1969.)

layer, and is presumably advantageous because otherwise the respiratory reflexes might be set up by irritant food at the back of the mouth.

As with the receptors in the lower respiratory tract, those in the epipharynx are rapidly adapting, irregular in firing and give a pronounced off-response to mechanical stimulation. They have myelinated afferent fibres.

### Laryngeal epithelial receptors

Earlier studies of these endings (*e.g.* Andrew, 1956; Sampson and Eyzaguirre, 1964; Storey, 1968; Suzuki and Kirchner, 1968) have recently been extended considerably (Boushey *et al.*, 1974). There are at least three groups of receptors in the cat, each of which is inhibited by weak solutions of local anaesthetic applied topically. There seem to be few histological studies of laryngeal nervous receptors.

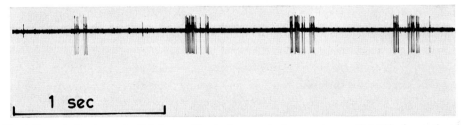

Fig. 4. Record of action potentials from a fibre in the superior laryngeal nerve (S.L.N.) of a paralyzed, artificially ventilated cat. It shows the effect of stroking the receptive field of a rapidly adapting receptor with a cotton thread. Note the irregular discharge. (From Boushey *et al.*, 1974.)

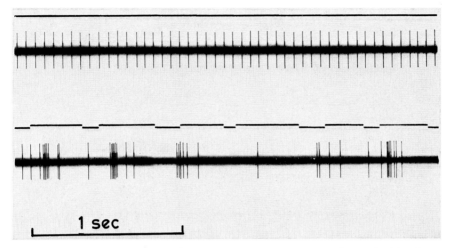

Fig. 5. The effect of a thread drawn across the receptive field of a continuously firing laryngeal afferent fibre in the S.L.N. Upper record: control tracing. Lower record: with each signal (upward movement of the trace) a thread was drawn across the receptive field. This alternately stimulated and inhibited the fibre. Records continuous. Upper trace: signal; lower trace: action potentials. (From Boushey *et al.*, 1974.)

*(1) Group I laryngeal epithelial receptors*

These have no spontaneous discharge under experimental conditions, but when activated have irregular, rather rapidly adapting discharges (Fig. 4). They have A$\delta$ afferent nerve fibres, and can fire with spike intervals as short as 2 msec. They are sensitive to mechanical stimulation with a catheter or thread, but not to dust. They are stimulated by the chemical irritants tested, including cigarette smoke and 5% carbon dioxide, but not by histamine.

*(2) Group II laryngeal epithelial receptors*

These have a regular spontaneous discharge when the larynx is open (average frequency, 37 impulses/sec). When stimulated they are not very rapidly adapting. They have A$\delta$ afferent fibres and can discharge with spike intervals of 4 msec. They are sensitive to mechanical stimulation with a catheter or a thread (Fig. 5), but not to dust. They are rather insensitive to chemical irritants (except ammonia), and are inhibited by carbon dioxide and often by cigarette smoke. They are not affected by histamine.

*(3) Laryngeal epithelial receptors with non-myelinated fibres*

Preliminary studies suggest that these may play a part in the responses to inhaled irritants. They may be the respiratory tract equivalent to the alveolar nociceptive (type J) receptors described by Paintal (1969) which are also stimulated by inhalation of irritant gases.

*References p. 251*

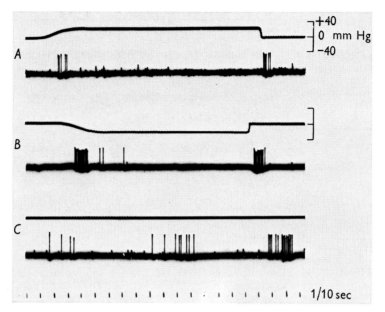

Fig. 6. Action potentials (lower traces) from a rapidly adapting receptor in the trachea of a cat. Upper traces: intratracheal pressure. Inflation (A) and deflation (B) of the trachea causes rapidly adapting discharges from the receptor. In C, the tracheal epithelium was gently touched with a catheter, causing further activity. (From Widdicombe, 1954b.)

## Large airway "cough" receptors

In structure these are terminal arborizations which extend under and between the columnar epithelial cells (Fig. 2) with fine endings that reach almost to the ciliary layer (Fillenz and Widdicombe, 1971). They have myelinated afferent nerve fibres which join the vagus nerves. The receptors are concentrated at the carina and points of branching of the larger bronchi, which are the sites in the lower airways most sensitive for eliciting the cough reflex (Widdicombe, 1954a and b).

These receptors have no spontaneous discharge in quiet breathing, but are stimulated by: (1) large inflations and deflations of the lungs, which presumably deform the epithelium; (2) intraluminal foreign bodies such as dust or a catheter; (3) inhaled chemical irritants such as ammonia, ethyl ether vapour or sulphur dioxide and (4) injections of histamine. The receptors are very rapidly adapting, have irregular discharges and show a clear off-response to mechanical stimulation (Fig. 6) (Widdicombe, 1954b). The relative anatomical simplicity of the trachea allows these endings to be identified with confidence with the epithelial receptors studied histologically.

## Lung irritant receptors

These have been investigated more extensively than those in the larger airways. They are virtually identical histologically, but their response to stimulation and the reflexes they induce show several distinctions. Koller (1968) and Homberger (1968)

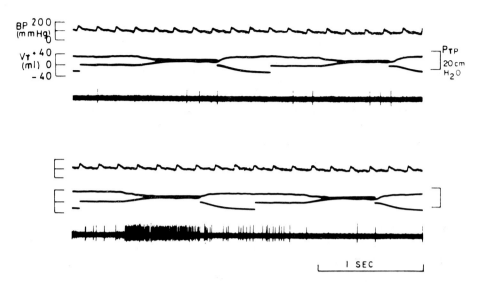

Fig. 7. Response of a lung irritant receptor to inhalation of carbon dust. Traces from above down: systemic arterial blood pressure (B.P.), transpulmonary pressure ($P_{TP}$), tidal volume ($V_T$) zeroing at points of zero air flow, and action potentials in a single vagal nerve fibre from a lung irritant receptor. Upper record: control showing slow spontaneous discharge. Lower record: during inhalation of dust, showing maximum stimulation of the receptor. The rabbit was paralyzed, artificially ventilated and vagotomized. (From Sellick and Widdicombe, 1971.)

called them "collapse" or "deflation" receptors, but they also respond to many other interventions, and the term "specific deflation receptor" had been applied to a different group of alveolar receptors (Paintal, 1955). The expression "irritant receptors" was first used in 1963 (Nadel and Widdicombe, 1963) and will be preferred here.

Lung irritant receptors are like the cough receptors in showing irregular rapidly adapting discharges, but do not usually give an off-response. They are more sensitive to chemical irritants and to various acute pulmonary pathological changes. They may show a weak discharge in quiet breathing, in the inflation or deflation phases or both. Their properties have been reviewed by Koller (1975), Mills *et al.* (1970), Fillenz and Widdicombe (1971), Luck (1970) and Widdicombe (1974). They are stimulated by: (1) large inflations and deflations, including pneumothorax and hyperpnoea; (2) intraluminal mechanical irritants such as dust or a catheter (Fig. 7); (3) contraction of underlying smooth muscle by drugs such as histamine; (4) inhalation of chemical irritants such as ammonia, sulphur dioxide and cigarette smoke and (5) pathological lung conditions such as anaphylaxis, pulmonary congestion, oedema and microembolism. They are sensitized by decreases in lung compliance which would lead to a larger mechanical pull on the bronchial wall during breathing. They have vagal afferent myelinated fibres in the A$\delta$ range.

It is obvious from these results that lung irritant receptors are very sensitive to changes in their mechanical environment — for example, a speck of dust on the epithelium can produce a vigorous stimulation. They also respond to many chemical substances, whether inhaled chemicals or endogenous active substances released

*References p. 251*

from the lungs. We do not know whether mechanical and chemical stimuli have a final common pathway before the receptor membrane is activated, or whether the afferent types of stimuli act at different sites in the receptor complex.

There is no evidence that the receptors are influenced by motor nerves to the epithelium, but there are two possibilities for "feed-back". The receptors cause reflex bronchoconstriction and are stimulated by bronchoconstriction, and they cause hyperpnoea and are activated in hyperpnoea. These "positive feed-backs" may be important in clinical conditions such as asthma (Widdicombe, 1970).

## CONCLUSIONS

We know from histological and physiological experiments that the respiratory tract is lined with nervous receptors in the epithelium which respond not only to inhaled mechanical and chemical irritants but also to local changes induced by a variety of physiological and pathological conditions. In some sites, the epipharynx, trachea and bronchi, it is possible to identify histologically the appearance of the receptors which have been studied physiologically. The reflex actions of these receptors have been studied extensively (Fillenz and Widdicombe, 1971; Widdicombe, 1964 and 1974; Tomori et al., 1973; Koller, 1973).

However, the areas about which we need more and precise information are depressingly large. For no receptor do we know exactly what, in its physical and chemical surroundings, can be responsible for setting up a receptor and resultant action potential. The inter-relationship between chemical and mechanical stimuli is completely obscure. The role of a mucous lining which might stimulate mechanically or protect chemically the receptor is indirectly supported by some experiments, but has not been clarified. The distinction between receptors in squamous cell epithelium and those in columnar cell epithelium is indicated by histological pictures and by physiological studies. A further complexity is that in some sites, for example the larynx, there are at least three groups of epithelial receptor which respond directly to mechanical and chemical irritation, and the reflex interaction of these three types is obscure.

## SUMMARY

The histological appearance of nervous receptors in the respiratory tract epithelium is reviewed. Their physiological behaviour, based on recording action potentials from single afferent nerve fibres from the receptors, shows many features in common. Most are rapidly adapting with irregular discharges, and have myelinated nerve fibres. They respond to mechanical and chemical irritant stimuli, and to various disease processes in the lungs and respiratory tract. The possible interaction of mechanical and chemical stimulations is discussed, together with the reflexes initiated by the receptors and their possible role in physiological and pathological conditions.

## REFERENCES

ANDREW, B. L. (1956) A functional analysis of the myelinated fibres of the superior laryngeal nerve of the rat. *J. Physiol. (Lond.)*, **133**, 420–432.

BOUSHEY, H. A., RICHARDSON, P. S., WIDDICOMBE, J. G. AND WISE, J. C. M. (1974) The response of laryngeal afferent fibres to mechanical and chemical stimuli. *J. Physiol. (Lond.)*, **240**, 153–175.

FILLENZ, M. AND WIDDICOMBE, J. G. (1971) Receptors of the lungs and airways. In E. NEIL, (Ed.), *Enteroceptors*. Springer, Heidelberg, pp. 82–112.

HOMBERGER, A. C. (1968) Beitrag zum Nachweis von Kollapsafferenzen im Lungenvagus des Kaninchens. *Helv. physiol. pharmacol. Acta*, **26**, 97–118.

KOLLER, E. A. (1968) Atmung und Kreislauf im anaphylaktischen Asthma bronchiale des Meerschweinchens. III. Die lungenveränderungen im Asthmaanfall und die inspiratorische Reaktion. *Helv. physiol. pharmacol. Acta*, **26**, 153–170.

KOLLER, E. A. (1973) Afferent vagal impulses in anaphylactic bronchial asthma. *Acta neurobiol. exp.*, **33**, 51–56.

LUCK, J. C. (1970) Afferent vagal fibres with an expiratory discharge in the rabbit. *J. Physiol. (Lond.)*, **211**, 63–75.

MILLS, J. E., SELLICK, H. AND WIDDICOMBE, J. G. (1970) Epithelial irritant receptors in the lungs. In R. PORTER (Ed.), *Breathing, Breuer-Hering Centenary Symposium*. Churchill, London. pp.77–82.

NADEL, J. A. AND WIDDICOMBE, J. G. (1963) Reflex control of airway size. *Ann. N.Y Acad. Sci.*, **109**, 712–722.

NAIL, B. S., STERLING, G. M. AND WIDDICOMBE, J. G. (1969) Epipharyngeal receptors responding to mechanical stimulation. *J. Physiol. (Lond.)*, **204**, 91–98.

PAINTAL, A. S. (1955) Impulses in vagal afferent fibres from specific pulmonary deflation receptors. The response of these receptors to phenyl diguanide, potato starch, 5-hydroxytryptamine and nicotine, and their role in respiratory and cardiovascular reflexes. *Quart. J. exp. Physiol.*, **40**, 89–111.

PAINTAL, A. S. (1969) Mechanism of stimulation of type J pulmonary receptors. *J. Physiol. (Lond.)*, **203**, 511–532.

SAMPSON, C. AND EYZAGUIRRE, C. (1964) Some functional characteristics of the mechanoreceptors in the larynx of the cat. *J. Neurophysiol.*, **27**, 464–480.

SELLICK, H. AND WIDDICOMBE, J. G. (1971) Stimulation of lung irritant receptors by cigarette smoke, carbon dust, and histamine aerosol. *J. appl. Physiol.*, **31**, 15–19.

STOREY, A. T. (1968) A functional analysis of sensory units innervating epiglottis and larynx. *Exp. Neurol.*, **20**, 366–383.

SUZUKI, M. AND KIRCHNER, J. A. (1968) Afferent nerve fibres in the external branch of the superior laryngeal nerve in the cat. *Ann. Otol. (St Louis)*, **77**, 1059–1070.

TOMORI, Z., JAVORKA, K. AND STRANSKY, A. (1973) Reflex responses to stimulation of the upper respiratory tract. *Acta neurobiol. exp.*, **33**, 57–69.

TOMORI, Z. AND WIDDICOMBE, J. G. (1969) Muscular, bronchomotor and cardiovascular reflexes elicited by mechanical stimulation of the respiratory tract. *J. Physiol. (Lond.)*, **200**, 25–50.

WIDDICOMBE, J. G. (1954a) Respiratory reflexes from the trachea and bronchi of the cat. *J. Physiol. (Lond.)*, **123**, 55–70.

WIDDICOMBE, J. G. (1954b) Receptors in the trachea and bronchi of the cat. *J. Physiol. (Lond.)*, **123**, 71–104.

WIDDICOMBE, J. G. (1964) Respiratory reflexes. In *Handbook of Physiology—Respiration I*. American Physiol. Soc., Washington, D.C. pp. 585–630.

WIDDICOMBE, J. G. (1970) Reflex mechanisms in bronchial obstruction. In *Bronchitis III*. Royal Van Gorcum, Assem. pp. 288–294.

WIDDICOMBE, J. G. (1974) Reflexes from the lungs in the control of breathing. In R. J. LINDEN (Ed.), *Recent Advances in Physiology. Ninth Ed.* Churchill Livingstone, Edinburgh. pp. 239–278.

## DISCUSSION

CAUNA: I am not asking the question, but I want to comment on the innervation I have studied in the laryngeal aspect of the epiglottis some 15 years ago in man, and I can assure you that this is an area with a density of nerve endings exceeding any other area that I have seen. The nerve fibers that supplied these endings range from very fine to very thick indeed nerve endings, right beneath epithelium and forming nests of complicated terminals and protruding through the surface, and there are very fine nerve fibers which appear to be playing the termination of our straight-line endings which again form a very dense net beneath epithelium.

PERL: I have a question regarding the responses of your lung irritant receptors. You showed rather remarkably strong vigorous responses to the carbon particle in contact, yet the responses to some other agents which one presumed being also considerably irritating to the laryngeal epithelium were less.

WIDDICOMBE: It was the kind of typical example one publishes. In other words, the most dramatic one. In fact we have applied dust to, I forget the total number of receptors, but the last number was two and showed that increase in discharge is statistically significant of the group but often there is not an immediate vigorous discharge like that but a rather slow build up of the activity as if the receptor had to be stimulated by more than one particle of dust settling in the neighborhood.

IGGO: I think you restricted your description to mammalian receptors. That is why I would like to comment that in birds there are receptors which appear to have a specific sensitivity to carbon dioxide. Many of your responses showed that the effect of carbon dioxide appeared not to be specific.

WIDDICOMBE: Yes, one of the reasons that we looked for the action of carbon dioxide was because of the results you mentioned; we have only receptors which are inhibited by carbon dioxide and as the receptor inhibits breathing, if you inhibit the receptors which inhibit breathing, you get a stimulation of breathing. Our results are consistent with the bird experiments since carbon dioxide inhibits stretch receptors which inhibit breathing in the mammals. But I think, that as far as the analogy goes, in the case of the bird the receptors seem to be deep in the lung, and because the bird lung does not distend on inflation so they are not physiologically mechanosensitive. Whether or not they have the same phylogenetic origin in development, nobody knows. There are similarities but there are also big differences. For example, the bird receptors are completely inhibited by $CO_2$ but not in the cat; but in the cat the laryngeal ones are completely inhibited, but the lung ones are not inhibited. In the bird there are no laryngeal $CO_2$ responses.

GLEBOVSKY: Concerning the report of Professor Widdicombe on irritant receptors of the respiratory tract, I would like to note good arguments adduced for the important role which these receptors play in acquisition of the defensive respiratory reflexes in pathology. However, the role of irritant receptors in the regulation of normal respiration is not quite clear yet. I think that the role of the dynamics of lung deflation, stimulation and inflation were underestimated. In the mechanoreceptors' stimulation several factors may be involved: decrease during the expiration in stimulation of stretch receptors of the lung and the decrease in the inhibitory effect of impulses from the receptors on expiration phase. Secondly, probably it is a hypothesis that reduced impulse discharge of the lung stretch receptors stimulate the inspiration similarly to frequency phenomena described in detail by Koller and Ferrer, 1968. Thirdly, I think the lung irritant receptors Professor Widdicombe mentioned might be probably involved in such stimulation of the irritant receptors.

WIDDICOMBE: I have only a comment. I entirely agree with the interpretation that the action of irritant receptors on the expiratory phase is very important. I think they have been neglected by respiratory physiologists who have done many experiments to study what inflation of the lung does to the inspiratory phase but tended to ignore the effect of afferent discharge during expiratory phase. And I think this is important.

# Resetting as a General Functional Property of Cardiovascular Mechanoreceptors (Experimental Study of Mechanoreceptors in the Aorta and Auricles)

E. P. ANYUKHOVSKY, G. G. BELOSHAPKO AND F. P. YASINOVSKAYA

*U.S.S.R. AMS Cardiological Institute, Moscow (U.S.S.R.)*

It is well known that increased arterial pressure results, in the long run, in the resetting of mechanoreceptors in the aortic arch and in the carotid sinus, which means that in spite of high pressure the activity of the baroreceptors remains at the same level as in the normal state (McCubbin *et al.*, 1956; Kreiger and Marseillan, 1966; Aars, 1968a; Angell-James, 1970).

Mechanisms of baroreceptor resetting are not yet clear. The most widely accepted hypothesis is that based on the fact that baroreceptors are receptors of distension. According to this hypothesis, resetting of baroreceptors in hypertension is caused by changes in the distensibility of vessels (Neil, 1962; Peterson, 1962; Markov, 1967; Aars, 1968a). This hypothesis has been proved only indirectly. Experiments where strips (Aars, 1968b) or segments (Jones *et al.*, 1967; Angell-James, 1973) of rabbits' aorta were used revealed decreased distensibility of the aorta in hypertensive animals.

In order to check the hypothesis directly it is necessary to compare the activity of aortic baroreceptors in the normal state and in hypertension at the same level of deformation of the aorta.

Our experiments were performed on "aortic arch–aortic nerve" preparations isolated in normal rabbits and in rabbits with renal hypertension. The relationships between integrated activity in left aortic nerve and aortic pressure and distension were studied.

Rabbits (2.5–3 kg) of both sexes were used in the experiments. The preparation was isolated from the vessel in the following way. The innominate and left subclavian arteries, as well as the descending aorta were ligated. A brass cannula connected to a thin glass pipe was introduced into the aortic orifice through the left ventricle. The system was filled with the animal's heparinized blood. The pressure in the preparation was changed by means of vertical displacement of the mercury container. The shift of the blood–mercury border pointed to the volume of the blood perfused into the preparation. Given the volume of the preparation it is easy to calculate its radius since up to 200 mm Hg deformation of a vessel due to pressure hardly affects its length (Remington *et al.*, 1948; Patel *et al.*, 1961).

The aortic nerve activity was assessed with the help of a specially designed integrator which produced at its output impulses with amplitudes in proportion to the electrical activity of input signals summed for a selected period of integration.

*References p. 259–260*

254 E. P. ANYUKHOVSKY *et al.*

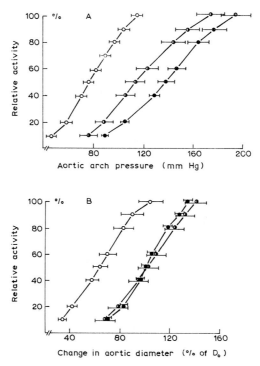

Fig. 1. Graph showing the relationship between aortic nerve activity (expressed as a per cent of the maximum activity), aortic arch pressure (A) and aortic distension (B) in the normal (open circles), 2–4 weeks hypertension (semi-solid circles) and 8–10 weeks hypertension (solid circles) animals. $D_0$ aortic diameter at zero pressure. Each point represents the mean value of a group of animals. Horizontal lines represent ± S.E.

Hypertensive animals were divided into two groups depending on the term of illness in order to study the dynamics of the interrelation of the mentioned factors. Experimenting with an isolated aortic arch preparation makes it possible to study the activity of aortic baroreceptors along a sufficiently wide range of pressures and thus to establish accurately thresholds of baroreceptor excitation as well as those values of aortic pressure and distension where activity of baroreceptors becomes maximum (points of inflection). Besides, this experimental technique excludes the possibility of neural and humoral influences of the baroreceptor area and thus makes it possible to reveal the effect of the mechanical factor by itself.

Increased arterial pressure developed in rabbits as a result of renal hypertension. For this aim, one kidney was removed and the renal artery of the remaining kidney was partly squeezed with a clamp. In the group of animals with the post-operative term of 0.5–1.0 month (8 animals) arterial systolic pressure varied from 145 to 185 mm Hg (mean value 160 mm Hg). In animals with the post-operative term of 2.0–2.5 months (10 rabbits) the pressure varied from 150 to 195 mm Hg (mean value 170 mm Hg). These terms of hypertension we named early and late hypertension. Eleven rabbits with a mean arterial systolic pressure value of 110 mm Hg comprised a control group.

The dependence of aortic nerve activity on aortic pressure in normal and hypertensive rabbits is shown in Fig. 1A. As can be seen, curves for hypertensive animals are shifted to the right, *i.e.* into the region of higher pressures, as compared with normals. The curve for animals with late hypertension is located more to the right than that for those with early hypertension. The threshold value in the normals was $46 \pm 4$ mm Hg; in early hypertension — $76 \pm 7$ mm Hg ($P < 0.0025$) and in late hypertension — $82 \pm 2$ mm Hg ($P < 0.001$). Pressures corresponding to the points of inflection were: in the normals — $115 \pm 4$ mm Hg; in early hypertension — $175 \pm 11$ mmHg ($P < 0.001$) and in late hypertension — $195 \pm 12$ mm Hg ($P < 0.001$).

To answer the question whether resetting of aortic baroreceptors is the result of increased stiffness of the aorta, we determined the dependence of activity in the aortic nerve on distension of the aorta. Relative deformation of a body is estimated by the ratio of the increase in the body's dimensions to its dimensions in an untensed state. Thus, we took as a measure of aortic deformation the ratio of increase of aortic diameter to its diameter at zero pressure.

In Fig. 1B curves relating activity in the aortic nerve of hypertensive animals with distension of the aorta are shifted to the right, *i.e.* into the region of stronger distensions of the aorta as compared with the norm. Values of aortic deformation at threshold pressure were: in the normals — $34 \pm 3\%$; in early hypertension — $68 \pm 8\%$ ($P < 0.001$) and in late hypertension — $69 \pm 4\%$ ($P < 0.001$). Deformation of the aorta corresponding to maximum activity in the nerve was: in the normals — $104 \pm 11\%$; in early hypertension — $142 \pm 2\%$ ($P < 0.001$) and in late hypertension — $133 \pm 3\%$ ($P < 0.01$).

It appears, therefore, that in hypertension a stronger than normal distension of the aorta is needed to obtain the same activity in the aortic nerve. Resetting of aortic baroreceptors in hypertension, thus, can not be explained merely by changes in the mechanical properties of the aorta. On the other hand, in Fig. 1B, the curves for animals with early and late hypertension practically coincide. This points to the fact that at equal levels of aortic deformation, activity in the aortic nerve is the same in animals with both early and late hypertension. It is thus likely that the shift of baroreceptor thresholds to the region of higher pressures in rabbits with late hypertension as compared with rabbits with early hypertension is the result of increased stiffness of the aorta in animals of the former group.

The dependence of aortic deformation on pressure is given in Fig. 2A. As can be seen in animals with early hypertension, tensility of the aorta equals that in the normals, while in animals with late hypertension its values are lower than normal.

What are the causes of baroreceptor resetting at early stages of hypertension?

This may be due to changes in elastic properties of the baroreceptor region itself and/or changes in the sensitivity of receptor endings (Abraham, 1967; Hilgenberg, 1967).

According to the most widely accepted theory of the physiological role of baroreceptors, vascular baroreceptors control the level of arterial pressure. It is assumed, correspondingly, that resetting of baroreceptor signals in hypertension assists in maintaining the high level of arterial pressure.

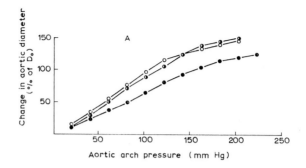

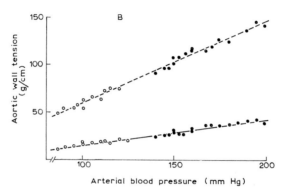

Fig. 2. A: graph showing the relationship between aortic distension and pressure in the normal (open circles), 2–4 weeks hypertension (semi-solid circles), and 8–10 weeks hypertension (solid circles) animals. Each point represents the mean value of a group of animals. Difference between aortic distension in normal and 8–10 weeks hypertension animals is statistically significant ($P < 0.005$). B: graph showing the relationship between the values of aortic wall tangential strain and initial arterial pressure in the normal (open circles) and hypertension (solid circles) animals. Continuous line corresponds to baroreceptor threshold pressure; the broken line corresponds to maximum activity pressure.

Khayutin (1967) has presented facts which disagree with the concept outlined above. In his opinion, baroreceptors participate in the selection of circulation parameters optimal for minimization of mechanical work of the heart. If we accept this point of view, the resetting of baroreceptors in hypertension can be considered as a transition to a new working regime adequate to the task of control. Deformation of the receptor region caused by the force applied to the region on the side of the vessel wall — tangential force $T = PR$ — stimulates baroreceptors. Dependence of the tangential force developing in the aortic wall at the threshold pressure and at the point of inflection on initial arterial pressure in all groups of experimental animals is shown in Fig. 2B. As can be seen points for animals with normal arterial pressure and for hypertensive animals are located practically on the same line. This suggests that aortic baroreceptor sensitivity is adjusted in correspondence with arterial pressure.

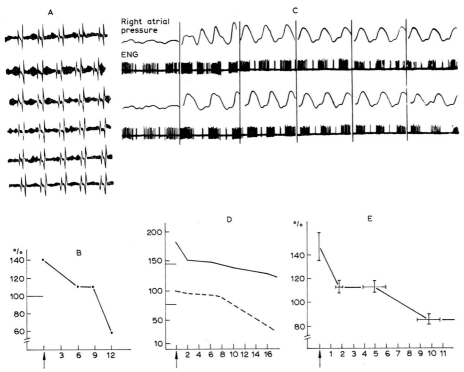

Fig. 3. A: activity in the right cardiac nerve branch resulting from distension of the right auricle produced by means of an umbrella-type dilator. From top to bottom: Initial ENG, ENG at the beginning of distension, ENG after 3, 6, 9, 12 min of distension. ENG = electroneurogram. B: a curve relating the intensity of impulses with the time of distension (the arrow indicates the moment of distension). C: activity of single auricle mechanoreceptor type B; below: activity of the same mechanoreceptor after repeated distension of auricle. D: activity of an auricle mechanoreceptor at the first (unbroken line) and repeated (broken line) distension of the auricle. Ordinate is the number of impulses in the filament during 1 respiratory cycle; abscissa is the time in minutes. E: a curve relating activity in single mechanoreceptors with the time of auricle distension. Ordinate is the activity in a filament in per cent of the initial level; abscissa is the time in minutes. Mean values for a group of experiments (10 filaments) and standard deviation of the means. The arrow indicates the moments of distension of the auricles.

It may be asked whether the resetting phenomenon is observed in the case of other cardiovascular mechanoreceptors, for example those in the auricles.

We found that prolonged distension of the auricles also resulted in decreased impulse activity of the corresponding mechanoreceptors. The experiments were performed on ether–chloralose anaesthetized cats, with distension of the right auricle by an umbrella-type dilator. Either the electroneurogram of the intact trunk innervating the right auricle or the activity of the vagus filaments leading to single auricle mechanoreceptors was recorded. Simultaneously we recorded the pressure in the right auricle.

As seen in Fig. 3A and 3B, the diastolic discharge in the nerve which innervates the right auricle is considerably increased at the moment of distension, and after

*References p. 259–260*

that it gradually decreases; however, it is still relatively high and only after 10–20 min (in different experiments) does the nerve's activity fall below the initial level.

Similar results were obtained in experiments where the activities of the vagus filaments leading to single mechanoreceptors were recorded. As seen in Fig. 3C and D, the activity of receptors firing during the diastole ("B-receptors", Paintal, 1953) is also sharply increased at the moment of distension — as may be judged by the number and frequency of impulses in a pack — and then falls while still exceeding the norm, and by 10–20 min passes below the initial level where it stays for more than half an hour. Repeated distension of the auricle (to the same extent) results in the same pattern of changes in the activity; however, the number and frequency of impulses in the pack are reduced. This obviously proves that mechanoreceptors in the auricle do indeed undergo resetting.

Similar results were obtained by Greenberg *et al.* (1973), who revealed reduced impulse characteristics of the left auricle mechanoreceptors in the case of chronic heart deficiency (pulmonary stenosis) as compared with characteristics of the intact auricle mechanoreceptors.

The phenomenon of resetting resulting from prolonged stimulation was established, therefore, for the mechanoreceptors of the carotid sinus, the aorta and the auricles. As was mentioned above, some authors believe that resetting of baroreceptors of the carotid sinus and aorta favours the development of hypertension, while resetting of the auricle mechanoreceptors in the case of heart deficiency leads to the deranged regulation of the volume of the circulating blood (Vinogradov *et al.*, 1971). On the other hand there is a point of view (Khayutin, 1967) according to which the resetting of baroreceptors in hypertension is, in fact, the resetting to a new working regime required by the goals of regulation — achievement of the optimum work of the heart. Our data seem to support the second hypothesis.

It is likely that the sympathetic nervous system is to a certain extent responsible for the transition of mechanoreceptors to a new range of pressures. Sampson and Mills (1970), Bagshaw and Peterson (1972) and Keith *et al.* (1974) showed that stimulation of the sympathetic nerve innervating the sinocarotid receptor region produces changes in the characteristics of the carotid sinus baroreceptors, both mechanical properties of the region and the sensitivity of the receptor endings being affected.

Zucker and Gilmore (1974) have demonstrated that the activities of the mechanoreceptors of the auricles, when the *ganglion stellatum* is stimulated are also reduced. It was found that this reduction of activity was due to a decrease of volume of the auricles. However, the influence of the sympathetic system in the resetting phenomenon is as yet problematic. Thus, in our preliminary experiments, undertaken in collaboration with Shatalov and Rodionov, it has been demonstrated that resetting may appear in immunosympathectomized rats suffering hypertension.

We may assume, therefore, that the region of linear dependence of mechanoreceptor activity on pressure or volume can shift as a result of changes in the parameters of arterial pressure or in the auricle diastolic volume. It is highly probable that resetting is the general functional property of cardiovascular mechanoreceptors.

## SUMMARY

The summed activity of the left aortic nerve, and the aortic diameter and pressure in both normal and renal hypertensive rabbits were investigated in isolated preparations of the aortic arch. It was shown that, in rabbits, a 2–4 week period of hypertension leads to resetting of aortic baroreceptors without changes in the distensibility of the aorta. In later stages of hypertension (8–10 weeks) the distensibility of the aorta decreases, which leads to a greater resetting of the baroreceptors. Similar results, *i.e.* decrease of activity of the auricle mechanoreceptors, were found on prolonged atrial distension of cats by means of an umbrella-type dilator. It may be supposed that resetting is a general property of the cardiovascular mechanoreceptors.

## REFERENCES

AARS, H. (1968a) Aortic baroreceptor activity in normal and in hypertensive rabbits. *Acta physiol. scand.*, **72**, 298–309.

AARS, H. (1968b) Static load–length characteristics of aortic strips from hypertensive rabbits. *Acta physiol. scand.*, **73**, 101–110.

ABRAHAM, Q. (1967) The structure of baroreceptors in pathological conditions in man. In P. KEZDI (Ed.), *Baroreceptors and Hypertension*. Pergamon Press, London. pp. 273–291.

ANGELL-JAMES, I. E. (1970) A comparison of the impulse activity in single aortic baroreceptor fibres in normal and in experimental renal hypertensive rabbits. *J. Physiol. (Lond.)*, **213**, 42–43.

ANGELL-JAMES, J. E. (1973) Characteristics of single left aortic and right subclavian baroreceptor fiber activity in rabbits with chronic renal hypertension. *Circulat. Res.*, **32**, 149–161.

BAGSHAW, I. AND PETERSON, L. K. (1972) Sympathetic control of mechanical properties of the canine carotid sinus. *Amer. J. Physiol.*, **222**, 1462–1468.

GREENBERG, T., RICHMOND, W., STOCKING, R., GUPTA, P., MEEHAN, J. AND HENRY, J. (1973) Impaired atrial receptor responses in dogs with heart failure due to tricuspid insufficiency and pulmonary artery stenosis. *Circulat. Res.*, **32**, 424–433.

HILGENBERG, F. (1967) Neurohistologic studies of the carotid sinus baroreceptors in hypertension. In P. KEZDI (Ed.), *Baroreceptors and Hypertension*. Pergamon Press, London. pp. 293–297.

JONES, A. W., PETERSON, L. H. AND FEIGEL, E. O. (1967) Vascular alterations in experimental hypertension. In P. KEZDI (Ed.), *Baroreceptors and Hypertension*. Pergamon Press, London. pp. 309–315.

KEITH, C., KIDD, C., MALPUS, C. H. AND PENNA, P. E. (1974) Reduction of baroreceptor impulse activity by sympathetic nerve stimulation. *J. Physiol. (Lond.)*, **238**, 61P.

KHAYUTIN, V. M. (1967) Development of presentation of carodial and carotid sinus zones. *Sechenov physiol. J. U.S.S.R.*, **53**, 1469–1475.

KREIGER, E. H. AND MARSEILLAN, R. F. (1966) Neural control in experimental renal hypertension. Role of baroreceptors and splanchnic fibres. *Acta physiol. lat.-amer.*, **16**, 343–352.

MARKOV, KH. M. (1967) On the role of carotid sinus and aortic arch baroreceptors in the pathogenesis of hypertension. *Vyestnik AMN S.S.S.R.*, **7**, 18–31.

MCCUBBIN, J. W., GREEN, J. H. AND PAGE, I. H. (1956) Baroreceptor function in chronic renal hypertension. *Circulat. Res.*, **4**, 205–210.

NEIL, E. (1962) Neural factors responsible for cardiovascular regulation. *Circulat. Res.*, **11**, 137–148.

PAINTAL, V. A. S. (1953) A study of right and left atrial receptors. *J. Physiol. (Lond.)*, **120**, 596–610.

PATEL, A. J., MALLOS, Q. J. AND FRY, D. J. (1961) Aortic mechanics in the living dog. *J. appl. Physiol.*, **16**, 293–299.

PETERSON, L. H. (1962) Some studies of the regulation of cardiovascular functions. *Arch. int. Pharmacodyn.*, **140**, 281–290.

REMINGTON, J. W., NOBACK, C. R., HAMILTON, W. F. AND GOLD, J. J. (1948) Volume elasticity characteristics of the human aorta and the prediction of the stroke volume from the pressure pulse. *Amer. J. Physiol.*, **153**, 298–308.

SAMPSON, S. R. AND MILLS, E. (1970) Effects of sympathetic stimulation on discharges of carotid sinus baroreceptors. *Amer. J. Physiol.*, **218**, 1650–1653.

VINOGRADOV, H. V., KRITSMAN, M. G., UDELNOV, M. E., SEREBROXSKAYA, YU, A., SYCHEVA, I. M., YASINOVSKAYA, F. P. AND KUZMINA, A. E. (1971) On the causes of fluid retention in cardiac insufficiency. *J. Cardiology U.S.S.R.*, **1**, 44–50.

ZUCKER, I. H. AND GILMORE, J. P. (1974) Evidence for an indirect sympathetic control of atrial stretch receptor discharge in the dog. *Circulat. Res.*, **34**, 441–446.

## DISCUSSION

SANTINI: How, according to your data does the sympathetic nervous system influence the activity of the receptors?

YASINOVSKAYA: So far we have not studied, as Peterson and co-authors have, the influence of activity of aortic baroreceptors, on the baroreceptors of the sinus caroticus and as you have in your work on the Pacinian corpuscle. But, on the basis of the above mentioned and other studies the sympathetic nervous system may influence the mechanical qualities of the receptor zone and/or the sensitivity of the receptors themselves.

WIDDICOMBE: I have not quite grasped your diagram about tangential forces. What does it signify?

YASINOVSKAYA: This is what the diagram meant to show: after every rabbit had its aortic pressure measured and its aortic zone isolated, we defined the threshold pressure at which receptor activity set in; we also defined the pressure at which the receptor activity reached its maximum. The diagram shows the tangential forces (T = PR) both at threshold pressure and at maximum pressure as related to initial pressure found in all the rabbits studied: those with normal blood pressure and those with hypertension. Since the points reflecting the threshold pressures tend to group along one line, as do the points reflecting the maximum activity pressure, we believe that the diagram could provide circumstantial evidence showing that the aortic baroreceptors are, if one may use such an expression, tuned to a certain range of pressures defined by the regulation demands.

SESSION V

# NOCICEPTOR MECHANISMS

# Sensitization of High Threshold Receptors with Unmyelinated (C) Afferent Fibers

E. R. PERL, T. KUMAZAWA\*, B. LYNN\*\* AND P. KENINS

*Department of Physiology, School of Medicine, University of North Carolina, Chapel Hill, N.C. 27514*
*(U.S.A.)*

Adrian and Zotterman (1926a and b) demonstrated that fatigue upon repeated activation by natural stimuli is a feature of somatic sense organ behavior. This fatigue, manifested by depression of response, varies in duration and magnitude according to the receptor type and the kind of stimulus. It is possibly related to the decrease or cessation of response during a constant stimulus, *i.e.* adaptation (see discussion by Burgess and Perl, 1973). The mechanisms underlying the depression of responsiveness are imperfectly understood, although a number of reasonable hypotheses have been advanced from Adrian and Zotterman's time onward. In this context, it is remarkable that polymodal nociceptors, one of the most common types of cutaneous sense organ with unmyelinated (C) afferent fibers, often show an enhanced rather than depressed responsiveness after activation; the increased response has been labeled *sensitization* (Bessou and Perl, 1969). Augmented activity upon repeated excitation is particularly noteworthy since the also common C mechanoreceptors exhibit an exceptional degree of fatigue (Bessou *et al.*, 1971). Sensitization of the polymodal nociceptors (and perhaps other high threshold sense organs) has characteristics suggesting an important bearing upon somatic sensation, particularly pain (Perl, 1972).

## METHODS

The activity of primary sensory units with unmyelinated fibers was recorded from fine bundles dissected from the central end of cut cutaneous nerves of anesthetized cats, monkeys, and rabbits. Splitting of filaments was carried out until the activity of a single fiber conducting at C velocity (on electrical stimulation of the whole nerve peripherally) was of relatively large amplitude and sufficiently distinctive shape and size so that it could be unequivocally identified in the recording. Sensory units forming the basis of this report conducted at less than 1.1 m/sec. The electrical activity

---

\* Present address: Department of Physiology, School of Medicine, Nagoya University, Nagoya, Japan.
\*\* Department of Physiology, University College London, London, Great Britain.

*References p. 275–276*

recorded from the filament was amplified and then observed on an oscilloscope and a direct writing oscillograph; amplified nerve potentials and measures of the stimulus were stored on analogue magnetic tape. In most instances the recording from the single C-fiber afferent unit required no special treatment for unequivocal identification. Analyses of the quantitative discharge were performed using either a special purpose instantaneous frequency display device (Ortec-4672) or programs of the type described by Schmittroth in Bessou and Perl (1969) for a digital computer–graphic system (DEC-PDP/11-Evans and Sutherland LDS-2 system).

Receptive units were identified according to criteria described in Bessou and Perl (1969) and Bessou *et al.* (1971). In general, these involved the use of semi-quantitative mechanical stimulation, non-noxious cooling and localized skin heating. Tests of the receptors for alterations in responsiveness were made by using quanti-tatively controlled mechanical stimulation and a programmable heat stimulator. The latter utilized either a thermode of approximately 3 sq.mm contact diameter or a focused infrared source. Control of the thermode or the radiant source was through a feedback loop from a small (0.4 mm diameter) thermistor placed at the tip of the thermode or in contact with the center of the receptive field heated by the radiant source. In experiments on perfused preparations, the major arterial and venous supplies to a skin area were cannulated. The skin area to be studied was completely cut free with blood vessels above the arteriole or venule dimension ligated. In prepa-rations left *in situ*, a stopcock arrangement permitted switching between blood from the animal's cardiovascular circulation or an artificial perfusate to be used. In many experiments the isolated skin or rabbit ear was perfused *in vitro* in a chamber per-mitting protection of exposed tissue under a layer of mineral oil.

### RESULTS

Polymodal nociceptors are common in hairy skin and, in many nerves, are a pre-dominant cutaneous receptive unit with a C afferent fiber. Characteristically they have elevated thresholds for all forms of natural stimulation when compared to other sensory elements generally accepted to be mechano- or thermoreceptive in type (Bessou and Perl, 1969). Threshold for otherwise identical mechanical stimuli range from five to several hundred times those of low threshold mechanoreceptors with either myelinated or C-afferent fibers; frank damage is necessary to excite more than a few impulses in a number of polymodal units. In addition, polymodal nociceptors typically scale their response in proportion to progressively graded mechanical stimuli of noxious and tissue-damaging intensity; this latter feature distinguishes them from low threshold mechanoreceptors which saturate or block with such intense stimula-tion (Burgess and Perl, 1973). Fig. 1A shows the just threshold responses of a poly-modal nociceptor to 0.8 g of force exerted by a punctate stimulator, an intensity some 40 to 80 times the threshold value for typical cutaneous mechanoreceptors with either C or A afferent fibers. The increased intensity of stimulation represented by 4.4 g of force exerted by a similar punctate stimulator produced a greater response, as is

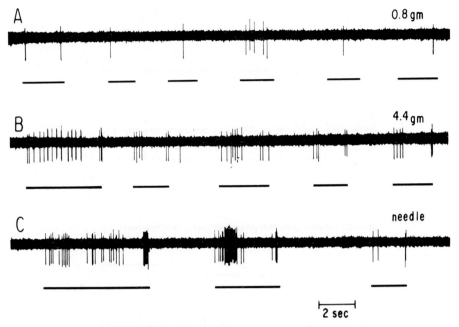

Fig. 1. Excitation of a cat polymodal nociceptor by punctate mechanical stimuli. Bars under traces mark approximate time and duration of skin pressure; all stimulation was at one spot. A: stimulation by flexible probe bending with 0.8 g force. B: stimulation by flexible probe bending at 4.4 g force. C: stimulation with sharp, rigid needle at a force sufficient to penetrate the skin. Note responses in B and C evoked as the mechanical stimulus was withdrawn. (From Bessou and Perl, 1969.)

illustrated in Fig. 1B; this stimulus level on repeated application produced abrasion of the skin surface. An overtly damaging stimulus, needle pressure of sufficient force to penetrate the epidermal surface (Fig. 1C), evoked still more impulses and a higher frequency of discharge.

Polymodal receptors give consistent responses to noxious heat applied to the uninjured skin surface. In Fig. 2A and B, step changes in temperature of a contact thermode centered on the receptive field of the unit illustrated in Fig. 1 produced a threshold response at about 45 °C and a vigorous response to the next (5 °C) increase of temperature. The latter level (just over 50 °C) is unequivocally noxious since prolonged or repeated stimuli at this thermode temperature are followed by local swelling and/or erythema of the skin. Fig. 2C and D illustrate the observation basic to sensitization of polymodal receptors: a second heating to 45 °C evoked a vigorous response in comparison to the threshold activity shown in Fig. 2A. Admittedly, the test illustrated by Fig. 2C has an equivocal feature since the temperature change carrying the thermode to 45 °C was greater than the one in Fig. 2A. For this reason all tests for alterations in responsiveness of receptors of the type to be described subsequently were done with stimulus sequences which carefully replicated one another in terms of rates and magnitude of temperature change.

Polymodal C fiber units also respond to chemical irritation of the intact skin. An example of a typical, low frequency but persisting response to a drop of dilute

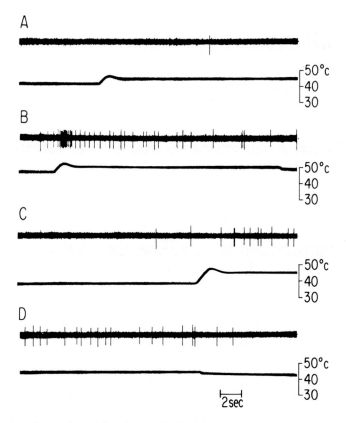

Fig. 2. Excitation of cat polymodal nociceptor (C fiber) by heat. Same receptor as in Fig. 1. Upper trace of each pair is the electrical activity in the nerve filament; lower trace shows the temperature of a thermode contacting approximately 3 sq.mm. A: first heating above 40 °C; B: 10 sec after end of A. C and D: continuous records starting approximately 1.5 min after B, during which the thermode had passively cooled. (From Bessou and Perl, 1969.)

hydrochloric acid is shown in Fig. 3. The discharges in Fig. 3 are graphed as a function of time in a format displaying the inverse of successive intervals between impulses on the vertical axis as a function of time of occurrence, a type of display which has proved particularly useful for illustrating patterns of discharge. The broad responsiveness illustrated by Figs. 1–3 is unusual for a receptor from the hairy skin of cat; no other sensory units in this kind of skin are known which give vigorous responses on mechanical, heat and irritant chemical stimulation.

The phenomenon of sensitization is illustrated by the responses plotted in Fig. 4 for a primate polymodal nociceptor. Identical heating cycles (of the form shown by the bottom trace in Fig. 4) were repeated every 200 msec; the thermode temperature was increased by 5 °C steps to a maximum of 52 °C, after which it was rapidly cooled and held at the starting temperature of approximately 30 °C until the next sequence (200 msec later). Fig. 4A graphically shows the response the first time the receptor was stimulated, Fig. 4B the response to the third heating cycle, and Fig. 4C that to the fifth stimulation cycle. The results in Fig. 4 make clear the progressive increase in

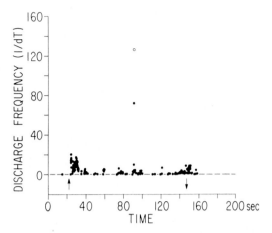

Fig. 3. Excitation of a cat polymodal nociceptor by dilute hydrochloric acid. Each impulse is marked by a dot, positioned vertically according to the reciprocal of the interval between it and the previous impulse. The horizontal axis shows time from an arbitrary beginning. The dot was placed along the time axis at the time of occurrence of the second impulse. The upward directed arrow marks application of a drop of dilute HCl to the receptive field. The downward arrow marks wash of the acid by a stream of water. (From Bessou and Perl, 1969.)

the total number and maximal frequency of discharges evoked by the third and fifth cycles of stimulation as compared to that elicited by the initial test. Careful examination of Fig. 4 also shows a progressive lowering of threshold with discharge appearing at lower temperatures in Fig. 4B and C than in Fig. 4A. In addition, an afterdischarge, representing the development of background activity, can be seen in Fig. 4C as impulses subsequent to the end of the heating sequence.

Polymodal nociceptors, with receptive fields in unstimulated and uninjured hairy skin, do not ordinarily exhibit background activity. After noxious stimulation, however, most polymodal units develop a persisting, ongoing discharge. The evolution of a substantial background discharge is illustrated in Fig. 5A for a feline polymodal receptor; skin heating in a smoothly increasing fashion over a period of many seconds evoked the first discharges at about 42 °C with a gradual increase in activity with increasing temperature and the appearance of bursts of activity (indicated by dots at the baseline and at higher frequency levels at nearly the same horizontal position). After a maximal temperature of just over 50 °C the thermode was allowed to cool passively and for some seconds there was no discharge; at a temperature well below the initial threshold level a low frequency irregular series of impulses appeared and continued even though the temperature had fallen to non-noxious levels. The correlation between temperature (on the horizontal axis) and discharge frequency (on the vertical axis) is shown in Fig. 5B for the first 150 sec of the sequence illustrated in Fig. 5A. Fig. 5C shows a similar correlation for the initial 150 sec of the next and identical heating sequence (not illustrated); a greater number of impulses and a higher maximal frequency is apparent. The amount and kind of background activity shown by Fig. 5 was often seen with polymodal receptors following vigorous excitation by one or more cycles of heating.

*References p. 275–276*

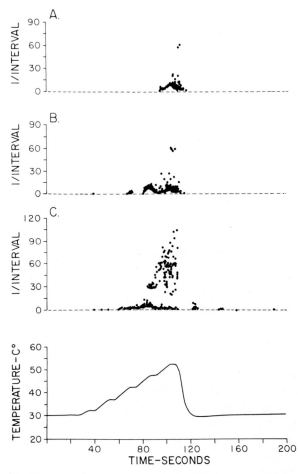

Fig. 4. Augmentation of discharge of a primate polymodal nociceptor (C fiber) with repeated cycles of noxious heating. The lower graph indicates the heating cycle (heating steps from approximately 32 °C to 52 °C in about 1 min followed by a rapid cooling to 30 °C. The cycle was repeated automatically every 200 msec. Graphs A, B and C are plotted as in Fig. 3. Each graph has been normalized to coincide with the same point in the temperature cycle. A: first heating cycle. B: third heating cycle. C: fifth heating cycle. (From Kumazawa and Perl, 1975.)

Changes in magnitude of response and threshold are shown in another fashion for five primate polymodal receptors in Fig. 6. Separate symbols indicate the activity produced by each receptor during repeated heating and cooling cycles of the form and temperature range illustrated in Fig. 4. The number of discharges produced by each cycle are plotted in Fig. 6A; the total impulse activity for the different examples increased over that recorded in the first test from about 150 % to large multiples in successive sequences of stimulation. In Fig. 6B the threshold, *i.e.* the lowest temperature for an unambiguous response during each heating cycle, is plotted as a function of time, a heating series being repeated once every 3 min. Estimation of threshold in the presence of background discharge can be difficult and has to be judged on the basis of the appearance of pairs or a number of impulses in close association with the

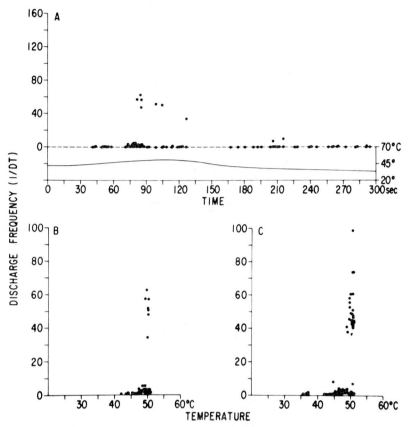

Fig. 5. Initiation of a background discharge of a cat polymodal nociceptor. A: plot of discharge as in Fig. 3 as a function of time. The time course of heating and cooling is indicated by the trace below the dashed line. Right vertical scale applied to the temperature record. B: a replot of the data from the first 150 sec of A — dots indicate the reciprocal of the interval between successive pairs of impulses on the ordinate as a function of the thermode temperature (abscissa). C: a plot of discharge frequency *versus* temperature as in B for the equivalent 150 sec period in a repeat (second) heating cycle as for A. (From Perl, 1972.)

rising phase of temperature changes; the five units of Fig. 6 were chosen for illustration since their threshold responses were clear-cut. These five receptors show a progressive decrease in threshold temperature; in some cases the threshold moved from the noxious level (over 45 °C) to a value within the physiological range (under 40 °C). As illustrated in Fig. 6 the degree of sensitization varied from receptor to receptor; it could be enhanced or diminished by the stimulus conditions. Heating of the skin to temperatures which severely damaged the skin (70 °C and above) often abolished evoked responses for varying periods, although background discharge might appear or remain. In some instances sensitization was manifest only by an increased response at a given temperature and not by a discernible change in threshold.

So far sensitization has been described relative to heat stimuli because this proved to be the most reliable manner of demonstrating it. Enhanced responsiveness was sometimes seen for some polymodal units following repeated, damaging mechanical

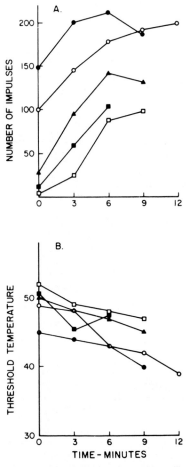

Fig. 6. Changes in response of primate polymodal nociceptors on successive tests. A: the total number of impulses generated by each of five receptors upon successive identical temperature cycles of the form shown in Fig. 4. A cycle repeated every 3 min. Each symbol shows the results for one receptor. Heating was with the thermode contacting approximately 3 sq.mm of skin. Vertical axis indicates a total number of impulses generated during the active heating phase. B: data from the five receptors of A plotting threshold temperature (see text). The first heating cycle plotted at zero time, the next at 3 min, the third at 6 min, etc. Symbols identifying a given receptor correspond to those used in A. (From Kumazawa and Perl, 1975.)

stimulation of the skin; it also was manifest by the appearance of background discharge and an apparent lowering of threshold. On the other hand, less destructive mechanical excitation of polymodal receptors showed that they too exhibit the adaptation and fatigue typical of other mechanically excitable sense organs. Sensitization by heat stimuli was associated with decreased thresholds for mechanical stimulaation in less than half of the polymodal elements so tested (Bessou and Perl, 1969).

Heightened responsiveness to heat stimuli has appeared within 30 sec after heat excitation. It may have even a shorter latency but we have not had the means of reliably assessing threshold and response more quickly. Once sensitization appears,

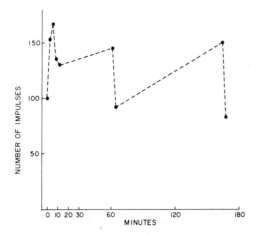

Fig. 7. Activity generated in a primate polymodal nociceptor by successive identical heat stimulations. Each dot indicates the total number of impulses during a heating cycle of the form illustrated in Fig. 4. The horizontal position of the dot marks the time after the first cycle (at zero time). After an initial sequence of five tests at 3-min intervals, delays between tests varied as indicated. (From Kumazawa and Perl, 1975.)

it can last for long periods. Increased responses relative to an initial test in repeated, identical heating series have been observed for over 3 hr. Some polymodal nociceptors, while showing augmented responses on repeated heating or repeated noxious mechanical stimulation, also exhibited evidence of a fatigue-like effect. An indication of the long duration of enhanced responsiveness and an apparent interaction between mechanisms leading to fatigue and those related to sensitization are illustrated in Fig. 7 for heating cycles of the form used in Fig. 4. The data for Fig. 7 was collected by using heating sequences repeated at various intervals with the results plotted as the total number of discharges during each cycle. The second test, 3 min after the first yielded an approximately 50% increase in the number of impulses, with a third test 3 min after the second resulting in a still larger response. Some diminution from the maximal response occurred after further tests (9 and 12 min). Prolonged rests (45 and 105 min) were associated with responses comparable to those seen on the second test, while a cycle 3 min after each of the latter resulted in less activity than observed in the initial test. The observations shown in Fig. 7 are consistent with many others which suggest that a large number of impulses from a polymodal nociceptor is followed by relative depression as seen with fatigue, sensitization notwithstanding.

   Our observations suggest that the process leading to sensitization is local, but can spread to nearby regions. Many experiments were done with stimulators of limited dimensions. A small thermode (about 3 sq.mm) can produce sensitization of a polymodal unit with a receptive field directly under it without causing the appearance of background discharge in other units isolated later in the experiment with receptive fields 1 cm or more away; the latter can be sensitized by stimuli directly applied to their receptive areas. Variability from one receptor to another has made it difficult to determine if effects were present which were subthreshold for the appearance of background discharge or submaximal for augmenting responses. On the other hand, massive damage or extensive stimulation appears to lead to diffusion of the sensitizing process. Repeated heat stimulation over a number of loci with punctate thermodes or a skin heating involving a larger area (50–200 sq.mm) was found to be associated with background discharge in polymodal units outside the area directly stimulated. When large areas of the skin were mobilized to permit control of the circulation or artificial perfusion, units with the characteristics of polymodal nociceptors some distance away from the cut skin edges showed both considerable background discharge and more vigorous responses at low skin temperatures than is typical for preparations with lesser surgery. In addition, polymodal units from skin subject to extensive stimulation or surgery may not show further enhancement of their already vigorous responses. Sensitization may be due to a process which is only capable of increasing responsiveness up to a certain level.

The latter observations suggested the possibility that the spread of effect from an injured portion of the skin might be due to a diffusible substance. A chemical intermediary as a link between tissue damage and pain has been suggested a number of times in the past and a variety of chemical agents have been proposed as the mediator over the years (reviewed by Keele and Armstrong, 1964 and by Lim, 1970). To explore this possibility, we have attempted to modify the environment of the skin containing receptive fields of identified receptors. Under conditions in which most of the circulation to the skin comes from an arterial perfusion using modified Kreb's or Locke's solution, polymodal nociceptors behave essentially as they do in undamaged skin normally supplied by blood; they have little background discharge while exhibiting a pronounced enhancement of response on successive heating. In contrast, as mentioned above, the trauma associated with total isolation and artificial fluid perfusion regularly causes a general sensitization of polymodal units. Consequently, we have turned to another preparation — the rabbit ear — in which the isolation procedures could be performed some distance from the receptive fields of cutaneous sense organs.

A preliminary survey of the cutaneous receptors with C afferent fibers of the rabbit ear yields the same general types previously determined for the cat (Bessou and Perl, 1969) and monkey (Kumazawa and Perl, 1975); polymodal nociceptors are very common, although significant numbers of C mechanoreceptors and thermo-receptors (warm and cool types) are also present. The rabbit polymodal nociceptors have essentially the same characteristics as those of the cat; these include elevated thresholds for mechanical and heat stimuli with almost no response to large cooling transients until sensitization was produced. Increased responsiveness and development of background discharge upon repeated heating to noxious temperature is readily demonstrable for polymodal units of the rabbit's ear, as is illustrated by Fig. 8 for pooled results from several units in ears with a normal blood circulation. Fig. 8A plots the average number of discharges for successive 5-sec periods (filled circles) in the standardized heating–cooling cycle shown on the lowermost graph. This method of analysis was used to account for variability in unit to unit behavior and provided a baseline for manipulation of conditions. Fig. 8B

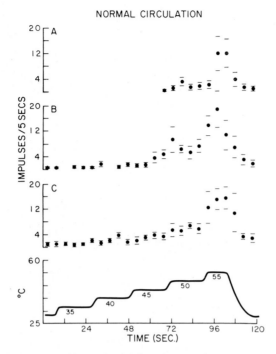

Fig. 8. Averaged responses to C fiber polymodal nociceptors from rabbit ear to repeated heating cycles in preparations with normal blood concentration. A standardized pattern of stepwise heating in 5 °C increments from 35 °C to 55 °C was used; impulses were summed at 5-sec intervals sequenced relative to the heating cycle. Heating cycles were repeated at 5-min intervals. Each filled circle plots the average of the results from different units; the short horizontal lines above and below the filled circles show the standard deviation for that mean. A: first heating, 5 units. B: second heating, 4 units. C: third heating, 3 units.

and C gives observations for the second and third heating cycles respectively. Similarly, the features described as sensitization were readily apparent in isolated rabbit ears perfused with an artificial solution containing $10^{-2}$ g/liter serotonin and $10^{-4}$ g/liter epinephrine, as shown in Fig. 9 for pooled data from 10 polymodal units in a format similar to that used for Fig. 8. Fig. 9A, B and C gives the mean number of impulses recorded during the first, second and third heating cycles respectively. No significant change in the responsiveness of the polymodal receptors has been evident due to the addition of either epinephrine or serotonin in concentrations sufficient to eliminate edema for the isolated and perfused preparations. The latter observation leads to the belief that serotonin is a poor candidate for the agent causing sensitization and background discharge.

The use of the perfused ear preparation has made several other points clear. First of all, it is apparent that the process leading to sensitization and the evocation of background discharge in polymodal receptors is not dependent upon some modification of complex organic substances borne to the stimulated region in the blood, since it can be shown to occur in ears totally perfused by an artificial solution not containing such material. Secondly, removal of either potassium or calcium from the perfusion fluid produces a consistent appearance of background discharge in poly-

*References p. 275–276*

274    E. R. PERL *et al.*

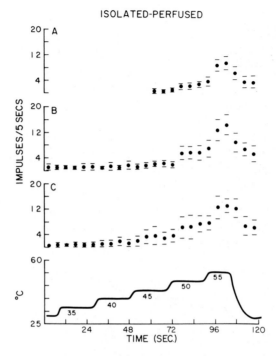

Fig. 9. Averaged responses of C fiber polymodal nociceptors from isolated rabbit's ears perfused
with modified Kreb's solution containing $10^{-2}$ g/liter serotonin and $10^{-4}$ g/liter epinephrine. Plots
made as in Fig. 8. A: first heating, 10 units. B: second heating, 10 units. C: third heating, 9 units.

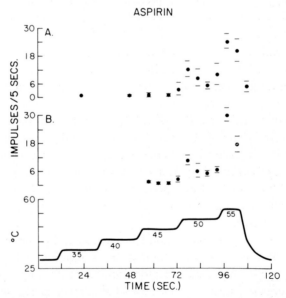

Fig. 10. Averaged responses of C fiber polymodal nociceptors from isolated rabbit's ears perfused
with modified Kreb's solution containing $10^{-2}$ g/liter serotonin and $10^{-4}$ g/liter epinephrine. Plots
made as in Fig. 8. A: first heating, 4 units. B: heating during perfusion (started 10–30 min earlier)
with acetylsalicylic acid $5 \times 10^{-1}$ g/liter added, 4 units.

modal receptors and an apparent enhancement of response to the first test as if the receptors were already sensitized. Thirdly, additional buffering of the perfusion fluid against a drop in pH has no discernible effect upon the development of the signs of sensitization. Fourthly, neither antihistaminic agents nor relatively high concentrations of agents acting on prostaglandin synthesis, such as acetylsalicyclic acid or indomethacin, produce dramatic effects upon background discharge or heightened responsiveness. Fig. 10A shows the average response of 4 units from isolated rabbit ear to heating of their receptive fields and Fig. 10B those recorded with $5 \times 10^{-1}$ g/liter acetylsalicyclic acid added to the perfusion fluid. Perfusion for 20 min with this solution produces no detectable changes. The one positive clue to date from the perfused skin studies is that a substance behaving like a protein fragment or a polypeptide seems to be present in the effluent perfusate after a heat stimulus of the type used, but its link to the altered polymodal behavior is still to be proven.

## SUMMARY

Polymodal nociceptors are a dominant cutaneous C-fiber sense organ of mammals. They are characterized by relatively high thresholds for mechanical and thermal stimuli and respond vigorously only to noxious levels of heat, mechanical and chemical stimuli. Noxious stimulation of the receptive field of polymodal nociceptors, particularly by heat, results in an enhanced responsiveness, lowered threshold and the development of background activity; these changes have been labeled sensitization. Sensitization develops in less than one minute and can last for hours. The process of sensitization, while exhibiting localization, is capable of spreading. Demonstrable evidence of spread of sensitization appears related to the degree of skin damage. Sensitization develops in skin preparations perfused with artificial solutions not containing proteins or protein fragments. Serotonin, antihistaminic and antiprostaglandin agents do not cause major modifications in the development of sensitization.

## ACKNOWLEDGEMENTS

This work was supported by USPHS Grant NS 10321. Support of the computer and service facilities were provided by USPHS Grant NS 11132, USPHS RR05406 and a grant from the Alfred P. Sloan Foundation.

## REFERENCES

ADRIAN, E. D. AND ZOTTERMAN, Y. (1926a) The impulses produced by sensory nerve-endings. Part 2. The response of a single end-organ. *J. Physiol. (Lond.)*, **61**, 151–171.
ADRIAN, E. D. AND ZOTTERMAN, Y. (1926b) The impulses produced by sensory nerve endings. Part 3. Impulses set up by touch and pressure. *J. Physiol. (Lond.)*, **61**, 465–583.
BESSOU, P., BESSOU, P. R., PERL, E. R. AND TAYLOR, C. B. (1971) Dynamic properties of mechanoreceptors with unmyelinated (C) fibers. *J. Neurophysiol.*, **34**, 116–131.

BESSOU, P. AND PERL, E. R. (1969) Response of cutaneous sensory units with unmyelinated fibers to noxious stimuli. *J. Neurophysiol.*, **32**, 1025–1043.

BURGESS, P. R. AND PERL, E. R. (1973) Cutaneous mechanoreceptors and nociceptors. In A. IGGO (Ed.), *Handbook of Sensory Physiology, Vol. II.* Springer, Berlin. pp. 29–78.

KEELE, C. A. AND ARMSTRONG, D. (1964) *Substances Producing Pain and Itch.* Edward Arnold, London.

KUMAZAWA, T. AND PERL, E. R. (1975) Primary cutaneous sensory units with unmyelinated (C) fibers. Submitted for publication.

LIM, R. K. (1974) Pain. *Ann. Rev. Physiol.*, **32**, 269–288.

PERL, E. R. (1972) Mode of action of nociceptors. In S. HIRSH AND Y. ZOTTERMAN (Eds.), *Cervical Pain.* Pergamon Press, Oxford. pp. 157–164.

## DISCUSSION

WIDDICOMBE: Can I use my privileged position to make a comment. The receptors one finds in the epithelium of the respiratory tract, which we called irritant receptors have several features in common with those that you described in the skin. They seem to be polymodal and they seem to be nociceptive. They can be sensitized by repeated noxious stimulation and the threshold is changed so that they produce a continuous discharge. So, perhaps what you described probably has a more general application to receptors than just to the skin.

PERL: My intention was to describe a phenomenon which probably has a wide distribution because I know that at least muscle C-fiber nociceptor sensitizes. But it is interesting that this is not a characteristic of all receptors, nor is it characteristic of all nociceptors. There are some nociceptors that do not produce any obvious sensitization. It may be that under different conditions or under special conditions all nociceptors can be sensitized. We know some nociceptors do not respond promptly to heat, at least in non-injured skin, and are much more difficult to sensitize. Perhaps only some of them can be sensitized.

KENSHALO: I enjoyed listening to your very elegant work. What might be called the steady-state response following the maintenance of 50–55 °C heating? I know that at this period the response becomes quite small, perhaps, one or two impulses/sec. Now, if one is allowed to assume that this is an analog of the human pain sensation, some other works from Hardy's laboratory and others, seem to indicate that in forearms at 50–55 °C the pain sensation builds up rather than diminishes with the maintenance of the temperature. Are there other kinds of nociceptors that you work with that might account for this or might support the persisting pain sensation.

PERL: In an attempt to demonstrate the sensitization phenomenon we deliberately held the duration of stimuli to about 10–15 sec at the highest temperature. If you hold the thermode temperature at 50 °C for 30 sec cycling of activity occurs with discharge nearly stopping followed by periods when bursts approach those seen in some phasic responses. Certainly if the thermode is in contact with the skin and held at this temperature for a long period of time one finds an effect which is a bit more consistent with what you might expect from human experience. I also have to point out that those temperatures in our figure are thermode temperatures and probably do not really represent skin temperatures. We know that the skin surface temperature is lower. And the temperature below the skin is still lower. We can only state the thermode temperature for that particular experiment.

HENSEL: May I ask two questions. You have shown the receptor at the beginning of your presentation that responded to cooling as well as to mechanical stimulation. May I ask: did you exclude the possibility that your mechanical stimulus was in fact a cold stimulus, because we found that some cold receptors are extremely sensitive even when touching with a hair. This stimulus can be a cold stimulus, not a mechanical one. If you warm up the hair a little bit, this inhibits the discharge. The second question: I found some difficulties with a definition of a nociceptor from mechanical stimulation from a difference of the response between a blunt and a sharp stimulus. A sharp point also is a very much stronger mechanical stimulus in terms of deformations or in terms of force or surface area.

PERL: The cooling question I think we can dispose of easily. You can very easily adapt the cooling response of C-mechanoreceptors and still obtain the mechanical response. The C-mechano-receptors are responsive to a uniquely limited range of moving stimuli, they are velocity detectors in Dr. Burgess' classification so that their cooling responses in fact are never as vigorous as the mechanical responses and if we go through the question of using the neutral temperatures with those receptors, it is clear that they are quite different from thermal receptors and from nociceptors. On the question of a nociceptor: originally when Dr. Burgess and I tried to define a nociceptor we used Sherrington's definition of "noxious" to mean "tissue damaging". In a case of these nociceptors, we labeled them that because they grade responses with stimuli which range from very strong to those that are producing clear-cut damage of the skin. We label only such elements nociceptors. In a case of the response you saw that needle was penetrating the skin and was obviously producing damage. Yet, the response was no greater for the C-mechanoreceptors for such obviously increased mechanical stimuli in terms of shearing force as one gets with the less strong distorting stimulus.

KHAJUTIN: You showed the response of a nociceptor with the force of 0.8 g. What is the surface of you mechanical stimulator?

PERL: About 1/4 mm in diameter.

KHAJUTIN: What is the diameter of thermode compared with the area occupied by the receptor?

PERL: The thermode was in fact designed for those receptors. It covers approximately 3 sq.mm, which covers most of the receptor area of these receptors. Receptors can actually be excited using a very small mechanical stimuli, best from the area of about a 100 $\mu$m across. But you can also excite them if you give some lesser response from an area of about 2 or 1.5 mm across. We designed the thermode to fit the larger areas.

KHAJUTIN: How many C-fibers could you put in this area?

PERL: Obviously we are not studying C-fibers, we are studying C-fiber receptors. What is known about the branching of sense organs in the skin suggests that certain unmyelinated fibers may have a spray of endings which occupy 100–150 $\mu$m and this would be perhaps a first estimation of the area of a nociceptor. We have seen two of these as close together as 2 mm.

# The Effect of Focused Ultrasound on the Skin and Deep Nerve Structures of Man and Animal

L. R. GAVRILOV***, G. V. GERSUNI*, O. B. ILYINSKY**,
M. G. SIROTYUK***, E. M. TSIRULNIKOV* AND E. E. SHCHEKANOV*

*Sechenov Institute of Evolutionary Physiology and Biochemistry, **I. P. Pavlov Institute of Physiology
Academy of Sciences of the U.S.S.R., Leningrad (U.S.S.R.) and ***Acoustical Institute, Academy of
Sciences of the U.S.S.R., Moscow (U.S.S.R.)

## INTRODUCTION

Among various factors that affect the receptors, the mechanical forces are of special importance. Modern techniques allow one to operate with mechanical oscillations of a significantly higher frequency and intensity than natural conditions can produce. High frequency ultrasonic oscillations (MHz) allow a considerable mechanical energy to be concentrated in various organs and tissues on the body surface as well as in the deep structures. The present study deals with the influence of focused ultrasound on the receptor and nerve structures of the organism.

Up to now focused ultrasound has mainly been used for lesion production in the brain of men and animals (for review see Gavrilov, 1971). However, it seemed valuable to use the ultrasound for stimulation of nerve structures. It has previously been shown that stimulation of the human arm with short focused ultrasound stimuli results in tactile, temperature and pain sensations, *i.e.* ones characteristic for a natural stimulation (Gavrilov *et al.*, 1972, 1973a and b). In the present work we studied the nature of, and conditions for, appearance of these sensations, special attention being paid to the factors which determine sensations of different modality. The effect of focused ultrasound on some receptor structures of animals was also studied.

## METHODS

Experiments were performed on the human arm immersed in distilled water together with the transducer. The water temperature was 30, 35 and 40 °C. To provide fixation, the arm was placed in a special casting made of silumin, its shape repeating the shape of the arm. The position of the focusing transducer with respect to the arm was controlled by a coordinate device. The transducer focal length (70 mm) allowed the focal region to enter arm tissues until it left them on the opposite side.

Transducers from concave piezoceramic plates of barium titanate were used to obtain ultrasound stimuli (Fig. 1a). The transducer focal region with the highest intensity of ultrasound is represented as an ellipsoid of rotation with intensity de-

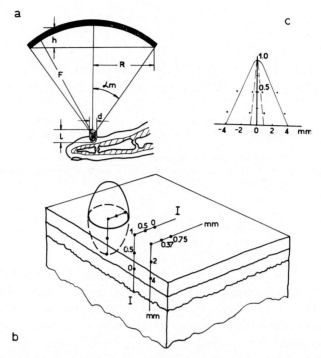

Fig. 1. a: geometrical characteristics of spherical transducer. Focal region center within finger skin. R, transducer radius; F, focal length; $\alpha_m$, convergence angle; h, depth; l and d, length and diameter of focal region, respectively. b: the position of the focal region when stimulating the skin spots. The axes: I, the ultrasound intensity in relative units; mm, the distance from the focal region center. Frequency, 1.95 MHz. c: intensity distribution in the focal region. Abscissa: distance from the focal region center in mm. Ordinate: ultrasound intensity in relative units. Dashed line is the calculated intensity in the focal plane and solid line, that in the axial plane. Dots show experimental recordings. Frequency, 1.95 MHz.

TABLE I

THE FOCAL REGION SIZES OF THE ULTRASOUND TRANSDUCERS

| $f(MHz)$ | $d(mm)$ | $l(mm)$ | $S(sq.mm)$ | $V(cu.mm)$ |
|---|---|---|---|---|
| 0.48 | 6.4 | 34 | 32 | 725 |
| 0.887 | 3.4 | 18 | 9.1 | 110 |
| 1.95 | 1.5 | 8 | 1.8 | 9.6 |
| 2.67 | 1.1 | 6 | 1.0 | 4.0 |

creasing from the center to the periphery (Fig. 1b and c). Table I shows the calculated focal regions of the transducers for frequencies used, where f is the ultrasound frequency and d, l, s and v are the diameter, length, square and volume, respectively, of the focal region within the limits of the main diffraction maximum. Although this maximum, determined by points where the ultrasound intensity diminishes to zero, is relatively large (Table I), the region where the intensity approximates its peak value

| Spot number on the drawing | The number of test in the spot | The ultrasound threshold intensity, W/cm$^2$ | | | | | | | |
|---|---|---|---|---|---|---|---|---|---|
| | | for sensation in the skin | | | | for sensation deep under the skin | | | |
| | | touch | warmth | cold | pain | touch | warmth | cold | pain |
| *Finger* | | | | | | | | | |
| I | I | 20 | – | – | 200 | | | | |
| 2 | I | 44 | – | – | 180 | | | | |
| | 2 | 18 | – | – | 180 | | | | |
| 3 | I | 15 | – | – | 140 | | | | |
| *Palm* | | | | | | | | | |
| 4 | I | 75 | 385 | 980 | – | | | | |
| 5 | I | 80 | – | 880 | 900 | | | | |
| | 2 | 80 | – | – | 680 | | | | |
| 6 | I | 80 | – | 980 | 1180 | | | | |
| 7 | I | 27 | 680 | – | – | | | | |
| 8 | I | 60 | 980 | – | 1380 | | | | |
| | 2 | 55 | – | 980 | – | | | | |
| 9 | I | 44 | – | – | 880 | | | | |
| | 2 | 27 | 980 | – | – | | | | |
| | 3 | | | | | – | – | – | 520 |
| | 4 | | | | | – | – | – | 650 |
| | 5 | | | | | – | – | – | 520 |
| I0 | I | + | – | – | – | | | | |
| | 2 | | | | | – | – | – | – |
| | 3 | | | | | – | – | – | – |
| | 4 | | | | | – | – | – | – |
| II | I | + | – | – | – | | | | |
| | 2 | | | | | – | – | – | – |
| *Forearm* | | | | | | | | | |
| I2 | I | 85 | – | 1100 | – | | | | |

Fig. 2. A schematic drawing of the arm of subject N3, with spots studied at a frequency of 0.887 MHz. The Table gives the ultrasound intensities corresponding to threshold sensations in the spots studied. A dash denotes that the sensation of a given modality was absent.

is considerably less: for the frequency of 2.67 MHz it is equal to portions of mm.

In the present study ultrasound stimuli of various intensities were used with frequencies of 0.48, 0.887, 1.95 and 2.67 MHz and durations of 1, 10 and 100 msec. Experiments were carried out on seven subjects, more than 300 spots on the skin of fingers, palm and forearm being investigated. Altogether about 600 experiments were performed, including repeated tests in one and the same skin spot and experiments involving immersion of the focal region into the deep layers of the arm tissue. When the stimulus was applied to the spot, the nature of sensation evoked was described and thresholds were determined with an ascending series of stimulus intensity. Experiments were immediately stopped after the first pain sensation appeared. The spots studied were marked on the skin and then transferred to special "charts", which

*References p. 291*

represented the life-size arm photographs. The scheme of one of these charts (reduced scale) is shown in Fig. 2.

Voltages on the focusing transducer having been measured in the experiment, the associated ultrasound intensities in the focal region were taken from a calibration curve. The ultrasound intensities thus obtained were then used for calculation of the other parameters to characterize the propagation of ultrasound within the medium by the conventional acoustic formula (Bergmann, 1954):

$$I = \frac{1}{2} \rho C (2\pi f A)^2 = \frac{1}{2} \rho C V^2 = \frac{P^2}{2\rho C}.$$

where I is the intensity, f is the ultrasound frequency, A is the displacement amplitude, V is the particle velocity amplitude, P is the sound pressure amplitude, $\rho$ is the medium density and C is the sound velocity within the medium.

In some series of experiments the appearance of cavitation in tissues was assessed by measuring of 1/2 subharmonics (Gavrilov *et al.*, 1973b). Also, the value of tissue temperature increase ($\Delta T$) due to absorption of ultrasound energy was calculated by the following formula (Pond, 1970):

$$\Delta T = \frac{\mu I_0}{J \rho C_P} \cdot e^{-\mu d} \cdot t \cdot A(t)$$

where $\mu$ is the intensity absorption coefficient in tissues, linearly depending on ultrasound frequency, $I_0$ is the ultrasound intensity in the focal region (without allowance for absorption in the medium), d is the depth of irradiated area under the skin surface, t is the ultrasound stimulus duration, J is the mechanical equivalent of heat, $\rho$ and $C_p$ are the tissue density and specific heat respectively and A(t) is a coefficient, taking into account the effect of thermal conductivity.

### RESULTS

When the focal region was within the skin layer or at a depth below the skin, the subject experienced various sensations depending on the focal region location, the ultrasound stimulus intensity and duration, and water temperature (Gavrilov *et al.*, 1972, 1973a and b). With the focal region in the skin, ultrasound was found to be capable of producing sensations of different modality. With gradually increasing intensity the first sensations to appear were ones resembling a slight local touch, stroke, shake, rupture of a falling water drop and push. Such sensations were classed as tactile. With higher intensity in some spots following the tactile sensation there appeared a sensation of warmth or cold, resembling a touch with a small heated or cooled object; sometimes it was compared with the spreading of a drop of either heated or cooled liquid along the skin surface. With still higher intensities the sensation appeared as pain. It proved possible to obtain all these sensation modalities in one and the same spot on the skin by increasing the stimulus intensity (Fig. 2), whereas in some other spots there appeared under the same conditions sensations of

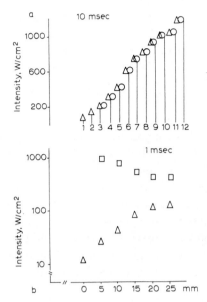

Fig. 3. a: an illustration of an experiment with the center of the focal region within the skin. Triangles: the tactile sensations; circles: the cold sensations. Figures from left to right denote the ordinal number of stimulus (stimuli presented while determining the tactile threshold by the method of limits not shown). The subject was N3 and the spot N4 from Fig. 2. Frequency, 0.887 MHz. b: changes in thresholds for tactile (triangles) and pain (squares) sensations when immersing the center of the focal region under the skin. Abscissa: the immersion depth. Subject N2; frequency 0.887 MHz. Note that tactile sensations were projected by the subject into the skin whereas the pain sensations were projected into the soft tissues.

only one or two modalities, *e.g.* tactile and temperature (Fig. 3a), or temperature alone, *etc.* With the focal region deep under the skin only pain sensations occurred (Fig. 2).

### Tactile sensations

Of all the sensations the tactile ones were associated with stimuli of the lowest intensity. Increasing stimulus duration from 1 to 100 msec failed to change reliably the associated thresholds. Increasing water temperature from 30 °C to 40 °C resulted in a decrease of the thresholds. Also, tactile thresholds increased on transferring the focal region from fingers to forearm. They also increased with immersion of the focal region center into the soft tissues (Fig. 3b); with the focal region entirely in the soft subcutaneous tissues, the tactile sensations vanished. It should be noted that if the focal region was projected through tissues, for instance between the thumb and the forefinger into the other side of the arm, tactile sensations reappeared, but with a higher threshold. Such increased thresholds were apparently due to the tissue attenuation of ultrasound.

With a stimulus duration of 100 msec and more, the tactile sensations appeared in response to the beginning and the end of the stimulus. For instance, the stimulus of

400 msec duration evoked the same sensations as two stimuli each of 10 msec duration, spaced at 380 msec (Gavrilov *et al.*, 1972). Thus, there is every reason to suppose that these tactile sensations are mediated by rapidly adapting structures.

### Temperature sensations

In some spots with increasing ultrasound intensity the tactile sensation was followed by temperature sensation (the subject felt warmth or cold). The sensation was most pronounced at the place of stimulation but could also spread. Similarly to the tactile sensation, the temperature one vanished when the focal region was under the skin. Warmth sensation reappeared on the skin of the opposite side of the arm after the focal region had been projected through the tissues. We failed to obtain cold sensation when projecting the focal region through the tissues into the opposite side of the arm.

Thresholds were found to increase with shifting the focal region from fingers to forearm; they decreased with increasing stimulus duration. The lowest thresholds were with a water temperature of 35 °C; they increased when water temperature was either 30 °C or 40 °C.

Focused ultrasound stimuli could evoke sensations both of warmth and cold depending on the temperature of water. Stimulation was applied to so-called "warmth" and "cold" spots on the skin surface which were determined by means of thermodes with a tip diameter of 1 mm. With water temperature of 30 °C the stimuli evoked mostly cold sensations; with 35 °C — both cold and warmth sensations; and with 40 °C — mostly warmth sensations (Fig. 6b).

### Pain sensations

With further increasing of the intensity of stimuli there appeared the pain sensation, which occurred more often with stimuli of 10–100 msec duration than with shorter stimuli (1 msec). Unlike the sensations of the other modalities, the pain appeared with the focal region not only in the skin but also in muscles, bones and joints. According to the localization of the focal region center there were observed four types of the pain sensations (Gavrilov *et al.*, 1973b).

(1) Focal region center within the skin. Sensation of a sharp localized burning pain, similar to a sharp pain from pricking a hand with a needle.

(2) Focal region center in soft tissues beneath the skin. Sensation of pain at a depth under skin, not so sharp and localized as in case 1 but more unpleasant.

(3) Focal region center projected into the bone. The pain is even less localized than in case 2, and still more unpleasant. Sensation of this kind seems to be associated with the periosteum. The pain quickly spread far along the bone and then came back to the place of stimulation.

(4) Focal region center in a joint. Sensation is similar to the pain in the periosteum but still more unpleasant. It also spread quickly, though within the joint only and then also came back to the place of stimulation.

The ultrasound threshold intensity was the highest in case 1 and the lowest in case 4.

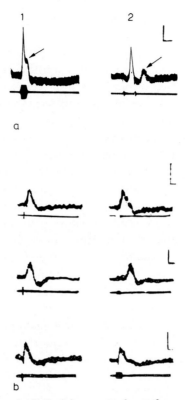

Fig. 4. a: the responses of two single Pacinian corpuscles to focused ultrasound stimulation at a frequency of 0.48 MHz. 1: a response to a single stimulus with intensity of 10 W/sq.cm and duration of 1 msec; 2: responses to spaced stimuli with intensity 6 W/sq.cm and duration 0.1 msec. The arrows indicate the receptor potentials. Calibration: 50 μV; 2.5 msec. b: evoked potentials in the auditory area of the frog's midbrain. The left column shows stimulation of the labyrinth with focused ultrasound (frequency 0.48 MHz, stimulus duration 1 msec). The right column shows responses to sound stimuli of optimal frequency (20 msec duration). The lines each represent the data of one experiment. Stimulus intensity was 20 dB above the threshold. The top tracing is the evoked potentials and the bottom tracing the stimulus. Calibration: 100 μV; 25 msec.

It increased with shifting the focal region from fingers to forearm, both on the skin and in the deep tissues.

### Other sensations

Focused ultrasound could evoke tickling and itching sensations as well. Thresholds for the tickling sensation were approximately the same as for the warmth sensation, though always a little lower. Itching thresholds were of the same magnitude as the pain thresholds, being invariably lower also. Sometimes the sensations of warmth or cold were replaced by the tickling sensation, and the pain sensation in the skin was often followed by the itching sensation.

*References p. 291*

*Effect of ultrasound on receptor structures of animals*

The tactile thresholds in man are thought to be mediated by highly sensitive rapidly adapting skin receptors, for instance, Pacinian corpuscles (Lindblom and Lund, 1966). Tactile sensations as observed in our work also seem to be due to the activity of rapidly adapting structures. It was therefore of interest to study the effect of ultrasound on single Pacinian corpuscles. In our experiments we applied the focused ultrasound stimulation to Pacinian corpuscles dissected from the cat's mesentery. Receptor and spike potentials were registered (Fig. 4a). With the ultrasound frequency of 0.48 MHz the threshold was 0.6–1.6 W/sq.cm, which corresponded to 0.03–0.05 $\mu$m for the particle displacement amplitude. With the same frequency the tactile threshold in man was 8–10 W/sq.cm (0.1–0.12 $\mu$m).

In the present study we also studied the action of focused ultrasound on the inner ear, the stimulation being applied to the labyrinth of a frog. Evoked potentials with characteristics similar to the responses to short sound stimuli were registered in the auditory region of the midbrain (Fig. 4b). Excitation of labyrinth receptors by ultrasound stimuli with a frequency of 0.48 MHz occurred with small intensities of 0.01–0.1 W/sq.cm (0.004–0.01 $\mu$m).

Thus, the stimulation with focused ultrasound could result in excitation not only of surface, but also of deep-lying mechanoreceptor structures whose activation is thought of as being responsible for the appearance of certain sensations.

DISCUSSION

The biological effect of focused ultrasound may be due to various factors: medium displacement in the focal region, cavitation and radiation pressure; it may also be due to such physicochemical phenomena as increased diffusion across biological membranes, heating of the tissues while absorbing ultrasound etc. To determine the relative contribution of ultrasound stimulus parameters, their threshold values have been compared at different frequencies. From ultrasound intensities so determined we calculated the medium displacement amplitude in the focal region (A, $\mu$m),

TABLE II

THE NUMBER OF THE SPOTS INVESTIGATED AND THE NUMBER OF TESTS (INCLUDING THE REPEATED TESTS FOR THE SAME SPOT) WITH TWO SUBJECTS: ULTRASOUND STIMULATION OF VARIOUS FREQUENCIES

|  |  | Number of spots/Number of tests | | | |
|---|---|---|---|---|---|
| $f(MHz)$ | | 0.48 | 0.887 | 1.95 | 2.67 |
| Subject N2 | Fingers | 5/8 | 4/6 | 21/23 | 4/9 |
| | Palm | 11/16 | 14/31 | 30/42 | 16/36 |
| Subject N3 | Fingers | 5/7 | 3/4 | 14/14 | 5/6 |
| | Palm | 7/15 | 8/18 | 14/15 | 9/21 |

## TABLE III

PARAMETERS OF ULTRASOUND STIMULI OF 1 msec DURATION ASSOCIATED WITH APPEARANCE OF THRESHOLD SENSATION (WATER TEMPERATURE: 35°C)

| Parameters | $I(W/sq.cm)$ | | | | $A(\mu m)$ | | | | $P(atmos)$ | | | | $V(m/sec)$ | | | | $\Delta T(°C)$ | | | |
|---|---|---|---|---|---|---|---|---|---|---|---|---|---|---|---|---|---|---|---|---|
| $f(MHz)$ | 0.48 | 0.887 | 1.95 | 2.67 | 0.48 | 0.887 | 1.95 | 2.67 | 0.48 | 0.887 | 1.95 | 2.67 | 0.48 | 0.887 | 1.95 | 2.67 | 0.48 | 0.887 | 1.95 | 2.67 |
| **Sensations** | | | | | | | | | | | | | | | | | | | | |
| **Tactile** | | | | | | | | | | | | | | | | | | | | |
| finger | 8 | 15 | 80 | 120 | 0.1 | 0.08 | 0.08 | 0.08 | 4.9 | 6.7 | 15.5 | 19 | 0.3 | 0.45 | 1 | 1.35 | $2 \times 10^{-4}$ | $0.6 \times 10^{-3}$ | $7.5 \times 10^{-3}$ | 0.015 |
| palm | 16 | 80 | 250 | 350 | 0.15 | 0.18 | 0.15 | 0.13 | 6.9 | 15.5 | 27 | 32 | 0.45 | 1 | 1.85 | 2.2 | $4 \times 10^{-4}$ | $3.5 \times 10^{-3}$ | $2.4 \times 10^{-2}$ | 0.045 |
| **Warmth** | | | | | | | | | | | | | | | | | | | | |
| finger | 55 | 90 | 1420 | 3200 | 0.28 | 0.2 | 0.35 | 0.4 | 13 | 16.5 | 65 | 98 | 0.85 | 1.1 | 4.3 | 6.7 | $1.3 \times 10^{-3}$ | $4 \times 10^{-3}$ | 0.14 | 0.41 |
| palm | 130 | 820 | 2940 | 4500 | 0.43 | 0.6 | 0.5 | 0.47 | 20 | 50 | 93 | 116 | 1.3 | 3.3 | 6.1 | 8 | $3.1 \times 10^{-3}$ | $3.5 \times 10^{-2}$ | 0.28 | 0.59 |
| **Cold** | | | | | | | | | | | | | | | | | | | | |
| finger | — | — | — | — | — | — | — | — | — | — | — | — | — | — | — | — | — | — | — | — |
| palm | 130 | 820 | 2000 | 3000 | 0.43 | 0.6 | 0.42 | 0.38 | 20 | 50 | 78 | 95 | 1.3 | 3.3 | 5.1 | 6.4 | $3.1 \times 10^{-3}$ | $3.5 \times 10^{-2}$ | 0.19 | 0.39 |
| **Pain** | | | | | | | | | | | | | | | | | | | | |
| finger | 55 | 140 | 2860 | — | 0.28 | 0.24 | 0.5 | — | 13 | 21 | 93 | — | 0.85 | 1.35 | 6.1 | — | $1.3 \times 10^{-3}$ | $6 \times 10^{-3}$ | 0.27 | — |
| palm | 290 | 350 | — | 3000 | 0.64 | 0.39 | — | 0.38 | 29 | 32 | — | 95 | 1.9 | 2.2 | — | 6.4 | $7 \times 10^{-3}$ | $1.5 \times 10^{-2}$ | — | 0.39 |

*References p. 291*

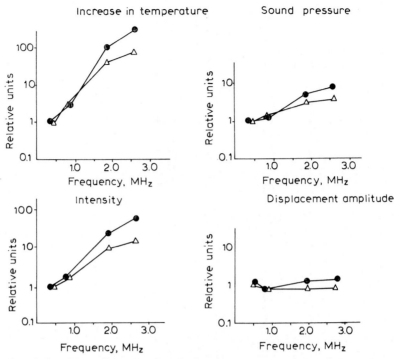

Fig. 5. The relative changes in parameters of ultrasound with frequency of a stimulus of 1 msec duration to produce threshold sensations from the fingers: tactile (triangles) and warmth (filled circles). Abscissa: ultrasound frequency; ordinate: relative changes in parameters (the parameter value at a frequency of 0.48 MHz is taken as unity).

acoustic pressure amplitude (P, atmos), particle velocity amplitude (V, m/sec) and increase in temperature in the focal region ($\Delta T \degree C$).

Given in Table III are the values of the above parameters for the ultrasound stimuli of 1 msec duration; they were calculated from the lowest intensities observed in two subjects (the total number of experiments in this set is given in Table II). It is reasonable to assume that the lowest thresholds involve some conditions which are more optimal for stimulus action upon the receptor structures, *e.g.* due to a more precise coincidence of the focal region center with a sensitive structure. Because of this the comparison of the lowest thresholds is more informative than the conventional procedure of calculating the mean and confidence intervals. It turned out that on stimulation with focused ultrasound of different frequencies the more or less identical medium displacement amplitudes in the focal region corresponded to the same threshold sensations (Table III). Other parameters characterizing the ultrasound propagation in the medium varied more significantly, in some cases by several orders (Fig. 5). Thus it can be supposed that the main active factor of ultrasound is a mechanical displacement of the medium in the focal region. At present there are no certain facts to say unambiguously whether the medium displacements are alternately occurring with ultrasound frequency or result from the transformation of alternating displacement. The fact that the long-lasting ultrasound stimuli resulted in the tactile

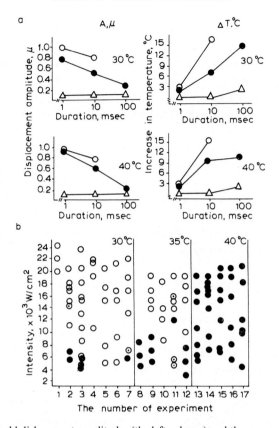

Fig. 6. a: the threshold dislacement amplitudes (the left column) and the corresponding temperature increase in the focal region (the right column) *versus* stimulus duration. Triangles, tactile sensations; empty and filled circles, cold and warmth sensations, respectively. The numerals to the right of the plots are bath water temperatures. Subject N1; ultrasound frequency 2.67 MHz. b: the relation between the modality of the temperature sensation (cold–warmth) and medium temperature. Empty and filled circles: cold and warmth sensations, respectively (the other sensations not shown). Abscissa: the ordinal number of experiment. Top numerals are bath water temperatures. Subject N2, ultrasound frequency 2.67 MHz.

sensation only when they were switched on and off suggests the existence of rectification effects due to which the effective stimulus is the envelope rather than frequency. It is still obscure when and how this rectification occurs.

With some stimulus parameters (for instance, with a frequency of 2.67 MHz and duration of 100 msec) threshold sensations are accompanied by a significant increase (up to 10–15 °C) in tissue temperature in the focal region, and this can doubtlessly produce temperature sensations. Hence, the increase in temperature in the focal region should be considered under definite conditions as one of the effective factors of the ultrasound stimulus. Further positive evidence is the fact that with a frequency of 2.67 MHz and a stimulus duration of 100 msec there was practically no cold sensation (Fig. 6a), whereas a stimulus of 10 msec duration produced a clear sensation of cold in spite of a 15 °C increase in temperature. So the tissue heating was of significance only with stimulus durations of about 100 msec and longer. The mechanical

*References p. 291*

factor (displacement) and temperature factor (tissue heating) appear to work jointly here.

We failed to find any connection between cavitation and threshold pain sensation. As to threshold sensations of the other modalities, the working intensities here were too low for cavitation to appear.

As was noted above, the tactile threshold is little affected by stimulus duration; with longer stimuli the sensation of touch appears only as a response to onset and offset of a stimulus. Again, the tactile thresholds are close to thresholds for excitation of single Pacinian corpuscles. These facts suggest that the threshold tactile sensations associated with stimulation of focused ultrasound may be mediated by Pacinian corpuscles or certain structures with much the same properties. We have no clear idea yet concerning the structures whose stimulation results in the thermal and pain sensation. It is felt that the effect of ultrasound on the receptor units, as well as directly on their afferent nerve fibers, may be involved. This question, though, requires further study.

The fact that sensations of different modalities appear in separately located discrete spots on the skin, when stimulus strength is of a definite magnitude, suggests that the sensory nerve structures could well be specific. Again, as was shown above, stimulation of the same spots could result either in cold or in warmth sensations, depending on the medium temperature (Fig. 6b). It is of interest to note that in the old phenomenological theories of thermoreception (Weber, 1846; Hering, 1877), where temperature sensations were thought to be connected with the same structures, such a factor as the medium temperature was paid great attention. It seems that in the case of temperature reception the question concerning the interrelation of "biophysical" and "sensory" specificity (Hensel, 1973) is to be considered with due regard for this factor.

The data obtained in our work allow one to use focused ultrasound in order to further investigate various nerve structures including sensory structures.

SUMMARY

It has been demonstrated that a variety of nerve structures can be excited with focused ultrasound (US). Stimulation of the human arm with short stimuli results in various sensations similar to natural stimulation; with the center of the focal region within the skin the stimuli of increasing intensity produced sensations of touch, tickling, warmth, cold, itching and pain. When the center of the focal region is projected into the deep structures of the arm, only the pain sensations appear, their character depending upon the type of the tissue (soft tissues, bone, joints). Stimulation of the same spots could result either in cold or in warmth sensations. Electrophysiological experiments demonstrated that single mechanoreceptors — Pacinian corpuscles — and receptor structures of the frog's labyrinth can be excited by the focused US. It is supposed that tactile sensations are due to excitation of the skin mechanoreceptors, whereas the temperature and pain sensations may involve the direct excitation of the nerve fibers. The comparative investigation of parameters to characterize the US propagation in the medium resulted in the conclusion that the main active factor in US stimulation is of a mechanical nature, *i.e.* medium displacement in the focal region. With certain parameters of the stimulus the local heating of the tissue at the place of stimulation is also involved.

## REFERENCES

BERGMANN, L. (1954) *Der Ultraschall und seine Anwendung in Wissenschaft und Technik*. Hirzel, Zurich.
GAVRILOV, L. R. (1971) Local effect on tissues by high intensity focused ultrasound. *Acoust. J.*, **17**, 337–355 (in Russian).
GAVRILOV, L. R., GERSUNI, G. V., ILYINSKY, O. B., SIROTYUK, M. G., TSIRULNIKOV, E. M. AND TSUKERMAN, V. A. (1972) The study of skin sensitivity with the aid of focused ultrasound. *Sechenov physiol. J. U.S.S.R.*, **58**, 1366–1371 (in Russian).
GAVRILOV, L. R., GERSUNI, G. V., ILYINSKY, O. B., POPOVA, L. A., SIROTYUK, M. G. AND TSIRULNIKOV, E. M. (1973a) Stimulation of peripheral nerve structures in men by focused ultrasound. *Acoust. J.*, **19**, 519–523 (in Russian).
GAVRILOV, L. R., ILYINSKY, O. B., POPOVA, L. A., SIROTYUK, M. G., TSIRULNIKOV, E. M. AND SHCHEKANOV, E. E. (1973b) Pain sensations in men in response to focused ultrasound. In A. V. VALDMAN (Ed.), *Neural Mechanisms of Pain*. Leningrad. pp. 23–25. (In Russian.)
HENSEL, H. (1973) Cutaneous thermoreceptors. In A. IGGO (Ed.), *Handbook of Sensory Physiology, Vol. 2. Somatosensory System*. Springer, Berlin. pp. 79–110.
HERING, E. (1877) *Grundzüge einer Theorie des Temperatursinns, Sitzber*. Wien. Akad., **75**, 101–135.
LINDBLOM, U. AND LUND, J. (1966) The discharge from vibration-sensitive receptors in the monkey foot. *Exp. Neurol.*, **15**, 401–417.
POND, J. B. (1970) The role of heat in the production of ultrasonic focal lesions. *J. acoust. Soc. Amer.*, **47**, 1607–1611.
WEBER, E. H. (1846) Temperatursinn. In A. R. WAGNER (Ed.), *Handwort der Physiol., Vol. 3*, Vieweg, Braunschweig. pp. 549–556.

## DISCUSSION

MINUT-SOROKHTINA: In which way did the subjects describe the appearance of the temperature sensations? Was the tactile sensation maintained and added to by the temperature one, or did the tactile sensation cease and be changed for a temperature sensation?

TSIRULNIKOV: As a rule, the tactile sensations in our experiments were of a rather short duration. The temperature sensation appeared soon (fractions of a second) after cessation of the tactile one. In some spots tactile sensation failed to appear, the temperature (cold or warmth) sensation arising with no preceding tactile one.

CATTON: When you stimulated with ultrasound stimuli did you identify the points of stimulation to correlate with the ordinary touch stimuli so that you stimulated at the same place as with von Frey's hairs?

TSIRULNIKOV: Yes, we did. The spots to give the tactile sensations when stimulated with ultrasound were the same as tactile spots identified with the aid of von Frey's hairs. The spots to give the temperature sensations when stimulated with ultrasound were the same as those identified with a thermode.

LINDBLOM: Do you think that the deep pain sensation is caused by mechanical displacement or by an increase in temperature?

TSIRULNIKOV: With the ultrasound frequency relatively low, when the absorption coefficient, and hence the tissue heating, are relatively small, the deep pain sensation appears to be due to a mechanical factor. With high ultrasound frequencies and long stimuli the tissue heating is of a significant value and should be taken into account.

BURGESS: If the same sensory structures are responsible for warmth and cold then presumably you could stimulate a cold spot with an electrical stimulus, for example, rather than ultrasound, and by stimulating with the appropriate pattern you could change the sensation from cold to warmth by varying the pattern of the output from the receptor. Have you ever done an experiment of this kind?

TSIRULNIKOV: We made no such experiments and failed to find any in the literature. Experiments of this kind would be of great interest but they require temperature control both of the skin and surrounding medium. In our case the subject's arm being in the water, the skin temperature was conditioned by the water temperature.

# Chemosensitive Spinal Afferents: Thresholds of Specific and Nociceptive Reflexes as Compared with Thresholds of Excitation for Receptors and Axons

V. M. KHAYUTIN, L. A. BARAZ, E. V. LUKOSHKOVA, R. S. SONINA
AND P. E. CHERNILOVSKAYA

*Institute of Normal and Pathological Physiology, Academy of Medical Sciences, Moscow (U.S.S.R.)*

Many outstanding physiologists of the past assumed that there existed chemosensitive receptors that reacted to changes in the composition of internal environment — "an organic fluid that surrounds and feeds all the anatomical elements of the tissues" (Bernard, 1878). These conjectures were proved when Chernigovsky (1943) found that very small doses of $K^+$ ions, acetylcholine or histamine injected through capillaries into the interstitial space of small intestine or spleen caused a reflex rise of arterial pressure and augmentation of respiration. In subsequent research chemosensitive tissue receptors — free endings of thin spinal afferents — were discovered in practically every organ (Chernigovsky, 1960). Similar reflex effects (a rise in arterial pressure, augmentation of respiration) and a very close sensitivity of chemoreceptors in many organs led up to the hypothesis that tissue receptors signal the increase of functional activity of specific cells in organs and that they can be stimulated by metabolites causing functional hyperaemia (Khayutin, 1964). The authors of a similar hypothesis used the term "metabolic receptors" (Coote *et al.*, 1971). The hypothesis of tissue receptor function should be based on the data of their threshold sensitivity.

We first turned our attention to $K^+$ ions: they move from the active cells into interstitial space. Maybe tissue receptors, by reacting to the exit of $K^+$ ions, signal that the organ has intensified its function? How sensitive to $K^+$ ions are tissue receptors?

In cats under urethane anaesthesia we perfused the small intestine with donor's blood using a constant-flow pump. The nervous supply to the intestine was left intact. At certain moments an injector was switched on, which added an amount of $K^+$ ions to the donor's blood. As the blood supply was fixed, it was easy to estimate the increase of $K^+$ ions' concentration in the arterial blood. An increase by even 1 or 2 mmoles/l was sufficient for the recipient to react by a distinct reflex rise in arterial pressure. An increase by 4–8 mmoles/l evoked pressor reflexes of about 10–15 mm Hg (Baraz, 1961; Khayutin, 1964). On transition from rest to work there may be just such an increase in the $K^+$ ion concentration in the outflowing venous blood. We had reasons to conclude that $K^+$ ions may be among the stimuli adequate for chemosensitive tissue receptors.

*References p. 305–306*

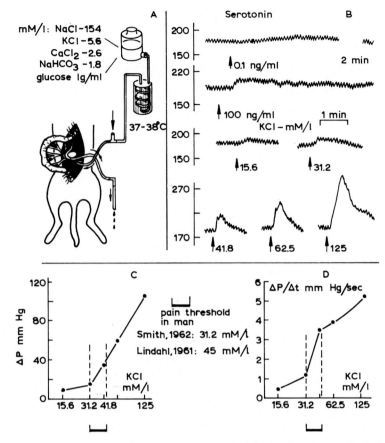

Fig. 1. Pressor reflexes evoked by K$^+$ ions and serotonin injection into humorally isolated small intestine in cat. Urethane anaesthesia.

It is common knowledge, however, that K$^+$ ions evoke pain. For differentiating the effects of substances in a range of concentrations from the threshold up to the algogenic ones we used Chernigovsky's method (1943). Cat's small intestine was perfused with Ringer–Locke's solution (Fig. 1A). The exact concentrations of the substances (1 ml in volume) added to the perfusion fluid on their reaching tissue receptors is not known, and further we give the concentration of the injected substance itself.

The lower row of records in Fig. 1B show a steep rise in arterial pressure in response to an increase of K$^+$ ion concentration above 31.2 mmoles/l. The latter concentration of K$^+$ ions in some people causes a slight pain (Smith, 1962). Fig. 1C shows that in the range of the chemalgia threshold (30–45 mmoles/l) the "logarithm of concentration–magnitude of pressor reflex" curve (the concentration–effect curve) becomes much more sharply inclined. Fig. 1D shows that the rate of the blood pressure rise grows still more steeply. The threshold for these effects, which probably reflect the nociceptive action of K$^+$ ions, is 15–30 times higher than for tissue receptor excitation.

Guzman *et al.* (1962) found that for a nociceptive effect it was necessary to inject 50–100 $\mu$g of serotonin (5-HT) into the arteries of internal organs or limbs. This is

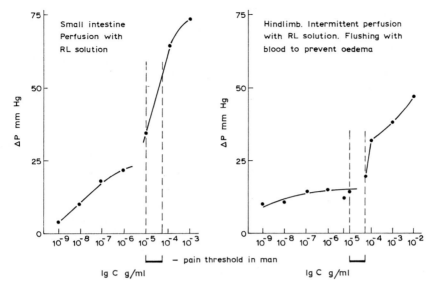

Fig. 2. Dependence of the reflex blood pressure rise on the concentration of acetylcholine acting on different receptive zones.

$0.5-1 \times 10^5$ times larger than the dose of 5-HT which is the threshold for tissue receptor excitation (Fig. 1B).

The huge difference in the sensitivity of tissue receptors and of the sensory apparatus, whose impulses evoke pain, is also typical for acetylcholine (Ach). Fig. 2 shows the concentration–effect curves for Ach injection into the vessels of the small intestine and the hindlimb. In both cases Ach excites tissue receptors already in concentrations of 1 ng/ml. It is the same for the epicardium of a vagotomized cat (Khayutin and Maliarenko, 1968). Thus we define the sensitivity of tissue receptors as the property of a certain common class of sensory endings. Otherwise it would seem that the extremely high sensitivity to 5-HT and Ach is a special property of chemosensitive receptors of the small intestine only.

Both the curves on Fig. 2 have two branches. The first branch corresponds to that range of concentrations in which there occurs a relatively small augmentation of the reflexes, but beginning from 10–50 μg/ml the reflexes start to grow very sharply. According to Keele and Armstrong (1964) this is the threshold for the algogenic effect of Ach. Consequently, Ach excites tissue receptors in concentrations $0.5-1 \times 10^4$ times lower than the threshold algogenic ones.

Bradykinin (BK) is quite as active a stimulus for tissue receptors as Ach (Sonina and Khayutin, 1966). It has a threshold concentration of 1 ng/ml. (Fig. 3). On increasing it 100 times reflexes still stay below 15 mm Hg, but on reaching a concentration of 0.5–1 μg/ml the animals usually react by a sharp (3–4-fold) increase of the reflex magnitude (Fig. 3A and B) and of the rate of the arterial pressure rise (Fig. 3C). The algogenic threshold for BK is 0.1–1 μg/ml (Elliot et al., 1960). Evidently the second branch of the curves (Fig. 3B and C) corresponds to concentrations that cause

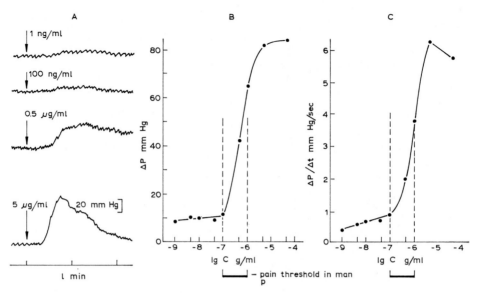

Fig. 3. Bradykinin-evoked pressor reflexes from the humorally isolated cat's small intestine. Chloralose—urethane anaesthesia. Dependence on bradykinin concentration of B: the magnitude of reflexes and C: the rate of arterial pressure rise.

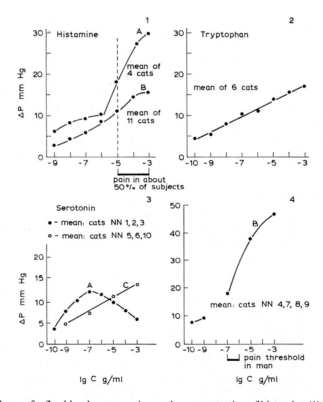

Fig. 4. Dependence of reflex blood pressure rise on the concentration of histamine (1), tryptophan (2) and serotonin (3 and 4) injected into cat's small intestine. Chloralose–urethane anaesthesia.

TABLE I

THRESHOLDS OF THE SPECIFIC AND NOCICEPTIVE REFLEXES EVOKED ON STIMULATION OF THE SMALL
INTESTINE REFLEXOGENIC ZONE IN CATS AS COMPARED WITH PAIN THRESHOLD IN MAN

| Substances | Threshold concentrations | | |
|---|---|---|---|
| | Specific reflex | Nociceptive reflex | Pain* |
| | ng/ml | μg/ml | |
| 1 Acetylcholine | 1 – 10 | 10 – 50 | 10 – 50 |
| 2 Methacholine | 1 – 10 | none up to 1000 | none up to 1000 |
| 3 Pilocarpine | 1 – 10 | none up to 1000 | none up to 1000 |
| 4 Carbachol | 1 – 10 | 500 | 250 – 750 |
| 5 Nicotine | 50 – 500 | 5 – 10 | 100 – 500 |
| 6 Subecholine | 1000 –10000 | 10 – 100 | —§ |
| 7 5-hydroxytryptamine | 0.1 | 1 – 100 | 0.1– 1 |
| 8 Tryptophan | 0.1–1 | none up to 1000 | none up to 1000 |
| 9 Bradykinin | 1 | 0.5 | 0.1– 1 |
| 10 Histamine | 1 – 10 | 10 –1000 | 10 –1000 |
| 11 Capsaicin | 0.001 | 0.01– 0.1 | 0.4** |
| | | mEq/litre | |
| 12 Potassium chloride | 2 – 4 | 30 – 40 | 15 – 30 |
| 13 Ammonium chloride | <15 | 125 – 150 | 150*** |
| 14 Sodium chloride | 185 | 350 – 400 | 300*** |

\* Application to blister base (Keele and Armstrong, 1964).
\*\* The conjunctiva (Heubner, 1925).
\*\*\* Intradermal injection (Lindahl, 1961).
§ Not studied.

pain in man. Tissue receptors, however, react to concentrations which are 500–1000 times smaller.

Especially sensitive people already began to feel pain when histamine was applied in a concentration of 10 μg/ml (Keele and Armstrong, 1964), but about half the subjects did not feel any pain in response to histamine in concentrations even 100 times higher. Whereas histamine on being injected into the intestinal vessels excites tissue receptors in concentrations of 0.1–1 ng/ml (Fig. 4, 1), only in every third animal did histamine in algogenic concentrations evoke comparatively large pressor reflexes (Fig. 4, 1, curve A). Curve B shows the results of all the rest of the experiments (Baraz and Khayutin, 1965).

Thus the chemosensitive small intestine receptors are more sensitive to 5-HT and BK by 3 orders, to Ach by 3.5–4 orders, and to histamine by 4–5 orders, than the sensory apparatus the impulses of which cause pain in man (Table I). On the other hand, the concentrations that correspond to the beginning of the second branch on the concentration–effect curves coincide with the threshold algogenic concentrations for each of these substances.

Evidently there are two kinds of pressor reflexes (Khayutin, 1964). The first kind arises in response to stimulation by substances with concentrations several orders lower than the algogenic ones. These reflexes may be termed as specific. The second kind are evoked by substances in algogenic concentrations. They are large and, what is especially important, have a high rate of arterial pressure rise. This may mean that this kind of reflex is nociceptive, *i.e.* represents the circulatory component of the defence reaction. Our conclusion is based on analogy proceeding from the fact that the effective concentrations, both for the second kind of reflex and for chemalgia, are the same. It was important to find proof of another kind; what mathematicians would call the argument from contraries. Let us assume that there is a substance that does not cause pain in man, but can excite tissue receptors. Such a substance would evoke only specific reflexes in animals, but no nociceptive ones.

Studying the algogenic effect of tryptamine derivatives Keele and Armstrong (1964) noticed that tryptophan does not cause pain even in concentrations as high as 1 mg/ml. On injection of tryptophan into the intestinal vessels we found that it already excited receptors in very low concentrations: 0.1 ng/ml (Fig. 4, 1), but even at such a high concentration as 1 mg/ml reflexes evoked by it do not exceed 15–25 mm Hg. In contrast to all the substances discussed above the tryptophan graph has no branch that corresponds to the second kind of reflex. It is evident that tryptophan, a non-algesic substance, evokes only specific reflexes.

5-HT, another tryptamine derivative, is algesic (Keele and Armstrong, 1964). It is natural to expect that the concentration–effect curve of 5-HT should have two branches, corresponding to specific and nociceptive reflexes (Baraz and Khayutin, 1965). In the first experiments we injected 5-HT into the intestinal vessels, raising each subsequent concentration 10 times. Against all expectations it turned out that 5-HT, on reaching algogenic concentration, evoked not bigger reflexes but, on the contrary, smaller ones (Fig. 4, 3, curve A). What is the reason for this phenomenon? As for man, 2–3 applications of 5-HT to the blister base are already sufficient for the sensory apparatus to lose its sensitivity to this substance (Keele and Armstrong, 1964). The induction of such a strong refractoriness made us, in subsequent experiments, use 5-HT in concentrations increasing 100-fold each time. The intervals between stimulation were prolonged to 30–60 min. Under these conditions in some cats the dependence of the magnitude of reflexes on the concentration of 5-HT is very like the expected one (Fig. 4, 4, curve B). In other animals, however, 5-HT-reactive structures evidently continued to be inactivated on repeated administration (Fig. 4, 3, curve C). This reveals the qualitative conformity of the properties of 5-HT-reactive structures of the nocireceptive sensory apparatus in animals and man. The same conformity is revealed in the similarity of the dynamic characteristics of pain sensation in man and nociceptive reflexes in animals. The recordings in Keele and Armstrong's experiments, by which the subjects endeavoured to express specific features of pain sensations, show that for 5-HT a long latent period is typical for pain development, a slow increase of pain intensity and prolonged action. Ach evokes pain quickly, and it also stops quickly. Exactly the same features are evident in the recordings of nociceptive pressor reflexes caused by 5-HT and Ach. We consider that such a coincidence points to a principle similarity of the properties of 5-HT- or Ach-reactive structures, the activation of which evokes pain in man and the defence reaction in animals.

Another pair of structurally similar substances, one of which is algesic and the other is not, are Ach and methacholine (Mch). Even in such a high concentration as

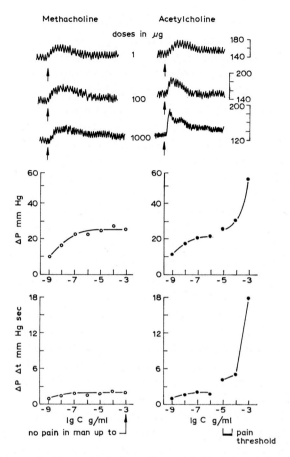

Fig. 5. Pressor reflexes evoked by methacholine and acetylcholine injected alternately into the small intestine vessels of the same animal. Chloralose–urethane anaesthesia.

1 mg/ml Mch does not cause pain (Keele and Armstrong, 1964). If the properties of the chemalgia apparatus in man and sensory units, the impulses of which are responsible for the defence reaction in animals, are identical, then Mch should not excite them and, consequently, not evoke nociceptive reflexes. It is possible, however, that Mch excites tissue receptors. Then it will evoke specific reflexes.

Fig. 5 shows the results of an experiment in which Ach and Mch were injected alternately into the intestinal vessels of one and the same cat. The threshold concentration of each of these substances was less than 1 ng/ml. The animal responded to equal concentrations of both substances by practically identical reflexes. Clearly the sensitivity of tissue receptors to Ach and Mch is the same. However, Mch at 1–10 $\mu$g/ml reaches the limit of its stimulating ability. Raising its concentration 10 times and, further, 100 times has no effect on the magnitude of the reflex and the rate of the arterial pressure rise. The intensity of the stimulating effect of Ach, in contrast, continues to grow with the rise in concentration. A reflex in response to 1 mg/ml of Ach is twice as large as the response to Mch in the same concentration. The rate of the arterial pressure rise is almost 10 times higher for Ach than for Mch.

Evidently Ach in concentrations of 10 $\mu$g/ml and higher is able to excite a certain sensory apparatus that is inaccessible to Mch. Furthermore, it is apparent that impulses, arising on stimulation of just this Ach-reactive apparatus, are responsible for nociceptive reflexes. What kind of an apparatus is it?

Methacholine is an M-cholinostructure activator and acetylcholine an M- and N-cholinostructure activator. Consequently, it appears that tissue-receptor discharges are caused by M-cholinostructure activation, whereas nociceptive reflexes arise as a result of N-cholinostructure activation. To check this assumption we compared the effect of another M-cholinostructure activator — pilocarpine — with that of subecholine, which is a selective N-cholinostructure activator (Riboloblev, 1957). We expected pilocarpine to activate only tissue receptors and, consequently, to evoke only specific reflexes just like Mch. Subecholine was expected to evoke nociceptive reflexes. Possibly it might slightly excite tissue receptors.

Our expectations were realized. It turned out that pilocarpine is just as highly active for tissue receptors as Mch. Pilocarpine reflexes grow, as a rule, slowly. The concentration–effect curve has only one branch. It remains to add that in Keele and Armstrong's (1964) experiments pilocarpine did not cause pain at up to 1 mg/ml. We know no data on the algogenic activity of subecholine. However, this powerful N-cholinostructure activator at up to 1–10 mg/ml does not evoke any reflexes at all. But in concentrations only 10 times higher than the threshold ones it already evokes a large and high-rate pressor, *i.e.* nociceptive, reflex.

Thus, pilocarpine and Mch — substances with primary action on M-cholinostructures — are able to evoke only specific reflexes. They excite tissue receptors in the same low concentrations as Ach and carbachol (Table I), both of which also have an M-cholinomimetic action. Nicotine is 5–50 times less effective for tissue receptors, while subecholine is 1000 times less effective. Thus, the excitation of tissue receptors by cholinomimetics is connected with activation of M-cholinostructures.

According to their activity as defence reaction initiators, these substances are arranged so: nicotine > acetylcholine ≥ subecholine > carbachol. Methacholine and pilocarpine are inactive. Consequently, excitation of the substrate responsible for the defence reaction is connected with N-cholinostructure activation. Keele and Armstrong (1964) came to the same conclusion concerning the substrate of chemalgia.

If chemosensitive tissue receptors and nocireceptors are different sensory units then evidently M-cholinostructures are located in tissue receptors, while N-cholinostructures are in nocireceptors. However, according to the "intensity theory", certain of the sensory units can function as specific receptors if a stimulus acts on their terminals, whereas, if its intensity reaches a level sufficient for direct excitation of the neurite itself, they begin to function as nocireceptors. Consequently, it is possible to assume that M-cholinostructures are located in the membranes of the terminals, while N-cholinostructures are in the membrane of the more proximal parts of the neurite. The grounds for the first assumption are that stimulation of just M-cholinostructures evokes specific reflexes. The second assumption is based on the following analogy.

Ritchie (1965) showed that in non-myelinated sympathetic axons — at the nervous trunk level — there are N-cholinostructures. Pilocarpine, Mch and other muscarino-mimetics do not depolarize these fibres. Nicotine, Ach and other nicotinomimetics, however, depolarize them, though not to such an extent as to evoke action potentials; but the preterminals of these axons respond to Ach and nicotine by generating such potentials. The cholinostructures of the preterminals of sympathetic axons are nicotinic (Ferry, 1963; Cabrera *et al.*, 1966). In our experiments (Khayutin *et al.*, 1970), as in the experiments of Hauesler *et al.* (1968), Ach evoked discharges in sympathetic preterminals already at 1 μg/ml.

If the preterminals of sympathetic axons respond to stimulation of N-cholino-structures by action potentials, then it is quite probable that the preterminals of thin (especially non-myelinated) spinal neurites are able to respond in the same way. In that case just the preterminal part of the neurite could be the source of signals which evoke the defence reflex and chemalgia.

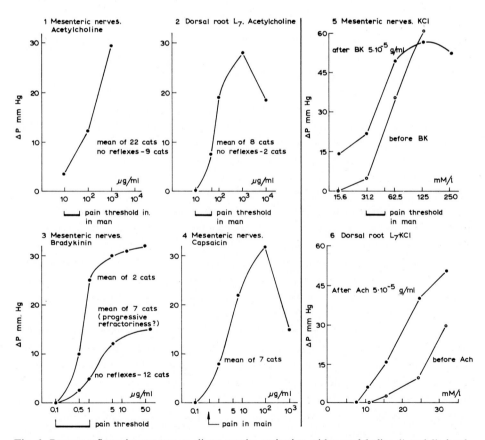

Fig. 6. Pressor reflexes in response to direct neurite excitation with acetylcholine (1 and 2), brady-kinin (3) and capsaicin (4). Sensitization of neurites to K$^+$ ion excitation by bradykinin (5) and acetylcholine (6). 1–4: mean results of a series of experiments, 5 and 6: results of individual experiments.

Such an hypothesis assumes that substances with algogenic action must excite preterminals of chemosensitive neurites and, what is important, in concentrations customary for the algogenic threshold. But it is impossible to study the action of algesic substances only on the preterminals without simultaneously exciting the terminals. Because of this we turned to experiments with application of stimuli to the dorsal root (Khayutin and Chernilovskaya, 1970), which was placed in a small chamber (Calma and Wright, 1947). In other experiments we prepared and then perfused part of the superior mesenteric artery with Ringer–Locke solution into which were added the stimulating substances (Baraz and Khayutin, 1961; Sonina and Khayutin, 1967; Baraz *et al.*, 1968). The latter reached the nerves surrounding this artery *via* the vasa nervorum.

Acting on the neurites of both the mesenteric nerves and the dorsal root Ach evokes pressor reflexes (Fig. 6, 1 and 2). The thresholds for pressor reflexes and for algogenic action coincide. In the most sensitive animals pressor reflexes reached 50–60 mm Hg. The pressure rise is steep. Consequently, Ach, on affecting neurites, is able to evoke nociceptive reflexes. Nonetheless, in certain animals it did not evoke any reflexes at all.

Subecholine excites the neurites of mesenteric nerves in the same concentrations that are active on injection into the intestinal vessels. Therefore there really are N-cholinostructures in these neurites.

BK excites mesenteric nerve neurites (Fig. 6, 3). The threshold concentrations for pressor reflexes and chemalgia coincide (Sonina and Khayutin, 1967), but in most animals the reflexes are small, or altogether absent. The dorsal root neurites are only slightly activated by BK, and then only in a concentration that is 10 times higher than the threshold algogenic one (Chernilovskaya, 1972).

Capsaicin affects tissue receptors in concentrations of 1 pg/ml. It evokes nociceptive reflexes at 0.01–1 $\mu$g/ml (Baraz *et al.*, 1968). The last concentration is the threshold for the activation of mesenteric nerve neurites (Fig. 6, 4).

Thus, all the algesic substances mentioned excite neurites directly and for each substance the concentrations sufficient for neurite activation coincide with their algesic thresholds. However, it is necessary to use 5–10 times higher concentrations to evoke an intensive and steep pressor reflex, *i.e.* a nociceptive one, from the neurites than on injection into the intestinal or hindlimb vessels. Further, the mean magnitude of the maximal reflex is less by 30% on action on the neurites, than on the receptor field. Lastly, Ach and BK do not excite the neurites in every animal.

All these phenomena, however, do not conflict with the hypothesis that the pre-terminal part of the neurite may function as a nocireceptor. They only show the different ability of different parts of the chemosensitive afferents to react to stimulating substances by generating action potentials. This ability decreases on moving from the terminals towards the dorsal roots. Sympathetic axons also have such a gradient. Their terminals generate action potentials in response to Ach, while their axons respond only by local depolarization.

The last is also characteristic for the Ach- and BK-sensitive mesenteric nerve neurites and dorsal roots. Already in such low concentrations as 10–100 ng/ml these substances, while not yet evoking reflexes, begin to raise the neurite sensitivity to $K^+$ ions (Sonina and Khayutin, 1967; Chernilovskaya, 1972). The sensitizing effect of Ach or BK lowers the excitation threshold of neurites to such a degree that they begin to respond to a subalgogenic concentration of $K^+$ ions (Fig. 6, 5 and 6, 6).

The $K^+$ ion excitation threshold for dorsal root neurites is about 20 mmoles/l (Khayutin and Chernilovskaya, 1970). This concentration is subalgogenic (Smith, 1962; Lindahl, 1961). After sensitizing by Ach or BK the threshold concentration of $K^+$ ions becomes twice as low (Chernilovskaya, 1972). In response to $K^+$ ions in concentrations of 20–25 mmoles/l there develops a steep pressor reflex of 30–40 mm Hg, $i.e.$ subalgogenic concentrations evoke a nociceptive reflex (Fig. 6, 6).

## CONCLUSIONS

Thus, non-algesic substances — tryptophan, methacholine and pilocarpine — evoke only specific reflexes on exciting sensory nerve endings in the organ (Figs. 4, 2 and 5). A lot of potentially algogenic substances when used in concentrations many orders lower than the algesic ones have the same effect (Table I). We have demonstrated, on the other hand, that certain of these substances ($K^+$, $NH_4^+$ and $Na^+$ ions, Ach, BK and capsaicin) are capable of exciting neurites directly (Fig. 6). This ability, however, is a necessary but not sufficient condition for the development of nociceptive reflexes.

After sensitization of the mesenteric nerve neurites or of dorsal roots with Ach or BK, $K^+$ ions begin to excite these neurites in subalgogenic concentrations, 10–15 mmoles/l (Fig. 6, 5 and 6), and although in this case the impulses are formed directly in the neurites themselves, animals respond to such stimulation with specific reflexes. To reach the threshold of activation of defence reaction central mechanisms it is necessary to raise the $K^+$ ion concentration up to 20–30 mmoles/l. The same goes for $Na^+$ ions. Specific reflexes in response to $Na^+$ ion injection into the mesenteric nerve blood supply or to application to dorsal roots were recorded at 185 mmoles/l, the threshold of activation of the most sensitive neurites. Nociceptive reflexes were evoked by $Na^+$ ions beginning only from 350–400 mmoles/l (Table I).

Consequently, for realization of nociceptive reflexes two conditions are indispensible: (1) the substance must be capable of exciting the neurite and (2) the resulting total afferent outflow must reach a certain critical intensity, sufficient for activating the central mechanisms of the defence reaction.

Though asserting that this reaction results from direct excitation of neurites we admit that these neurites belong to a certain type of afferent fibre. The first assertion is a point in common with the "intensity theory", and the second with the "specificity theory".

We assumed that preterminals of certain chemosensitive spinal afferents are capable of generating discharges of a higher frequency than their endings and that thanks to just this ability preterminals can function as nocireceptors. Our conclusion conflicts with the concept of specific nocireceptors as a special type of terminal structure.

## TABLE II

COMPARISON OF MINIMAL CONCENTRATIONS (nanogram/ml) FOR TISSUE RECEPTOR AND DIRECT NEURITE EXCITATION AND FOR PAIN IN MAN WITH THOSE USED FOR ELICITING ACTIVITY IN CAT'S SKIN AND MUSCLE NERVES

| Substances | Tissue receptor excitation | Direct neurite excitation | Pain in man (1) | Activity in nerves |
|---|---|---|---|---|
| Serotonin | 0.1–1 | — | $10^2$–$10^3$ | $10^4$–$10^5$ (2) |
| | | | | $1$–$40 \times 10^3$ (3; dose) |
| | | | | $0.25$–$1.5 \times 10^5$ (4) |
| | | | | $1.35 \times 10^4$–$10^5$ (5) |
| Bradykinin | 0.1–1 | $5 \times 10^2$ | $10^2$–$10^3$ | $0.25$–$1 \times 10^5$ (4) |
| | | | | $3$–$4 \times 10^5$ (3; impure; dose) |
| | | | | $2.6 \times 10^3$–$10^4$ (5) |
| Histamine | 1–10 | — | $10^4$–$10^6$ | up to $10^6$ (2) |
| | | | | $6.6 \times 10^3$–$2.3 \times 10^5$ (3; dose) |
| | | | | $0.9$–$1.8 \times 10^5$ (5) |
| Acetylcholine | 1–10 | $10^4$–$0.5 \times 10^5$ | $10^4$–$0.5 \times 10^5$ | $10^4$–$10^5$ (2) |
| | | | | $2$–$6 \times 10^4$ (3; dose) |

(1) Keele and Armstrong, 1964; (2) Douglas and Ritchie, 1959; (3) Fjällbrandt and Iggo, 1961; (4) Beck and Handwerker, 1974; (5) Mense and Schmidt, 1974.

Iggo (1974) and Perl (1971) have singled out thermal (polymodal) nocireceptors. These nocireceptors react not only to firm pressure, but also to an abrupt increase in skin temperature above 40 °C. But just what part of the sensory unit is the source of discharges arising on the thermal or mechanical stimulation that is used for nocireceptor identification? The free endings or the preterminal part of the neurite? Euler (1947) showed that heating the skin or muscle nerves up to 40–44 °C evokes in decerebrate cats nociceptive reflexes. We consider that this shows identical thermal excitability for the nerve trunk neurites that are excited by heating and for those skin "sensory units" that are thought to be specific thermonocireceptors.

It is illustrative to compare the threshold concentrations of certain endogenic substances, sufficient for exciting tissue receptors, for causing pain in man and for exciting neurites, with those concentrations of the same substances that were used to evoke discharges in afferent fibres on close arterial injection into skin and muscle. Table II shows that the latter concentrations coincide with the chemalgia and nociceptive reflex thresholds or are 10 or even 100 times higher. But we demonstrated that for Ach and BK the thresholds for neurite excitation and for pain coincide. Thus, at least for these two substances, electrophysiological studies describe the chemosensitive properties not of receptor endings, but of neurites.

In our opinion, the question of adequate stimuli for the so-called nociceptor units is still an open one. It is not ruled out that the terminals of at least some sensory units of this type may just turn out to be highly sensitive tissue chemoreceptors.

SUMMARY

The reflex rise of arterial pressure is an extremely sensitive indicator of tissue receptor excitation that is caused by endogenic substances. At the same time a study of the dependence of pressor reflex magnitude on the concentration of a number of substances discloses the presence of two types of reflex responses — the specific and the nociceptive reflexes. The first is the result of tissue receptor excitation, the second of direct stimulation of chemosensitive neurites.

REFERENCES

BARAZ, L. A. (1961) On the sensitivity of small intestine receptors to K ions. *Dokl. Acad. Nauk. SSSR, Otd. Biol.*, **140**, 1213–1216.

BARAZ, L. A. AND KHAYUTIN, V. M. (1961) Differentiation of the action of chemical agents on the receptors and sensory fibres of the small intestine. *Sechenov physiol. J. U.S.S.R.*, **47**, 1289–1297.

BARAZ, L. A. AND KHAYUTIN, V. M. (1965) Serotonin and histamine as exciters of self-regulatory and nociceptive vasomotor reflexes. In *Physiology and Pathology of the Cardiovascular System.* Institute of Normal and Path. Physiol. Acad. Med. Sci. of the USSR, Moscow. pp. 82–85.

BARAZ, L. A., MOLNAR, E. AND KHAYUTIN, V. M. (1968) Analysis of the stimulatory action of capsaicin on receptors and sensory fibres of the small intestine in the cat. *Acta physiol. Acad. Sci. hung.*, **33**, 225–235.

BECK, P. W. AND HANDWERKER, H. O. (1974) Bradykinin and serotonin effects on various types of cutaneous nerve fibres. *Pflügers Arch. ges. Physiol.*, **347**, 209–222.

BERNARD, C. (1878) *Leçons sur les Phénomènes de la Vie communs aux Animaux et aux Végétaux.* Ballière, Paris.

CABRERA, R., TORRANCE, R. W. AND VIVEROS, H. (1966) The action of acetylcholine and other drugs upon the terminal parts of the postganglionic sympathetic fibres. *Brit. J. Pharmacol.*, **27**, 51–63.

CALMA, I. AND WRIGHT, S. (1947) Effects of intrathecal injection of KCl and other solutions in cats. Excitatory action of K ions and posterior nerve root fibres. *J. Physiol. (Lond.)*, **106**, 211–235.

CHERNIGOVSKY, V. N. (1943) *The Afferent Systems of Internal Organs.* Navy Medical Academia, Kirov.

CHERNIGOVSKY, V. N. (1960) *The Interoceptors.* Medgiz, Moscow.

CHERNILOVSKAYA, P. E. (1969) Interoceptive and nociceptive pressor reflexes evoked by the action of KCl on hindlimb tissues. *Bull. exp. Biol. Med.*, **68**, 10–14.

CHERNILOVSKAYA, P. E. (1972) Sensitization of the fibres of posterior roots to the stimulating action of potassium ions caused by bradykinin and acetylcholine. *Bull. exp. Biol. Med.*, **73**, 3–6.

COOTE, J. H., HILTON, S. M. AND PEREZ-GONZALES, J. F. (1971) Reflex nature of the pressor response to muscular exercise. *J. Physiol. (Lond.)*, **224**, 173–186.

DOUGLAS, W. W. AND RITCHIE, J. M. (1959) The sensory functions of the non-myelinated afferent nerve fibres from the skin. In *Pain and Itch Nervous Mechanisms.* Churchill, London. pp. 26–39.

ELLIOT, D. E., HORTON, E. W. AND LEWIS, G. P. (1960) Actions of pure bradykinin. *J. Physiol. (Lond.)*, **153**, 473–480.

EULER, C. (1947) Selective responses to thermal stimulation of mammalian nerves. *Acta physiol. scand.*, **14**, Suppl. 45, 1–75.

FERRY, C. B. (1963) Sympathomimetic effect of acetylcholine on the spleen of the cat. *J. Physiol. (Lond.)*, **167**, 487–504.

FJÄLLBRANDT, N. AND IGGO, A. (1961) The effect of histamine, 5-hydroxytryptamine and acetylcholine on cutaneous afferent fibres. *J. Physiol. (Lond.)*, 156, 578–590.

GUZMAN, F., BRAUN, C. AND LIM, R. K. S. (1962) Visceral pain and the pseudoaffective response to intra-arterial injection of bradykinin and other algesic agents. *Arch. int. Pharmacodyn.*, **136**, 353–384.

HAUESLER, G., THOENEN, H., HAEFELY, W. AND HUERLIMAN, A. (1968) Electrical events in cardiac adrenergic nerves and noradrenaline release from the heart induced by acetylcholine and KCl. *Arch. Pharmakol.* **261**, 389–411.

HEUBNER, W. (1925) Zur Pharmakologie der Reizstoffe. *Arch. exp. Path. Pharmakol.* **107**, 129–154.

IGGO, A. (1974) Activation of cutaneous nocireceptors and their actions on dorsal horn neurons. *Advances in Neurology, Vol. 4.* Raven, New York. pp. 1–8.

KEELE, C. A. AND ARMSTRONG, D. (1964) *Substances Producing Pain and Itch.* Arnold, London.

KHAYUTIN, V. M. (1964) *Vasomotor Reflexes.* Nauka, Moscow.

KHAYUTIN, V. M. AND CHERNILOVSKAYA, P. E. (1970) Sensitivity of dorsal root fibres to K ions and the hypothesis of the peripheral mechanism of pain. *Bull. exp. Biol. Med.,* **69**, 3–6.

KHAYUTIN, V. M. AND MALIARENKO, YU. E. (1968) Heart and problems of visceral pain. *Circulation (Yerevan)*, **1**, 21–28.

KHAYUTIN, V. M., SHUR, V. L. AND MALIARENKO, YU. E. (1970) Excitation of sympathetic post-ganglionic fibres by KCl and acetylcholine action on epicardium. *Sechenov physiol. J. U.S.S.R.,* **56**, 84–94.

LINDAHL, O. (1961) Experimental skin pain induced by injection of water-soluble substances in humans. *Acta physiol. scand.,* **51**, Suppl. 179, 1–90.

MENSE, S. AND SCHMIDT, R. F. (1974) Activation of group IV afferent units from muscle by algesic agents. *Brain Res.,* **72**, 305–310.

PERL, E. R. (1971) Is pain a specific sensation? *J. psychiat. Res.,* **8**, 273–287.

RIBOLOVLEV, R. S. (1957) Connection between structure and action in fatty dicarbonic acids amino-esters. In M. IA. MICHELSON (Ed.), *Physiological Importance of Acetylcholine and a Search for New Drugs.* First Pavlov's Medical Institute, Leningrad. pp. 322–337.

RITCHIE, J. M. (1965) The action of acetylcholine and related drugs on mammalian non-myelinated nerve fibres. In *Pharmacology of Cholinergic and Adrenergic Transmissions.* Sec. Int. Pharmacol. Meet., Vol. 3. Pergamon Press, Oxford. pp. 55–71.

SMITH, R. (1962) The vocabulary of pain. In C. A. KEELE AND R. SMITH (Eds.), *Assessment of Pain in Man and Animals.* Livingstone, London. pp. 32–40.

SONINA, R. S. AND KHAYUTIN, V. M. (1966) Chemoreception and the nociceptive effects of bradykinin. *Sechenov physiol. J. U.S.S.R.,* **52**, 547–555.

SONINA, R. S. AND KHAYUTIN, V. M. (1967) Bradykinin-induced sensitization of afferent fibres to K ion excitation. *Sechenov physiol. J. U.S.S.R.,* **53**, 291–298.

# The Peripheral Mechanisms of Sensitization of Inflamed Tissues

L. N. SMOLIN

*The Institute of Normal and Pathological Physiology of the Academy of Medical Sciences, Moscow*
*(U.S.S.R.)*

It is common knowledge that a gentle touch to inflamed skin elicits pain instead of a tactile sensation. In spite of a long discussion the mechanisms of this phenomenon are poorly understood. In the present investigation an effort was made to elucidate whether this phenomenon is due, at least in part, to sensitization of mechanoreceptors in inflamed tissues. For this purpose the reaction of skin mechanoreceptors to tactile stimuli before and after the development of the inflammation was studied using the collision technique of Douglas and Ritchie (1957).

The experiments were performed on cats and dogs anaesthetized with Nembutal (40–60 mg/kg, i.p.). The inflammation of the skin region served by the saphenous nerve was evoked by a subcutaneous injection of turpentine or saturated solution of sodium chloride. To exclude or, at least, reduce the damage of the small saphenous nerve twigs to a minimum both of these phlogogenic agents were injected close to but not within the region of the skin served by the nerve. The saphenous nerve was cut near the groin, freed from the underlying tissue and immersed in liquid paraffin at about 30–35 °C. The antidromic compound action potential was recorded in

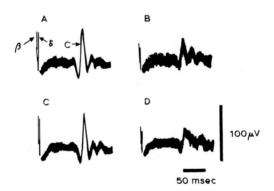

Fig. 1. Antidromic compound action potentials of the medullated (beta and delta) and non-medullated (C) fibres of a knee twig of the cat's saphenous nerve. Each record consists of five superimposed traces. Records were obtained before (A and B) and after (C and D) the development of the inflammation in the skin area supplied by the knee twig. Records A and C are controls taken before stroking and records B and D were taken while the skin supplied by the twig was stroked with a piece of cotton gauze. Note almost complete suppression of the second component of the C potential in D.

*References p. 309*

peripheral branches of the nerve by a pair of platinum electrodes. Light stroking of the skin with a blunt glass rod or a cotton gauze loosely held in the hand was used for tactile stimuli.

In accordance with the data of the other investigators, (Douglas and Ritchie, 1957; Stolwijk and Wexler, 1971), it was found that the tactile stimulation of the intact skin caused a profound fall in the amplitude of the beta, delta and the first component of the C potential, but little or no change in the amplitude of the second component of the C potential. These observations are illustrated in Fig. 1. The two upper records of Fig. 1 were taken before (A) and during (B) the light stroking of the intact skin area supplied by the saphenous nerve. It means that the tactile stimulation of the undamaged skin excites only those receptors which are innervated by the beta, delta and more rapidly propagating C fibres. On the contrary, the receptors supplied by the more slowly propagating non-medullated fibres which generate the second component of the C potential are not excited by the tactile stimulation of the intact skin. After the development of the inflammation the tactile stimuli set up exactly the same reduction in the amplitude of the beta and delta potentials as before the damage of the skin. Examples of such observations are given in the two bottom records of Fig. 1 taken before (C) and during (D) the light stroking of the inflamed skin area supplied by the saphenous nerve. The records show that tactile stimulation of the inflamed skin area (D) elicits the same reduction in size of the beta and delta potentials as stroking of the intact skin (B). It indicates the absence of any noticeable changes in the sensitivity of the mechanoreceptors supplied by the beta and delta fibres. In contrast, the sensitivity of the mechanoreceptors innervated by the C fibres greatly increased after the development of the inflammation; indeed, the tactile stimulation of the inflamed skin evoked an almost 1.5 times stronger effect on the amplitude of the first component of the C potential than before the damage and, what is particularly remarkable, the stroking of the inflamed skin began to depress the second component of the C potential (compare Fig. 1B with Fig. 1D). The latter decreased during tactile stimulation of the inflamed skin by an average of 63%. Moreover, as can be seen in Fig. 1D, stroking of the inflamed skin often almost completely abolished the second component of the C potential. In addition to sensitization, the receptors innervated by the C fibres acquired, after the development of the inflammation, the property to generate an extremely long after-discharge — about 1 min instead of the usual 5–10 sec.

Thus, the development of the inflammation is accompanied by an essential sensitization of the mechanoreceptors. The latter are presumably supplied only by the non-medullated fibres and mainly by the more slowly propagating ones which generate the second component of the C potential. According to Bessou and Perl (1969), these fibres innervate principally the polymodal nociceptors. This suggests that sensitization of the polymodal nociceptors may be one of the reasons of hyperalgesia. The other reason is the increase in the excitability of the central cells (Smolin and Samko, 1966).

SUMMARY

Responses of the cutaneous mechanoreceptors to tactile stimulation of the inflamed area of the skin were studied in acute experiments on cats and dogs using the collision technique of Douglas and Ritchie. It was established that development of the inflammation is accompanied by the marked sensitization, decrease in the rate of adaptation, and by the considerable prolongation of after-discharges in the receptors with non-medullated afferent fibres. These receptors are in all likelihood the polymodal nociceptors. Reaction of mechanoreceptors with medullated afferent fibres were not changed. It is assumed that sensitization of the polymodal nociceptors is one cause of the hyperalgesia of the inflamed tissues.

REFERENCES

BESSOU, P. AND PERL, E. R. (1969) Response of cutaneous sensory units with unmyelinated fibers to noxious stimuli. *J. Physiol. (Lond.)*, **32**, 1025–1043.
DOUGLAS, W. W. AND RITCHIE, J. M. (1957) Non-medullated fibres in the saphenous nerve which signal touch. *J. Physiol. (Lond.)*, **139**, 385–399.
SMOLIN, L. N. AND SAMKO, N. N. (1966) Central mechanism of hyperaesthesia. *Nature (Lond.)*, **211**, 1412–1413.
STOLWIJK, J. A. K. AND WEXLER, I. (1971) Peripheral nerve activity in response to heating the cat's skin. *J. Physiol. (Lond.)*, **214**, 377–392.

# Subject Index

**Somatosensory and visceral receptor mechanisms :** proceedings of
an international symposium held in Leningrad, U.S.S.R., on October 11-15, 1974 / edited by A. Iggo and O. B. Ilyinsky. —
Amsterdam ; New York : Elsevier Scientific Pub. Co., 1976.

314 p. : ill. ; 27 cm. — (Progress in brain research ; v. 43)

"Organised under the auspices of the I. P. Pavlov Institute of Physiology,
Academy of Sciences of the U.S.S.R."
Includes bibliographies and index.
ISBN 0-444-41342-1

1. Neural receptors—Congresses.   I. Iggo, Ainsley.   II. Il'inskiĭ, Oleg
Borisovich.   III. Akademiia nauk SSSR.   Institut Fiziologii imeni I. P. Pavlova.
/IV. Series.

(Continued on next card)

75-43677
MARC